Introduction to Health Care Management

Edited by

Sharon B. Buchbinder, RN, PhD

Professor and Chair
Department of Health Science
Towson University
Towson, MD

Nancy H. Shanks, PhD

Chair, Department of Health Professions
Professor and Coordinator, Health Care Management Program
Metropolitan State College of Denver
Denver, CO

JONES AND BARTLETT PUBLISHERS
Sudbury, Massachusetts
BOSTON   TORONTO   LONDON   SINGAPORE

World Headquarters

Jones and Bartlett Publishers
40 Tall Pine Drive
Sudbury, MA 01776
978-443-5000
info@jbpub.com
www.jbpub.com

Jones and Bartlett Publishers
Canada
6339 Ormindale Way
Mississauga, ON L5V 1J2
CANADA

Jones and Bartlett Publishers
International
Barb House, Barb Mews
London W6 7PA
UK

Jones and Bartlett's books and products are available through most bookstores and online booksellers. To contact Jones and Bartlett Publishers directly, call 800-832-0034, fax 978-443-8000, or visit our Web site at www.jbpub.com.

Substantial discounts on bulk quantities of Jones and Bartlett's publications are available to corporations, professional associations, and other qualified organizations. For details and specific discount information, contact the special sales department at Jones and Bartlett via the above contact information or send an email to specialsales@jbpub.com.

Library of Congress Cataloging-in-Publication Data

Not available at the time of printing.

ISBN-10: 0-7637-3473-X
ISBN-13: 978-0-7637-3473-2

Production Credits
Publisher: Michael Brown
Associate Editor: Kylah Goodfellow McNeill and Katey Birtcher
Production Director: Amy Rose
Production Editor: Renée Sekerak
Marketing Manager: Sophie Fleck
Manufacturing Buyer: Amy Bacus
Composition: Publishers' Design and Production Services, Inc.
Cover Design: Kristin E. Ohlin
Printing and Binding: Malloy, Inc.
Cover Printing: Malloy, Inc.

Printed in the United States of America
11 10 09 08 07   10 9 8 7 6 5 4 3 2

We dedicate this book to our loving husbands,
Dale Buchbinder and Rick Shanks—
Who coached, collaborated, and coerced us to:
"FINISH THE BOOK!"

Contents

FOREWORD xv
PREFACE xix
ACKNOWLEDGMENTS xxi

CHAPTER 1   Leadership 1
            Louis Rubino
            Leadership vs. Management 1
            Followership 3
            History of Leadership in the United States 4
            Contemporary Models 6
            Leadership Styles 10
            Leadership Competencies 11
            Leadership Protocols .12
            Governance 14
            Barriers and Challenges 15
            Ethical Responsibility .17
            Leaders Looking to the Future 18

CHAPTER 2   Management and Motivation 23
            Nancy H. Shanks
            Introduction 23
            Motivation—The Concept 24
            Theories of Motivation 25
            A Bit More about Incentives and Rewards 30
            Misconceptions about Motivation and
            Employee Satisfaction .31
            Motivational Strategies .33
            Conclusion 34

CHAPTER 3   Organizational Behavior and
Management Thinking 37
Sheila K. McGinnis

Introduction 38

The Field of Organizational Behavior 38

Organizational Behavior's Contribution
to Management 39

Key Topics in Organizational Behavior 39

Organizational Behavior Issues in Health
Organizations 40

How Thinking Influences Organizational
Behavior 41

Individual Perception and Thinking 42

Managing and Learning 48

Thinking and Sensemaking in Communication
and Problem Solving 49

Conclusion and Applications 51

CHAPTER 4   Strategic Planning 59
Susan Judd Casciani

Introduction 59

Purpose and Importance of Strategic Planning 60

The Planning Process 60

Situational Assessment 61

Strategy Tactical Plans 71

Rollout and Implementation 72

Monitoring and Control 73

Strategy Execution 75

Strategic Planning and Execution—The Role
of the Healthcare Manager 76

Conclusion 77

CHAPTER 5   **Performance Improvement in Health Care:**
The Quest to Achieve Quality 81
Grant T. Savage, Eric S. Williams

Introduction 81

Defining Quality in Health Care 82

Why Is Quality Important? 84

A Brief History of Quality and Performance
Improvement 86

Quality Assurance 86

The End Result System and the Flexner Report 87

The Joint Commission 88

QA Essentials 89

QA Assumptions and Actions 90

From Peer Review to Quality Improvement
Organizations 91

Professional Standards Review Organizations
(PSROs) Programs 91

Peer Review Organization (PRO) Program 92

Quality Improvement Organization (QIO)
Program 93

Continuous Quality Improvement 94

The Concept of CQI in Health Care 96

Applying CQI 99

Other Leading Quality Improvement Models 101

Key Quality Improvement Concepts 103

Quality Improvement Tools 106

System Thinking and Healthcare Quality
Improvement 108

Health Care as High Hazard Industry 111

Approaches to System Improvement 111

Assessing Healthcare System Improvement 115

Healthcare System Improvement Challenges 116

Developing a National Information
Technology Infrastructure 121

Conclusion 127

CHAPTER 6   **Information Technology** .137
Carla Wiggins

Introduction 137

Historical Overview 138

Health Information and Its Users 140

Health Information Technology
and Applications 142

The Role of the Health Manager 147

Challenges 150

Conclusion 152

CHAPTER 7   **Financing Health Care and Health Insurance** . . .155
Nancy H. Shanks, Suzanne Discenza, Ralph Charlip

Introduction 155

National Health Spending 156

Paying for Health Care 157

Introduction to Health Insurance 158

Brief History of Health Insurance 159

Characteristics of Health Insurance 160

Private Health Insurance Coverage 163

Consumer-Driven Health Plans 166

The Evolution of Social Insurance 169

The Convergence of Political Opportunity
and Leadership 169

Major Legislation 170

Major "Players" in the Social Insurance Arena 173

Statistics on Health Insurance Coverage
and Costs 187

Those Not Covered—The Uninsured 189
Conclusion 193

CHAPTER 8   Managing Costs and Revenues 197
             Suzanne Discenza
             Introduction 198
             What Is Financial Management and Why
             Is it Important? 198
             Ten Major Objectives of Financial
             Management 199
             Tax Status of Healthcare Organizations 200
             Financial Governance and Responsibility
             Structure 202
             Managing Reimbursements from Third-Party
             Payers 204
             What Are the Primary Methods of Payment
             Used by Private Health Plans for Reimbursing
             Providers? 204
             What Are the Primary Methods of Payment
             Used for Reimbursing Providers by Medicare
             and Medicaid? 207
             How Are Providers Reimbursed by Individuals
             with No Health Insurance? 209
             Controlling Costs and Cost Accounting 211
             Classifying Costs 211
             Allocating Costs 212
             Determining Product Costs 213
             Break-Even Analysis 213
             Setting Charges 214
             Other Determinants of Setting Charges
             and Prices 215
             Managing Working Capital 217
             Managing Accounts Receivable 219

Major Steps in Accounts Receivable
Management 220

Managing Materials and Inventory 221

Managing Budgets 224

Conclusion 228

CHAPTER 9   Managing Healthcare Professionals 231
Sharon B. Buchbinder, Dale Buchbinder

Introduction 231

Physicians 232

Registered Nurses 243

Licensed Practical Nurses/Licensed Vocational
Nurses 250

Nursing, Psychiatric, and Home Health Aides 251

Midlevel Practitioners 253

Allied Health Professionals 255

Conclusion 257

CHAPTER 10   The Strategic Management of
Human Resources 265
Jon M. Thompson

Introduction 266

Environmental Forces Affecting HR
Management 268

Understanding Employees as Drivers of
Organizational Performance 271

Key Functions of Human Resources
Management 272

Workforce Planning/Recruitment 275

Employee Retention 282

Conclusion 297

CHAPTER 11   Teamwork 303
Sharon B. Buchbinder, Jon M. Thompson

Introduction 303
What Is a Team? 304
The Challenge of Teamwork in Healthcare
Organizations 305
The Benefits of Effective Healthcare Teams 308
The Costs of Teamwork .310
Who's on the Team? 313
Team Communication 315
Methods of Managing Teams of Healthcare
Professionals 316
Conclusion 319

CHAPTER 12   **Cultural Competency and Diversity** 323
Joanna Basuray

Introduction 323
Cultural Frameworks in Healthcare
Management 326
Cultural Competency and Diversity Staff
Training 329
Cultural Competency at the Workplace 331
Conclusion 337

CHAPTER 13   **Ethics and Law** 343
Patricia M. Alt

Introduction 343
Ethical Concepts 344
Legal Concepts 346
Elements of a Contract .347

Types of Torts 347

Malpractice 349

Patient and Provider Rights and
Responsibilities 349

Legal/Ethical Concerns in Managed Care 351

Biomedical Concerns 353

Beginning- and End-of-life Care 353

Research in Healthcare Settings 354

Conclusion 355

CHAPTER 14   Fraud and Abuse 357
Maron J. Boohaker

Introduction 358

What Is Fraud and Abuse? 358

History 359

Operation Restore Trust 359

The Social Security Act and the
Criminal-Disclosure Provision 360

The Emergency Medical Treatment and
Active Labor Act 362

Hospital Compliance with EMTALA 363

The Balanced Budget Act of 1997 363

Antitrust Issues 364

Federal Enforcement Actions 364

Safe Harbor/Anti-Kickback Regulations 365

Anti-Kickback Statutes .365

Safe Harbor Laws 367

Stacked Penalties 369

Management Responsibility for Compliance
and Internal Controls 369

Corporate Compliance Programs 370

Conclusion 371

CHAPTER 15 **Healthcare Management Guidelines
and Case Studies** 375
Sharon B. Buchbinder, Donna M. Cox

Introduction 375

Guidelines 375

Team Structure and Process for Completion 377

Guidelines for Effective Participation 377

CASE STUDIES 383

Oops Is Not an Option 383

Building a Better MIS-Trap 384

The Case of the Complacent Employee 386

Managing Healthcare Professionals:
Mini-Case Studies 389

Negotiation in Action 391

The Merger of Two Competing Hospitals:
A Case Study 397

The Orchestra: A Narrative in a Minor Key 404

Labor and Delivery Dilemma 415

Sexual Harassment at the
Diabetics Clinic 416

Seaside Convalescent Care Center 421

Staffing at River Oaks Community Hospital:
Measure Twice, Cut Once 423

Heritage Valley Medical Center: Are Your
Managers Culturally Competent? 429

Humor Strategies in Healthcare Management
Education 433

Electronic Medical Records in a Rural Family
Practice Residency Program 438
Medication Errors Reporting at Community
Memorial Hospital 442

INDEX 449

Foreword

The discipline of healthcare management, while not particularly young, is a relative newcomer at the undergraduate level. Historically, persons wishing to be prepared for careers in hospital administration in the years immediately following World War II had to obtain a master's degree at one of just a small handful of universities that offered this type of curriculum. As the number of hospitals grew (thanks in part to the Hill-Burton Act), the need for professionally trained managers accelerated in response to this demand. In addition to hospitals, other forms of healthcare delivery and payment discovered that having managers who possessed the specialized knowledge of the field meant that new hires could immediately work with and understand the unique nuances that make health care fundamentally different from any other business enterprise. Whether the locus of practice was in physician practices, pharmaceuticals, insurance, or long-term care, graduates with healthcare management preparation were well positioned to quickly assume leadership roles in their organizations.

By the early 1970s, a new form appeared on the healthcare management education landscape. While the large and well established graduate degree granting programs continued to focus on hospital management, a small number of undergraduate degree programs began to emerge across the country. These degrees were much more diverse than the traditional residential programs that expected students to study at their respective schools full time. While some of the undergraduate programs fit this mold (and continue to do so), others were designed to meet the needs of a different type of learner with very different expectations. In many cases, the "typical" student was a full-time working adult who was attending school part-time. In others, the student was already working in the healthcare field in some sort of clinical capacity and needed to complete their degrees in order to advance within their organization. Other programs evolved to fill specific niches in physician practice and long-term care. However, regardless of where the program was located and who the students were, they all had one thing in common and that was preparing students for entry-level management jobs in their respective organizations. The Association of University Programs in Health Administration (AUPHA) brought undergraduate degree programs on board and in the 1980s began to offer what ultimately became certification, with the goal of creating a desired standard for curriculum, student support, and program infrastructure including adequate numbers of specifically trained faculty.

In 2006, undergraduate healthcare management education became a widely accepted method for preparing entry-level healthcare leaders. While many of the graduates from our programs ultimately seek their master's degrees, the vast majority either begin work or continue their careers in the field. Given this trend, undergraduate programs must be eminently practical. For too long the only textbooks on the market were either written for graduate programs, which while good, had a very strong theoretical focus, or alternatively for current managers who needed a "how-to" book that ended up being theory free. Undergraduate students needed something midway between these two extremes—the combination of both theory and application that would neither overwhelm nor create a collective yawn.

The book that you hold contains the work of a number of well known and important educators and scholars whose careers have recognized the vital importance of undergraduate healthcare management education. Drs. Buchbinder and Shanks have done a masterful job in selecting topics and authors and putting them together in a meaningful and coherent manner. Each chapter of the book is designed to give the student the core content that must become part of the repertoire of each and every healthcare manager, whether entry level or senior executive. Each of the chapters and accompanying cases serve to bring to life what it means to be a truly competent healthcare manager.

As you read this book, keep in mind two themes that are woven throughout and will be used in each and every professional setting you might find yourself in. First, healthcare management is at its core, a relationship business. Your ability to build, grow, and maintain relationships will be the key determinant to your future success. These relationships are all around you and will include management colleagues, clinicians, payers, patients, regulators, legislators, and uncounted other stakeholders. At the heart of effective relationships will be your willingness to listen carefully to others and to yourself. The second theme is that of organizational excellence. To quote my friend Quint Studer, people in the healthcare business are driven by "purpose, worthwhile work, and making a difference." In this time of continuous environmental change (some might even call it turbulence), what role do you have in creating and sustaining organizations that are truly excellent? For that matter, what does excellence mean to you and to those around you?—Excellence represents the "north star" that guides the actions of the organization and those within.

This textbook will be an invaluable guide as you seek to create the map that will guide you in your healthcare management career. Our job is to create and sustain the systems that allow dedicated and skilled clinicians to deliver the safest and highest quality patient care possible. I congratulate you on your decision to become a leader in the field and a hero to your community.

Leonard H. Friedman, PhD, MPH
Associate Professor and Coordinator
Health Management and Policy Program
Department of Public Health
Oregon State University
Corvallis, OR

Preface

Never underestimate the power of a good cup of coffee. The idea for this book came about in October, 2003, when Nancy Shanks and I sat down for java and breakfast and began to talk about the field of healthcare management, the role of educators, and the courses we were teaching. When the conversation turned to our introductory courses, we both said— almost in unison: "I'm not happy with the text I'm using." We were unhappy because the books that were available were either too advanced (or too simple) and had too few learning tools for students and professors. In addition, there was a dearth of case studies related to healthcare management in a wide variety of settings. As we emptied a pot of coffee, becoming giddy with caffeine, we took turns telling each other: "You should write a textbook!" At last, we agreed that we should write a textbook together.

We turned to our colleagues for their collective expertise and conducted an online survey of 37 healthcare management educators. Much like Goldilocks, our colleagues, too, had yet to find a textbook that was "Just right!" Like us, they found that many of the healthcare management textbooks were: too dense and over the head of the student; contained no appropriate case studies; too expensive; and didn't contain enough graphs, tables, charts, or figures. The same survey enabled us to identify which topic areas were critical for an introductory textbook in healthcare management.

After we shared the results of the survey with our colleagues, we sent out a call for chapter authors and case studies. Master teachers and researchers with expertise in each topic stepped forward and offered to assist us with this exciting project. Each contributor knew exactly what did or did not work in the classroom and was eager for a student-friendly, professor-friendly textbook. We are grateful to all our authors for their insightful, well-written chapters and realistic case studies. Without them, this dream textbook would not have become a reality.

This textbook will be useful to a wide variety of students and programs. Undergraduate students in healthcare management, nursing, public health, and allied health programs will find the writing to be engaging. In addition, students in graduate programs in discipline-specific areas, such as business administration, nursing, pharmacy, occupational therapy, public administration, and public health will find the materials theory-based and readily applicable to real-world settings. Along with lively writing and contents critical for a foundation in healthcare management, this book has the following features:

- Learning objectives and discussion questions for each chapter;
- Instructors' resources online for each chapter, including PowerPoint slides, sample syllabus, and test items;
- Fifteen case studies in a wide variety of settings, in an assortment of healthcare management topics; and,
- A case study guide, with rubrics for evaluation of student performance, enabling professors at every level of experience to hit the ground running on that first day of classes.

We hope you enjoy this book as much as we enjoyed bringing it together. May your classrooms be bursting with excited discussions, and may your coffee cup always be full.

Sharon B. Buchbinder, RN, PhD
Towson University

Nancy H. Shanks, PhD
Metropolitan State College of Denver

Acknowledgments

This book is the result of a 3-year process that involved the majority of the United States' leaders in excellence in undergraduate healthcare management education. We are deeply grateful to the Association of University Programs in Health Administration (AUPHA) faculty, members, and staff for all the support, both in time and expertise, in developing the proposal for this textbook and for providing us with excellent feedback at every step of the way.

In the beginning, Nancy and I met over coffee at a meeting: the AUPHA Undergraduate Workshop in Nashville in October of 2003. After consultation with our colleagues and friends, we decided to launch a survey to delineate the key topics to be covered and the deficiencies in the marketplace this book needed to address.

Lydia Reed, CEO of AUPHA, was instrumental in assisting us with getting this survey out to AUPHA Undergraduate Program Directors (PDs). The PDs, in turn, were generous and giving with their time and suggestions. Their guidance enabled us to avoid the beginner authors' dilemma of writing the right book—for the wrong audience. Thanks, thanks, and thanks again to our Undergraduate colleagues!

Louis Rubino, Chair of the AUPHA Undergraduate Program Committee, gave us a bully pulpit by providing us with time on the Undergraduate Program agenda to present the findings of our survey, to refine our proposal, and to get the word out that this book was coming. When we asked for contributors for both chapters and case studies, we were overwhelmed with the level of responsiveness from our colleagues.

Over 30 authors have made this contributed text a one-of-a-kind book. Not only are our authors experts in their disciplines and research niches, they are also practiced teachers and mentors. As we read each chapter and case study, we could hear the voices of each author. It has been a privilege and honor to work with each and everyone of them: Patricia Alt, Joanna

Basuray, Maron Boohaker, Dale Buchbinder, Susan Casciani, Emilie Celluci, Ralph Charlip, Donna Cox, Suzanne Discenza, Daniel Fahey, Mary Anne Franklin, Leonard Friedman, Brenda Freshman, Kenneth Johnson, Barry Gomberg, Dale Mapes, Audrey McDow, Sheila McGinnis, Spence Meighan (deceased), Karen Mithamo, Wayne Nelson, Dawn Oetjen, Woody Richardson, Velma Roberts, Lou Rubino, Grant Savage, Donna Slovensky, Rosalind Trieber, Carla Wiggins, Jon Thompson, and Eric Williams.

And, finally, and never too often, we thank our husbands, Dale Buchbinder and Rick Shanks, who listened to long telephone conversations about the book's progress, trailed us to meetings and dinners, and served us wine with our whines. We love you and could not have done this without you.

Contributors

EDITORS

Sharon B. Buchbinder, RN, PhD
Professor and Chair
Department of Health Science
Coordinator, Health Care Management Program
Towson University
Towson, MD

Nancy H. Shanks, PhD
Professor and Chair
Department of Health Professions
Coordinator, Health Care Management Program
Metropolitan State College of Denver
Denver, CO

CONTRIBUTORS

Patricia M. Alt, PhD
Professor
Department of Health Science
Towson University
Towson, MD

Joanna Basuray, RN, PhD
Professor
Department of Nursing
Towson University
Towson, MD

Maron Joseph Boohaker, MPH
Compliance Audit Manager
HealthSouth Corporation
Birmingham, AL

Dale Buchbinder, MD, FACS
Chairman, Department of Surgery and
Clinical Professor of Surgery
The University of Maryland Medical School
The Greater Baltimore Medical Center
Baltimore, MD

Susan Judd Casciani, MSHA, MBA
Director, Corporate Strategy
The Greater Baltimore Medical Center
Baltimore, MD

Leigh W. Cellucci, MBA, PhD
Director
Idaho Center for Disabilities Evaluation and
Assistant Professor, Health Care Administration
Idaho State University
Pocatello, ID

Ralph Charlip, FACHE, FAAMA
Director
Veterans' Administration Health Administration Center
Denver, CO

Suzanne Discenza, PhD
Associate Professor
Health Care Management
Director of Gerontology Programs
Department of Health Professions
Metropolitan State College of Denver
Denver, CO

Donna M. Cox, PhD
Associate Professor and Assistant Chair
Department of Health Science
Towson University
Director
Alcohol Tobacco and Other Drugs Prevention Center
Towson, MD

Daniel Fahey, PhD
Associate Professor
Health Science Department
California State University, San Bernardino
San Bernardino, CA

Mary Anne Franklin, EdD, MSA, LNFA
Division Head of Nursing and Allied Health
Louisiana State University at Eunice
Eunice, LA

Brenda Freshman, PhD
President and Senior Consultant
Social Logistics
Santa Monica, CA

Leonard H. Friedman, PhD, MPH
Associate Professor and Coordinator
Health Management and Policy Programs
Department of Public Health
Oregon State University
Corvallis, OR

Barry Gomberg, JD
Attorney-At-Law
Weber State University
Ogden, UT

Ken Johnson, PhD, CHES
Associate Professor and Associate Dean
Dumke College of Health Professions
Weber State University
Ogden, UT

Jennifer L. Krapfl, MHA, RN
Director
Physician Practice Management
Advocate HealthCare
Oak Brook, IL

Dale Mapes, MSA
Vice President of Human Resources and Support Services
Portneuf Regional Medical Center
Pocatello, ID

Audrey McDow, Senior
Department of Health Care Administration
Idaho State University
Pocatello, ID

Sheila K. McGinnis, PhD
Director, Health Administration Program
College of Allied Health Professions
Montana State University-Billings
Billings, MT

Karin Mithamo, Graduate Student
Department of Business
Idaho State University
Pocatello, ID

H. Wayne Nelson, PhD
Associate Professor
Department of Health Science
Towson University
Towson, MD

Dawn M. Oetjen, PhD
Associate Professor and Director of Graduate Studies
Health Services Administration Program
Department of Health Professions
University of Central Florida
Orlando, FL

Woody D. Richardson, PhD
Department of Marketing and Management
Miller College of Business
Ball State University
Muncie, IN

Velma Roberts, PhD
Assistant Professor
School of Allied Health Sciences
Healthcare Management Division
Florida A & M University
Tallahassee, FL

Louis Rubino, PhD, FACHE
Associate Professor
California State University, Northridge
Northridge, CA

Grant T. Savage, PhD
Chairman
Health Management and Informatics
Alumni Distinguished Professor
The Department of Health Management and Informatics (HMI)
University of Missouri—Columbia School of Medicine
Columbia, MO

Donna J. Slovensky, PhD, RHIA, FAHIMA
Professor and Director
School of Health Related Professions
University of Alabama at Birmingham
Birmingham, AL

Jon M. Thompson, PhD
Professor and Director
Health Services Administration Program
Department of Health Sciences
James Madison University
Harrisonburg, VA

Rosalind Trieber, MS, CHES
Trieber Associates, Inc.
Owings Mills, MD

Carla Wiggins, PhD
Professor and Chair
Health Care Administration
Acting Director
The Center for Executive Studies in Health Idaho State University
Idaho State University
Pocatello, ID

Eric S. Williams, PhD
Associate Professor
Minnie Miles Research Professor
University of Alabama
Tuscaloosa, AL

CHAPTER 1

Leadership

Louis Rubino

LEARNING OBJECTIVES

By the end of this chapter the student will be able to describe:

- The difference between leadership and management;
- Followership and why it's as important as leadership;
- The history of leadership in the United States from the 1920s to current times;
- Contemporary models of leadership;
- Leadership domains and competencies;
- Leadership styles;
- Old and new governance trends; and,
- Why healthcare leaders have a greater need for ethical behavior.

LEADERSHIP VS. MANAGEMENT

In any business setting, there must be leaders as well as managers. But are these the same people? Not necessarily. There are leaders who are good managers and there are managers who are good leaders, but usually neither case is the norm. In health care, this is especially important to recognize because of the need for both. Health care is unique in that it is a service industry that depends on a large number of highly trained personnel as well as trade workers. Whatever the setting, be it a hospital, a long-term care facility, an ambulatory care center, a medical device company, an insurance company, or some other healthcare sector, leaders as well as managers are needed to keep the organization moving in a forward direction and at the same time maintain current operations. This is done by leading and managing its people.

Leaders usually take a focus that is more external, whereas the focus of managers is more internal. Even though they need to be sure their healthcare facility is operating properly, leaders tend to spend the majority of their time communicating and aligning with outside groups that can benefit (partners, community, vendors) or influence (government, public agencies, media) their organizations (Figure 1-1). There is crossover between leaders and managers across the various areas even though a distinction remains for certain duties and responsibilities.

Usually the top person in the organization (e.g., Chief Executive Officer, Administrator, Director) has full and ultimate accountability. There

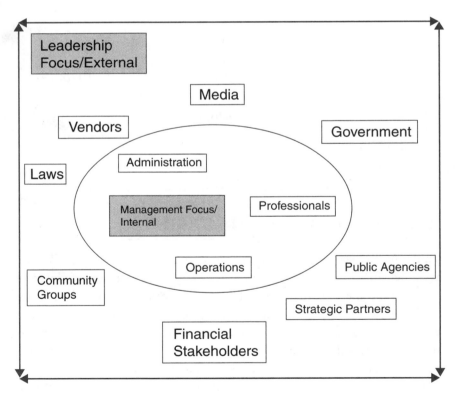

FIGURE 1-1 Leadership and Management Focus

Figure Note: Arrows represent continual interactions between all elements of the model.

TABLE 1-1 Leadership vs. Management Competencies

Leadership Competencies	Management Competencies
Setting Direction or Mission	Staffing Personnel
Motivating Stakeholders	Controlling Resources
Being Effective Spokesperson	Supervising Service Provided
Determining Strategies for Future	Overseeing Adherence to Regulations
Transforming Organization	Counseling Employees

are several managers reporting to this person, all of whom have various functional responsibilities (e.g., Chief Nursing Officer, Physician Director, Information Officer). These managers can certainly be leaders in their own areas but their focus will be more internal within the organization's operations.

Leaders have a particular set of competencies that are more forward thinking than managers. Leaders need to set a direction for the organization. They need to be able to motivate their employees, as well as other stakeholders, so that the business continues to exist and hopefully thrive in periods of change. No industry is as dynamic as health care with rapid change occurring due to the complexity of the system and government regulations. Leaders are needed to keep the entity on course and to maneuver around obstacles that come in its way, like a captain commanding his ship at sea. Managers must tend to the business at hand and make sure the staff is following proper procedures. They need a different set of competencies. See Table 1-1.

FOLLOWERSHIP

For every leader there must be a follower. Leaders must have someone they can lead in order to accomplish what they set out to do. Not everyone can be a leader nor should be one. Leaders should have certain recognizable traits that will help them take charge, but also followers must have a willingness to be led as well as the ability to do the task requested. True leaders inspire commitment from dedicated people.

Atchison (2003) wrote about this process in his book, *Followership*. He describes followership as complementary to leadership and recommends that it be recognized as a necessary component for an effective leader. A self-absorbed administrator will not make a good leader. A true leader will recognize the importance of getting respect, not simply compliance, from the people who follow. It is one thing to have people do what you say, but to have someone want to do it is another thing. The leader who understands this is on the way to greatness and will create a much more meaningful work environment. As Atchison says, "An executive title without followers has an illusion of power. These titled executives create a workplace without a soul."

HISTORY OF LEADERSHIP IN THE UNITED STATES

Leaders have been around since the beginning of man. We think of the strongest male becoming the leader of a caveman clan. In Plato's time, the Greeks began to talk about the concept of leadership and acknowledged the political system as critical for leaders to emerge in a society. In Germany during the late 19th century, first Sigmund Freud described leadership as unconscious exhibited behavior and later Max Weber identified how leadership is present in a bureaucracy through assigned roles. Formal leadership studies in the United States, though, have only been around for the last one hundred years (Sibbet, 1997).

We can look at the decades spanning the 20th century to see how leadership theories evolved, placing their center of attention on certain key components at different times (Northouse, 2004). These emphases often matched or were adapted from the changes occurring in the society.

With the industrialization of the United States in the 1920s, productivity was of paramount importance. Scientific management was introduced and researchers tried to determine which characteristics were identified with the most effective leaders based on their units having high productivity. **The Great Man Theory** was developed out of the idea that certain traits determined good leadership. The traits that were recognized as necessary for effective leaders were ones that were already inherent in the person, such as being male, being tall, being strong, and even being Caucasian. Even the idea that "you either got it or you don't" was supported by this theory, the notion being that a good leader had charisma. Behaviors were not considered important in determining what made a good leader. This theory discouraged anyone who did not have the specified traits from aspiring to a leadership position.

Fortunately, after two decades, businesses realized that leadership could be enhanced through certain conscious acts and researchers began to study which behaviors would produce better results. Resources were in short supply due to World War II and leaders were needed who could truly produce good results. This was the beginnings of the **Style Approach to Leadership**. Rather than looking at only the characteristics of the leader, researchers started to recognize the importance of two types of behaviors in successful leadership: completing tasks and creating good relationships. This theory states that leaders have differing degrees of concern over each of these behaviors and the best leaders would be fully attentive to both.

In the 1960s, American society had a renewed emphasis on helping all of its people and began a series of social programs that still remain today. The two that impact health care directly by providing essential services, are Medicare for the elderly (age 65 and over) and the disabled and Medicaid for the indigent population. The **Situational Approach to Leadership** then came into prominence and supported this national concern. This set of theories focused on the leader changing his/her behavior in certain situations in order to meet the needs of subordinates. This would imply a very fluid leadership process whereby one can adapt one's actions to an employee's needs at any given time.

Not much later, researchers believed that perhaps leaders should not have to change how they behaved in a work setting but instead the appropriate leaders should be selected from the very beginning. This is the **Contingency Theory of Leadership** and was very popular in the 1970s. Under this theory the focus was on both the leader's style as well as the situation in which the leader worked, thus building upon the two earlier groups of theories. This approach was further developed by what is known as **Path-Goal Theory of Leadership**. This theory still placed its attention on the leader's style and the work situation (subordinate characteristics and work task structure) but also recognized the importance of setting goals for employees. The leader was expected to remove any obstacles in order to provide the support necessary for them to achieve those goals.

In the later 1970s, the United States was coming out of a war in which many of its citizens did not think the country should have been involved. More concern was expressed over relationships as the society became more psychologically attuned to how people felt. The **Leader-Member Exchange Theory** evolved over the concern that leadership was being defined by the leader, the follower, and the context. This new way of looking at leadership focused on the interactions that occur between the leaders and the followers. This theory claimed that leaders could be more effective if they developed better relationships with their subordinates through high quality exchanges.

After Vietnam and a series of weak political leaders, Americans were looking for people to take charge who could really make a difference. Charismatic leaders came back into vogue, as demonstrated by the support shown to President Ronald Reagan, an actor turned politician. Unlike the Great Man Theory earlier in the century, this time the leader had to have certain skills to transform the organization through inspirational motivational efforts. Leadership was not centered upon transactional processes that tied rewards or corrective actions to performance. Rather, the transformational leader could significantly change an organization through its people by raising their consciousness, empowering them, and then providing the nurturing needed as they produced the results desired.

In the late 1980s, the United States started to look more globally for ways to have better production. Total Quality Management became a popular concept and arose from researchers studying Japanese principles of managing production lines. In the healthcare setting, this was embraced through a process still used today called Continuous Quality Improvement or Performance Improvement. In the decade to follow, leaders assigned subordinates to a series of work groups in order to focus on a particular area of production. Attention was placed on developing the team for higher level functioning as well as how a leader could create a work environment that could improve the performance of the team. Individual team members were expendable and the team entity was all important.

CONTEMPORARY MODELS

We have entered the 21st century with some of the greatest leadership challenges ever in the healthcare field. Critical position shortages, limited resources, and increased governmental regulations provide an environment that yearns for leaders who are attentive to the organization and its people, yet can still address the big picture. Several of today's leadership models relate well to the dynamism of the healthcare field and are presented here. Looking at these models, there seems to be a consistent pattern of self-aware leaders who are concerned for their employees, and understand the importance of meaningful work. Perhaps we can project for the 2000s, the Self-Actualized Leadership Theory, taking the term from Maslow's top level in his Hierarchy of Needs (Maslow, 1943). See Table 1-2.

Emotional Intelligence (EI)

Emotional Intelligence (EI) is a concept made famous by Daniel Goleman in the late 1990s. It suggests that there are a certain set of skills (intrapersonal and interpersonal) that a person needs to be well-adjusted in today's world. These skills include self-awareness (having a deep understanding of one's emotions, strengths, weaknesses, needs, and drives), self-regulation (a propensity for reflection, an ability to adapt to changes, the power to say no to impulsive urges), motivation (being driven to achieve, being passionate over profession, enjoying challenges), empathy (thoughtfully considering someone's feelings when interacting), and social skills (moving people in the direction you desire due to your ability to interact effectively) (Freshman & Rubino, 2002).

Since September 11, 2001, leaders have needed to be more understanding of their subordinates' world outside of the work environment. EI, when applied to leadership, suggests a more caring, confident, enthusiastic boss who can establish good relations with workers. Researchers have

---

TABLE 1-2 Leadership Theories in the United States

Period of Time	Leadership Theory	Leadership Focus
1920s and 1930s	Great Man Theory	Having certain inherent traits
1940s and 1950s	Style Approach	Task completion and developing relationships
1960s	Situational Approach	Needs of the subordinates
Early 1970s	Contingency and Path-Goal Theories	Both style and situation
Late 1970s	Leader-Member Exchange Theory	Interactions between leader and subordinate
1980s	Transformational Approach	Raising consciousness and empowering followers
1990s	Team Leadership	Team performance and development
2000s	Self-Actualized Leadership	Introspection and concern for meaningfulness

TABLE 1-3   Emotional Intelligence's Application to Healthcare Leadership

EI Dimension	Definition	Leadership Application
Self-Awareness	A deep understanding of one's emotions and drives	Knowing if your values are congruent to organization's
Self-Regulation	Adaptability to changes and control over impulses	Considering ethics of giving bribes to doctors
Motivation	Ability to enjoy challenges and being passionate toward work	Being optimistic even when census is low
Empathy	Social awareness skill, putting yourself in another's shoes	Setting a patient-centered vision for the organization
Social Skills	Supportive communication skills, abilities to influence and inspire	Having an excellent rapport with board

shown that EI can distinguish outstanding leaders and strong organizational performance (Goleman, 1998). For health care, this seems like a good fit. See Table 1-3.

Inspirational Leadership

This model's focus is on leaders who inspire by giving people what they need. This can be very different from what they want. Inspirational leaders are not perfect and in fact expose their weaknesses so people can relate to them better. As with emotional intelligence, empathy is recognized as important. **Inspirational leadership** supports the concept known as "tough empathy," which is when leaders care passionately about their employees and their work yet are prudent in what they provide in the way of support. Inspirational leaders will rely on intuition to act and use their uniqueness (e.g., expertise, personality, or even something as simple as a greeting) as a way to distinguish themselves in the leadership role (Goffee & Jones, 2000).

Diversity Leadership

Our new global society forces healthcare leaders to address matters of diversity whether it is with their patient base or with their employees. This commitment to diversity is necessary for today's leader to be successful. The environment must be assessed so that goals can be set that embrace the concept of diversity in matters such as employee hiring and promotional practices, patient communication, and governing board composition, to name a few. Strategies have to be developed that will make diversity work for the organization. The leader who recognizes the importance of diversity and designs its acceptance into the organizational culture will be most successful (Warden, 1999).

Servant Leadership

Many people view health care as a very special type of work. Individuals usually work in this setting because they want to help people. **Servant leadership** applies this concept to top administration's ability to lead, acknowledging that a healthcare leader is largely motivated by a desire to serve others. This leadership model breaks down the typical organizational hierarchy and professes the belief of building a community within an organization in which everyone contributes to the greater whole. A servant leader is highly collaborative and gives credit to others generously. This leader is sensitive to what motivates others and empowers all to win with shared goals and vision. Servant leaders use personal trust and respect to build bridges and use persuasion rather than positional authority to foster cooperation. This model works especially well in a not-for-profit setting since it continues the mission of fulfilling the community's needs rather than the organization's (Swearingen and Liberman, 2004).

Spirituality Leadership

Recently, the United States has experienced some very serious misrepresentations and misreporting by major healthcare companies as reported by U.S. governmental agencies (some examples being HealthSouth, Tenet, and Paracelsus Healthcare). Trying to claim a renewed sense of confidence in the system, a model of leadership has emerged that focuses on spirituality. This spiritual focus does not imply a certain set of religious beliefs, but emphasizes ethics, values, relationship skills, and the promotion of balance between work and self (Wolf, 2004). The goal under this model is to define our own uniqueness as human beings and to appreciate our spiritual depth. In this way, leaders can become more profound and at the same time productive. These leaders have a positive impact on their workers and create a working environment that supports all individuals in finding meaning in what they do (Table 1-4). They practice five common behaviors: 1) Challenge the process, 2) Inspire a shared vision, 3) Enable others to act, 4) Model the way, and 5) Encourage the heart, thus taking leadership to a new level (Strack & Fottler, 2002).

TABLE 1-4 Spirituality Leadership's Application

Behavior	Definition	Leadership Application
Challenge the process	Always striving to do better	Change management
Inspire a shared vision	Collective sense of purpose	Strategic orientation
Enable others to act	Meeting needs of followers to get results	Gaining trust and confidence to achieve goals
Model the way	Setting a personal example	Coaching to motivate
Encourage the heart	Developing others to find meaning in work	Encouraging personal development of followers

LEADERSHIP STYLES

Models give us a broad understanding of someone's leadership philosophy. Styles demonstrate a particular type of leadership behavior that is consistently used. Various authors have attempted to explain different leadership styles (McConnell, 2003; Schaeffer, 2002; and Goleman, 2000). Some styles are more appropriate to use with certain healthcare workers, depending on their education, training, competence, motivation, experience, and personal needs. The environment must also be considered when deciding which style is the best fit.

A **coercive leadership style** is when power is used inappropriately to get a desired response from a follower. This should probably not be used unless the leader is dealing with a very problematic subordinate or is in an emergency situation and needs immediate action. In healthcare settings over longer periods of time, three other leadership styles could be used more effectively: **participative, pacesetting, and coaching**.

Many healthcare workers are highly trained, specialized individuals who know much more about their area of expertise than their supervisor. Take the generally trained chief operating officer of a hospital who has several department managers (e.g., Radiology, Health Information Systems, Engineering) reporting to him/her. These managers will respond better and be more productive if the leader is participative in his/her style. Asking these managers for their input and giving them a voice in making decisions will let them know they are respected and valued.

A pacesetting style is when a leader sets high performance standards for his/her followers. This is very effective when the employees are self-

TABLE 1-5 Leadership Styles for Healthcare Personnel

Style	Definition	Application
Coercive	Demanding and power based	Problematic Employees
Participative	Soliciting input and allowing decision making	Most Followers
Pacesetting	Setting high performance standards	Highly Competent
Coaching	Focus on personal development	Top Level

motivated and highly competent like research scientists or intensive care nurses. A coaching style is recommended for the very top personnel in an organization. With this style, the leader focuses on the personal development of his/her followers rather than the work tasks. This should be reserved for followers the leader can trust and who have proven their competence. See Table 1-5.

LEADERSHIP COMPETENCIES

A leader needs certain skills, knowledge, and abilities to be successful. These are called competencies. The pressures of the healthcare industry have initiated the examination of a set of core competencies for a leader who works in a healthcare setting (Shewchuk, O'Connor, and Fine, 2005). Criticism has been directed at the educational institutions for not producing administrators who can begin managing effectively right out of school. Educational programs in health administration are working with the national coalition groups (e.g., Health Leadership Alliance and National Center for Healthcare Leadership) and healthcare administrative practitioners to come up with agreed upon competencies. Once identified, the programs can attempt to have their students learn how to develop these traits and behaviors.

Some of the competencies are technical, for example, having analytical skills, having a full understanding of the law, and being able to market and write. Some of the competencies are behavioral, for example, decisiveness, being entrepreneurial, and an ability to achieve a good work/life balance. As people move up in organizations, their behavioral competencies are a greater determinant of their success as leaders than their technical competencies (Hutton and Moulton, 2004). Another way to examine leadership

---

TABLE 1-6 Leadership Domains and Competencies

Domain: Functional and Technical	Domain: Self Development and Self Understanding
Competencies: Knowledge of Business/Business Acumen Strategic Vision Decision Making and Decision Quality Managerial Ethics and Values Problem Solving Change Management/Dealing with Ambiguity Systems Thinking Governance	Competencies: Self Awareness and Self Confidence Self Regulation and Personal Responsibility Honesty and Integrity Life Long Learning Motivation/Drive to Achieve Empathy and Compassion Flexibility Perseverance Work/Life Balance
Domain: Interpersonal	**Domain: Organizational**
Competencies: Communication Motivating Empowerment of Subordinates Management of Group Process Conflict Management and Resolution Negotiation Formal Presentations Social Interaction	Competencies: Organizational Design Team Building Priority Setting Political Savvy Managing and Measuring Performance Developing Others Human Resources Community and External Resources Managing Culture/Diversity

Source: Hilberman, Diana (Ed.), The 2004 ACHE-AUPHA Pedagogy Enhancement Work Group. June, 2005.

---

competencies is under four main groupings or domains. The Functional and Technical Domain is necessary but not sufficient for a competent leader. Three other domains provide competencies that are behavioral and relate both to the individual (Self Development and Self Understanding) and to other people (Interpersonal). A fourth set of competencies falls under the heading Organizational and has a broader perspective. See Table 1-6 for a full listing of the leadership competencies under the four domains.

LEADERSHIP PROTOCOLS

Healthcare administrators are expected to act a certain way. Leaders are role models for their organizations' employees and need to be aware that their actions are being watched at all times. Sometimes people at the top of an organization get caught up in what they are doing and do not realize the message they are sending throughout the workplace by their inappropriate behavior. Specific ways of serving in the role of a healthcare leader can be demonstrated and can provide the exemplary model needed to send the correct message to the employees. These appropriate ways in which a leader acts are called **protocols**.

There is not a shortage of information on what protocols should be followed by today's healthcare leader. Each year, researchers, teachers of health administration, practicing administrators, and consultants write books filled with their suggestions on how to be a great leader (for some recent examples see Manion, 2005: McGinn, 2005; and Spath, 2005). There are some key ways a person serving in a leadership role should act. These are described here and summarized in Table 1-7.

Professionalism is essential to good leadership. This can be manifested not only in the way people act but also in their mannerisms and their dress. A leader who comes to work in sloppy attire or exhibits obnoxious behavior will not gain respect from followers. Trust and respect are very important for a leader to acquire. Trust and respect must be a two-way exchange if a leader is to get followers to respond. Employees who do not trust their leader will consistently question certain aspects of their job. If they do not have respect for the leader, they will not care about doing a good job. This could lead to low productivity and bad service.

Even a leader's mood can affect workers. A boss who is confident, optimistic, and passionate about his/her work can instill the same qualities in the workers. Such enthusiasm is almost always infectious, and is passed on to others within the organization. The same can be said of a leader who is weak, negative, and obviously unenthusiastic about his/her work—these poor qualities can be acquired by others.

TABLE 1-7 Key Leadership Protocols

1. Professionalism
2. Reciprocal trust and respect
3. Confident, optimistic, and passionate
4. Being visible
5. Open communicator
6. Risk taker
7. Admitting fault

Leaders must be very visible throughout the organization. Having a presence can assure workers that the top people are "at the helm" and give a sense of stability and confidence in the business. Leaders must be open communicators. Harboring information that could have been shared with followers will cause ill feelings and a concern that other important matters are not being disclosed. Leaders also need to take calculated risks. They should be cautious, but not overly so, or they might lose an opportunity for the organization. And finally, leaders in today's world need to recognize that they are not perfect. Sometimes there will be errors in what is said or done. These must be acknowledged so they can be put aside and the leader can move on to more pressing current issues.

GOVERNANCE

Individuals are not the only ones to consider in leadership roles. There can be a group of people who collectively assume the responsibility for strategic oversight of a healthcare organization. The term **governance** describes this important function. Governing bodies can be organized in a variety of forms. In a hospital, this top accountable body is called a board of trustees for a not-for-profit setting, and a **board of directors** for a proprietary or profit setting. Since many physician offices, long-term care facilities, and other healthcare entities are set up as professional corporations, these organizations would also have a board of directors.

Governing boards are facing heightened scrutiny due to the failure of many large corporations in the last decade. The United States government recognizes the importance of a group of people who oversee corporate operations and give assurances for the fair and honest functioning of the business. Sarbanes-Oxley is a federal law enacted in 2002 to enforce this disclosure for proprietary companies. Many believe the not-for-profits should have the same requirements and are applying pressure for them to fall under similar rules of transparency. Financial records must be appropriately audited and signed off by top leaders. Operations need to be discussed more openly so as to remove any possibility of cover-up, fraud, or self-interest. Each governing board member has fiduciary responsibility to forgo his/her own personal interests and to make all decisions concerning the entity for the good of the organization.

Although healthcare boards are becoming smaller in size, they recognize the importance of the composition of their members. A selection of people from within the organization (e.g., system leaders, the management staff, physicians, etc.) should be balanced with outside members from the community (see Table 1-8). The trend is to appoint members who have certain expertise to assist the board in carrying out its duties. Also, having governing board members who do not have ties to the healthcare operations will reduce the possibility of conflicts of interests. Board meetings have gone from ones in which a large volume of information is presented for a "rubber stamp," to meetings that are well prepared, purposeful, and focused on truly important issues. A self assessment should be taken at least annually and any identified problem areas (including particular board members) addressed. This way, the governing board can review where it stands in its ability to give fair, open, and honest strategic oversight (Gautam, 2005).

BARRIERS AND CHALLENGES

The healthcare industry is as dynamic as it gets. The only constant is change. Healthcare leaders are confronted with many situations that must be contended with as they lead their organizations. Some can be considered barriers that, if not dealt with properly, will stymie the leader's capability. Certain other areas are challenges that must be addressed if the leader is to be successful. A few of the more critical ones in today's healthcare world are presented here. See Table 1-9.

Due to the complex healthcare system in the United States, many regulations and laws are in place that sometimes can inhibit innovative and

TABLE 1-8 Healthcare Governance Trends

Area	Old Way	New Trend
Size of board	Large (10 to 20 people)	Smaller (6 to 12 people)
Membership	Many members from within the organization	Many with a balance of members within and outside
Conflicts of interest	Some present, not disclosed	Must be disclosed but prefer none
Meetings	Voluminous, detailed	Strategic information and trends presented
Evaluations	If done, not taken too seriously	Taken seriously to identify and correct issues

---

TABLE 1-9 Key Healthcare Leadership
Barriers and Challenges

---

1. Laws and Regulations (Barrier)
2. Physicians (Challenge)
3. New Technology (Barrier)
4. Culture of Safety (Challenge)

---

creative business practices. Leaders must assure that the strategies developed for their entity comply with the current laws or else they jeopardize the long-term survivability of their organization. Leaders are expected to sometimes think "outside the box" to provide new ideas for the development of their business, yet this can be challenging when many constraints must be considered. Some good examples are the government's anti-trust requirements, which can affect developing partners; federal moratoriums on certain services, which can affect growing the business; and safe harbor requirements, which can affect physician relations. These, as well as other laws and regulations, can affect a healthcare leader's ability to lead.

The healthcare industry is unique in the way a major player in the arena, the physicians, are not always easily controlled by the medical organizations where they work (e.g., hospitals, insurance companies, long-term care facilities). Yet, this very influential group of stakeholders has substantial input over the volume of patients that a healthcare facility receives. This necessitates the healthcare leader to find ways to include the doctors in the process of setting a direction, monitoring the quality of care, and fulfilling other administrative functions. The wise healthcare leader will include physicians early on in any planning process. Doctors are usually busy with their own patients and practices, but if they are not looked to for their expertise and advice on certain important matters in the facilities where they work, then they will become disengaged. This could cause essential functions to be overlooked. It could also cause physicians to alter the referral patterns for their patients. Everybody would much rather work at a place where their opinions are requested and respected.

Technology is a costly requirement in any work setting. Information systems management and new medical equipment are especially expensive for the modern healthcare facility or practice due to the rapidly changing data collection requirements and medical advances in the field. Healthcare leaders must assess the capabilities of their entities for new technology and determine if their systems and equipment are a barrier to making future progress. Healthcare leaders cannot be successful if their organizations have antiquated systems and out-of-date support devices in today's high tech world. Computer hardware and clinical software must be integrated to provide the quality and cost information needed for an efficient medical organization. Electronic medical records, wireless devices, and computerized order entry systems, as well as advanced medical equipment and new age pharmaceuticals, will be items the leader must have in place in order to be able to lead his/her healthcare organization into the 21st century.

Safety concerns have traditionally been a management responsibility. However, it has become such an important issue in today's healthcare world that leaders must be involved in its oversight. A top-down direction must be given through the organization that mistakes will not be tolerated. Coordinated efforts must shift from following up on errors, to preventing their reoccurrence, to developing systems and mechanisms to prevent them from ever occurring. The Joint Commission on Accreditation of Healthcare Organizations (JCAHO) has recently proposed new leadership standards for all sectors, calling for the leaders in the healthcare entity to accept the responsibility for instilling a culture of safety. A systems approach is being recommended that will anticipate and prevent human errors, prevent errors from reaching the patient, and mitigate harm when they do (JCAHO, 2005).

ETHICAL RESPONSIBILITY

Ethics is exhibiting behavior and conduct that is appropriate in a certain setting. It is a matter of doing right vs. wrong. Ethics is especially important for healthcare leadership and requires two areas of focus. One area is **bioethics** and the actions a leader needs to consider as he/she relates to a patient. Another is **managerial** ethics. This involves business practices and doing things for the right reasons. A leader must assure an environment in which good ethical behavior is followed.

The American College of Healthcare Executives (ACHE) does an excellent job in educating its professional membership as to the ethical responsibilities of healthcare leaders (ACHE, 2005). Ethical responsibilities apply to several different constituencies: to the profession itself, to the patients and others served, to the organization, to the employees, and to the community and society at large (see Table 1-10). A healthcare leader who is concerned about an ethical workplace will not only model the appropriate behavior but will also have a zero tolerance for any deviation by a member of the organization. A Code of Ethics gives specific guidelines to be followed by individual members. An Integrity Agreement would address a commitment to follow ethical behavior by the organization.

LEADERS LOOKING TO THE FUTURE

Some people believe that leaders are born and one cannot be taught how to be a good leader. The growing trend though is that leaders can in fact be taught skills and behaviors that will help them to lead an organization effectively (Parks, 2005). In healthcare, many clinicians who do well at their job are promoted to supervisory positions. Yet, they do not have the management training which would help them in their new roles. For example, physicians, laboratory technologists, physical therapists, and nurses are pushed into management positions with no administrative training. We are doing a disservice to these clinicians and setting them up for failure.

Fortunately, this common occurrence has been recognized and many new programs have sprouted to address this need. Universities have devel-

TABLE 1-10 American College of Healthcare Executives Code of Ethics

Responsible Area	Sample Guidelines
To the Profession	Comply with laws Avoid any conflicts of interest Respect confidences
To the Patients or Others Served	Prevent discrimination Safeguard patient confidentiality Have process to evaluate quality of care
To the Organization	Allocate proper resources Improve standards of management Prevent fraud and abuse within
To the Employees	Allow free expression Ensure a safe workplace environment Follow nondiscrimination policies
To the Community and Society	Work to meet the needs of the community Provide appropriate access to services Advocate for healthy society

oped executive programs to attract medical personnel into a fast-track curriculum to attempt to give them the essential skills they need to be successful. Some schools have developed majors in Healthcare Leadership and some healthcare systems have started internal leadership training programs. This trend will continue into the future since healthcare services are expected to grow due to the aging population and thus there will be a need for more people to be in charge. In addition, leaders should continually be updated as to the qualities which make a good leader in the current environment, and therefore, professional development, provided through internal or external programs, should be encouraged.

Each of the different sectors in health care has a professional association that will support many aspects of its particular career path. These groups provide ongoing educational efforts to help their members lead their organizations. Also, professional associations are a good way to network with people in similar roles, a highly desirable process for healthcare leaders. Another benefit for leaders is that these groups provide up-to-date information about their chosen field. Most have student chapters, and early involvement in these organizations is highly recommended for any future healthcare leader. Table 1-11 lists some of these associations.

TABLE 1-11 Professional Associations

Name	Acronym	Targeted Career	Website
American College of Healthcare Executives	ACHE	Health Administrators	www.ache.org
Healthcare Financial Management Association	HFMA	Healthcare Chief Financial Officers	www.hfma.org
Association for University Programs in Health Administration	AUPHA	Health Administration Education Program Directors	www.aupha.org
Medical Group Management Association	MGMA	Medical Groups Administrators	www.mgma.org
American College of Health Care Administrators	ACHCA	Long-Term Care Administrators	www.achca.org
American Academy of Nursing	AAN	Nurse Leaders	www.aannet.org
American College of Physician Executives	ACPE	Physician Leaders	www.acpe.org

To prepare an organization for the future, its leader needs to be looking out for opportunities to partner with other entities. Health care in the United States is fragmented, and to be successful, different services need to be aligned and networks created that will allow patients to flow easily through the continuum of care. It is the astute leader who can determine who are the best partners and negotiate a way to have a win-win situation. Of course these efforts to develop partnerships must be in line with the organization's mission and vision, or the strategic direction will have to be reexamined.

A leader who is concerned about the future will stay on top of things in the healthcare industry. Reading newspapers, industry journals, and Web reports will keep the leader in-the-know and allow him/her to determine how changes in the field could impact the organization. A leader who remains current will be better positioned to act proactively and to provide the best chance for his/her organization to seize a fresh opportunity.

Finally, the healthcare leader who is concerned about the future, as well as today's business, must continuously reassess how he/she fits in the organization. Nothing could be worse than a disenchanted person trying to lead a group of followers without the motivation and enthusiasm needed by great leaders. A leader should consider his/her own succession planning so that the organization is not left at any time without a person to lead. Truly unselfish leaders think about their commitment to their followers and do their best to assure that consistent formidable leadership will be in place in the event of their departure. This final act will allow adequate time for a smooth transition and insure the passage of accountability so that the followers can realign themselves with the new leader.

DISCUSSION QUESTIONS

1. What is the difference between leadership and management?

2. What is followership? Why is it as important as leadership?

3. Are leaders born or are they trained? How has the history of leadership in the United States evolved to reflect this question?

4. List and describe the contemporary models of leadership. What distinguishes them from past models?

skills, knowledge, abilities
table 1-6

5. What are the leadership domains and competencies? Can you be a good leader and not have all the competencies listed in this model?

6. Why do healthcare leaders have a higher need for ethical behavior than might be expected in other settings? *difficult decisions to be made*

REFERENCES

American College of Healthcare Executives. (2005). *Annual report and reference guide.*

Atchison, T. A. (2003). *Followership: a practical guide to aligning leaders and followers.* Chicago: Health Administration Press.

Freshman, B., & Rubino, L. (2002). Emotional intelligence: a core competency for health care administrators. *The Health Care Manager, 20,* 1–9.

Gautam, K. (2005). Transforming hospital board meetings: guidelines for comprehensive change. *Hospital Topics: Research and Perspectives on Healthcare, 83*(3), 25–31.

Goffee, R., & Jones, G. (2000, September). Why should anyone be led by you? *Harvard Business Review,* 62–70.

Goleman, D. (1998, December). What makes a leader? *Harvard Business Review,* 93–102.

Goleman, D. (2000, March-April). Leadership that gets results. *Harvard Business Review,* 79–90.

Hilberman, D. (Ed.) (2005, June). *Final report: pedagogy enhancement project on leadership skills for healthcare management.* The 2004 ACHE-AUPHA Pedagogy Enhancement Work Group. Association of University Programs in Health Administration.

Hutton, D., & Moulton, S. (2004). Behavioral competencies for health care leaders. *Best of H&HN OnLine.* American Hospital Association, 15–18.

Joint Commission on Accreditation of Healthcare Organizations. (2005). Critical Access Hospitals Leadership Standards Field Review.

Manion, J. (2005). *From management to leadership: practical strategies for health care leaders (2nd ed.).* San Francisco: Jossey-Bass.

Maslow, A. H. (1943). A theory of human motivation. *Psychological Review, 50,* 370–396.

McConnell, C. (2003). Accepting leadership responsibility: preparing yourself to lead honestly, humanely, and effectively. *The Health Care Manager, 22*(4), 361–374.

McGinn, P. (2005). *Leading others, managing yourself.* Chicago: Health Administration Press.

Northouse, P. (2004). *Leadership: theory and practice.* Thousand Oaks, CA: Sage Publications.

Parks, S. (2005). *Leadership can be taught: a bold approach for a complex world.* Boston: Harvard Business School Press.

Schaeffer, L. (2002, October). The leadership journey. *Harvard Business Review*, 3–7.

Shewchuk, R., O'Connor, S., & Fine, D. (2005). Building an understanding of the competencies needed for health administration practice. *Journal of Healthcare Management, 50*(1), 32–47.

Sibbet, D. (1997, September-October). 75 years of management ideas and practice 1922–1997. *Harvard Business Review Supplement*.

Spath, P. (2005). *Leading your healthcare organization to excellence: a guide to using the Baldrige criteria*. Chicago: Health Administration Press.

Strack, G., & Fottler, M. (2002). Spirituality and effective leadership in healthcare: is there a connection? *Frontiers of Health Services Management, 18*(4), 3–18.

Swearingen, S., & Liberman, A. (2004). Nursing leadership: serving those who serve others. *The Health Care Manager, 23*(2), 100–109.

Warden, G. (1999). Leadership diversity. *Journal of Healthcare Management, 44*(6), 421–422.

Wolf, E. (2004). Spiritual leadership: a new model. *Healthcare Executive, 19*(2), 22–25.

Additional Websites to Explore

National Center for Healthcare Leadership	www.nchl.org
Health Leadership Council	www.hlc.org
National Public Health Leadership Institute	www.phli.org
World Health Organization Leadership Service	www.who.int/health_leadership
Health Leaders Media	www.healthleaders.com
Institute for Diversity of Health Management	www.diversityconnection.org
Healthcare Leadership Alliance Competency Directory	http://www.healthcareleadershipalliance.org/

CHAPTER 2

Management and Motivation

Nancy H. Shanks

LEARNING OBJECTIVES

By the end of this chapter the student will be able to:

- Frame the context for understanding the concept of motivation, particularly who and what motivates employees;
- Provide an overview of the different theories of motivation;
- Identify extrinsic and intrinsic factors that impact motivation;
- Assess misconceptions about motivation; and,
- Suggest strategies to enhance employee motivation.

INTRODUCTION

Managers are continually challenged to motivate a workforce to do two things. The first challenge is to motivate employees to work toward helping the organization achieve its goals. The second is to motivate employees to work toward achieving their own personal goals.

Meeting the needs and achieving the goals of both the employer and the employee is often difficult for managers in all types of organizations. In health care, however, this is often more difficult, in part as a result of the complexity of healthcare organizations, but also as a function of the wide array of employees who are employed by or work collaboratively with healthcare providers in delivering and paying for care. The types of workers run the gamut from highly trained and highly skilled technical and clinical staff members to relatively unskilled workers. To be successful, healthcare managers need to be able to manage and motivate this wide array of employees.

MOTIVATION—THE CONCEPT

According to *Webster's New Collegiate Dictionary*, a motive is "something (a need or desire) that causes a person to act." **Motivate**, in turn, means "to provide with a motive," and motivation is defined as "the act or process of motivating." Thus, **motivation** is the act or process of providing a motive that causes a person to take some action. In most cases motivation comes from some need that leads to behavior that results in some type of reward when the need is fulfilled. This definition raises a couple of basic questions.

What are Rewards?

Rewards can take two forms. They can be either intrinsic/internal rewards or extrinsic/external ones. **Intrinsic rewards** are derived from within the individual. For a healthcare employee this could mean taking pride and feeling good about a job well done (e.g., providing excellent patient care). **Extrinsic rewards** pertain to rewards that are given by another person, such as a healthcare organization giving bonuses to teams of workers when quality and patient satisfaction are demonstrated to be exceptional.

Who Motivates Employees?

While rewards may serve as incentives and those who bestow rewards may seek to use them as motivators, the real motivation to act comes from within the individual. Managers do exert a significant amount of influence over their employees, but they do not have the power to force a person to act. They can work to provide various types of incentives in an effort to influence an employee in any number of ways, such as by changing job descriptions, rearranging work schedules, improving working conditions, reconfiguring teams, and a host of other activities, as will be discussed later in this chapter. While these may have an impact on an employee's level of motivation and willingness to act, when all is said and done, it is the employee's decision to take action or not. In discussing management and motivation, it will be important to continually remember the roles of both managers and employees in the process of motivation.

Is Everybody Motivated?

As managers, we often assume that employees are motivated or will respond to inducements from managers. While this is perhaps a logical and rational approach from the manager's perspective, it is critical to understand that this is not always the case. While the majority of employees do, in fact, want to do a good job and are motivated by any number of factors, others may not share that same drive or high level of motivation. Those folks may merely be putting in time and may be more motivated by other things, such as family, school, hobbies, or other interests. Keeping this in mind is useful in helping managers understand employee behaviors that seem to be counter-productive.

THEORIES OF MOTIVATION

Psychologists have studied human motivation extensively and have derived a variety of theories about what motivates people. This section briefly highlights the motivational theories that are regularly discussed in management textbooks. These include theories that focus on motivation being a function of 1) employee needs of various types, 2) extrinsic factors, and 3) intrinsic factors. Each set of theories will be discussed below.

Needs-Based Theories of Motivation

- **Maslow's Hierarchy of Need**—Maslow (1954) postulated a hierarchy of needs that progresses from the lowest, subsistence-level needs to the highest level of self-awareness and actualization. Once each level has been met, the theory is that an individual will be motivated by and strive to progress to satisfy the next higher level of need. The five levels in Maslow's hierarchy are
  - **Physiological needs**—including food, water, sexual drive, and other subsistence-related needs;
  - **Safety needs**—including shelter, a safe home environment, employment, a healthy and safe work environment, access to health care, money, and other basic necessities;

- **Belonging needs**—including the desire for social contact and interaction, friendship, affection, and various types of support;
- **Esteem needs**—including status, recognition, and positive regard; and,
- **Self-actualization needs**—including the desire for achievement, personal growth and development, and autonomy.

The movement from one level to the next was termed **satisfaction progression** by Maslow, and it was assumed that over time individuals were motivated to continually progress upward through these levels. While useful from a theoretical perspective, most individuals do not view their needs in this way, making this approach to motivation a bit unrealistic.

- **Alderfer's ERG Theory**—The three components identified by Alderfer (1972) drew upon Maslow's theory, but also suggested that individuals were motivated to move forward and backward through the levels in terms of motivators. He reduced Maslow's levels from five to the following three:
  - **Existence**—which related to Maslow's first two needs, thus combining the physiological and safety needs into one level;
  - **Relatedness**—which addressed the belonging needs; and,
  - **Growth**—which pertains to the last two needs, thereby combining esteem and self-actualization.

Alderfer also added his **frustration-regression principle**, which postulated that individuals would move in and out of the various levels, depending upon the extent to which their needs were being met. This approach is deemed by students of management to be more logical and similar to many individuals' world views.

- **Herzberg's Two Factor Theory**—Herzberg (2003) further modified Maslow's needs theory and consolidated down to two areas of needs that motivated employees. These were termed
  - **Hygienes**—These were characterized as lower level motivators and included, for example, "company policy and administration, supervision, interpersonal relationships, working conditions, salary, status, and security" (p. 5).
  - **Motivators**—These emphasized higher level factors and focused on aspects of work, such as "achievement, recognition for achieve-

ment, the work itself, responsibility and growth or advancement" (p. 5).

Herzberg's is an easily understood approach that suggests that individuals have desires beyond the hygienes and that motivators are very important to them.

- **McClelland's Acquired Needs Theory**—The idea here is that needs are acquired throughout life. That is, needs are not innate, but are learned or developed as a result of one's life experiences (McClelland, 1985). This theory focuses on three types of needs:
  - **Need for achievement**—which emphasizes the desires for success, for mastering tasks, and for attaining goals;
  - **Need for affiliation**—which focuses on the desire for relationships and associations with others; and,
  - **Need for power**—which relates to the desires for responsibility for, control of, and authority over others.

All four of these theories approach needs from a somewhat different perspective and are helpful in understanding employee motivation on the basis of needs. However, other theories of motivation also have been posited and require consideration.

Extrinsic Factor Theories of Motivation

Another approach to understanding motivation focuses on external factors and their role in understanding employee motivation. The best known of these is:

- **Reinforcement Theory**—B.F. Skinner (1953) studied human behavior and proposed that individuals are motivated when their behaviors are reinforced. His theory is comprised of four types of reinforcement. The first two are associated with achieving desirable behaviors, while the last two address undesirable behaviors:
  - **Positive reinforcement**—relates to taking action that rewards positive behaviors;
  - **Avoidance learning**—occurs when actions are taken to reward behaviors that avoid undesirable or negative behaviors. This is sometimes referred to as **negative reinforcement**;

- **Punishment**—includes actions designed to reduce undesirable behaviors by creating negative consequences for the individual; and,
- **Extinction**—represents the removal of positive rewards for undesirable behaviors.

The primary criticism of the reinforcement approach is that it fails to account for employees' abilities to think critically and reason, both of which are important aspects of human motivation. While reinforcement theory may be applicable in animals, it doesn't account for the higher level of cognition that occurs in humans.

Intrinsic Factor Theories of Motivation

Theories that are based on intrinsic or endogenous factors focus on internal thought processes and perceptions about motivation. Several of these are highlighted below:

- **Adam's Equity Theory**—which proposes that individuals are motivated when they perceive that they are treated equitably in comparison to others within the organization (Adams, 1963);
- **Vroom's Expectancy Theory**—which addresses the expectations of individuals and hypothesizes that they are motivated by performance and the expected outcomes of their own behaviors (Vroom, 1964); and,
- **Locke's Goal Setting Theory**—which hypothesizes that by establishing goals individuals are motivated to take action to achieve those goals (Locke & Latham, 1990).

While each of these theories deals with a particular aspect of motivation, it seems unrealistic to address them in isolation, since these factors often do come into play in and are important to employee motivation at one time or another.

Management Theories of Motivation

Other approaches to motivation are driven by aspects of management, such as productivity, human resources, and other considerations. Most notable in this regard are the following:

- **Scientific Management Theory**—Frederick Taylor's ideas, put into practice by the Gilbreths in the film *Cheaper by the Dozen*, focused on studying job processes, determining the most efficient means of performing them, and in turn rewarding employees for their productivity and hard work. This theory assumes that people are motivated and able to continually work harder and more efficiently and that employees should be paid on the basis of the amount and quality of the work performed. Over time, this approach is limited by the capacity of employees to continue to increase the quantity of work produced without sacrificing the quality.

- **McGregor's Theory X and Theory Y**—This approach again draws upon the work of Herzberg and develops a human resources management approach to motivation. This theory first classifies managers into one of two groups. Theory X managers view employees as unmotivated and disliking of work. Under the Theory X approach the manager's role is to focus on the hygienes and to control and direct employees; it assumes that employees are mainly concerned about safety. In contrast, Theory Y managers focus on Herzberg's motivators and work to assist employees in achieving these higher levels. In assessing this theory, researchers have found that approaching motivation from this either/or perspective is short-sighted.

- **Ouchi's Theory Z**—This theory is rooted in the idea that employees who are involved in and committed to an organization will be motivated to increase productivity. Based on the Japanese approach to management and motivation, Theory Z managers provide rewards, such as long-term employment, promotion from within, participatory management, and other techniques to motivate employees (Ouchi, 1981).

While all of these theories are helpful in understanding management and motivation from a conceptual perspective, it is important to recognize that most managers draw upon a combination of needs, extrinsic factors, and intrinsic factors in an effort to help motivate employees, to help employees meet their own personal needs and goals, and ultimately to achieve effectiveness and balance within the organization. Managers typically take into account most of the aspects upon which these theories focus. That is, expectancy, goal setting, performance, feedback, equity, satisfaction, commitment, and other characteristics are considered in the process of motivating employees.

A BIT MORE ABOUT INCENTIVES AND REWARDS

Throughout this chapter we have discussed what motivates employees. As the previous discussion indicates, motivation for employees results from a combination of incentives that take the form of extrinsic and intrinsic rewards. These topics warrant a bit more discussion.

Extrinsic Rewards

There are a host of external things that managers can provide that may serve as incentives for employees to increase their productivity. These include:

- Money—in the form of pay, bonuses, stock options, etc.
- Benefits—also in many different forms, including health insurance, vacation, sick leave, retirement accounts, etc. Increasingly benefits are offered under some form of cafeteria plans, allowing employees flexibility in what can be selected and in the management of their own benefit package.
- Flexible schedules.
- Job responsibilities and duties.
- Promotions.
- Changes in status—conveyed either by changes in job titles or in new and different job responsibilities.
- Supervision of others.
- Praise and feedback.
- A good boss.
- A strong leader.
- Other inspirational people.
- A nurturing organizational culture.

As this list demonstrates, extrinsic rewards are all tangible types of rewards. Intrinsic rewards stand in marked contrast to these.

Intrinsic Rewards

Intrinsic rewards are internal to the individual and are in many ways less tangible. In fact, they are highly subjective, in that they represent how the individual perceives and feels about work and its value. Five types of intrinsic rewards that have been summarized by Manion (2005) include:

- **Healthy relationships**—in which employees are able to develop a sense of connection with others in the workplace.
- **Meaningful work**—where employees feel that they make a difference in people's lives. This is typically a motivator for people to enter and stay employed in the healthcare industry. This type of work is viewed as that in which the meaningful tasks outweigh the meaningless. This reinforces the mantra Herzberg first espoused in 1968, and revisited in a 2003 issue of the *Harvard Business Review*, in which he stated: "Forget praise. Forget punishment. Forget cash. You need to make their jobs more interesting." As paperwork in health care has increased, managers need to be aware that such tasks detract from the meaningfulness quotient.
- **Competence**—where employees are encouraged to develop skills that enable them to perform at or above standards, preferably the latter.
- **Choice**—where employees are encouraged to participate in the organization in various ways, such as by expressing their views and opinions, sharing in decision making, and finding other ways to facilitate participatory approaches to problem solving, goal setting and the like.
- **Progress**—where managers find ways to hold employees accountable, facilitate their ability to make headway towards completing their assigned tasks, and celebrate when progress is made toward completing important milestones within a project.

Intrinsic rewards, coupled with extrinsic ones, lead to high personal satisfaction and serve as motivators for most employees.

MISCONCEPTIONS ABOUT MOTIVATION AND EMPLOYEE SATISFACTION

Managers tend to have many misconceptions about motivation. As health-care managers, it is important to assess and understand such misconceptions in an effort to become more effective managers and to not perpetuate myths about motivation. For example, research indicates that managers typically make incorrect assumptions about what motivates their employees. Morse (2003) states that "managers are not as good at judging employee motivation as they think they are. In fact, people from all walks of life seem to consistently misunderstand what drives employee motivation." The following is an enumeration of many of these misconceptions.

- *Although I'm not motivated by extrinsic rewards, others are.* This idea is discussed by Morse (2003) in his review of Chip Heath's study of intrinsic and extrinsic rewards. The conclusion is that an "extrinsic incentive bias" exists and is, in fact, wide-spread among managers and employees. That is, individuals assume that others are driven more by extrinsic rewards than intrinsic ones. This has been shown to be a false assumption.

- *All motivation is intrinsic.* Managers need to remember that typically a combination of factors motivates employees, not just one type of extrinsic or intrinsic reward (Manion, 2005, p. 283).

- *Some people just are not motivated.* Everyone is motivated by something; the problem for managers is that "that something" may not be directed toward the job. This creates challenges for managers who must try to redirect the employees' energies toward job-related behaviors (Manion, 2005, p. 283).

- *People are motivated by money.* Compensation motivates only to a point; that is, when compensation isn't high enough or is considered to be inequitable, it's a de-motivator. In contrast, when it is too high, it also seems to be a de-motivator, what Atchison calls the "golden handcuffs," and results in individual performance being tempered to protect the higher compensation level. Generally, employees tend to rank pay as less important than other motivators. This is supported by the 1999 Hay Group study, where 500,000 employees ranked fair pay and benefits as the least important of 10 motivating factors that keep them committed to staying with their companies. The bottom line from Atchison's perspective is that "as soon as money is predictable, it is an entitlement, not a motivator" (2003, p.21).

- *Motivation is manipulation.* Manipulation carries negative implications; in contrast motivation is positive and benefits both management and the employee (Manion, 2005).

- *One-size-fits-all reward and recognition programs motivate staff.* People, being people, are different, act in different ways, and are motivated by different things. Tailoring rewards and recognition is viewed as a way to focus on and understand the individual and his/her unique qualities (Atchison, 2003, p. 21).

- *Motivational people are born, not made.* Studies show that people aren't born to motivate. In fact, Manion states "anyone can become an effective motivator. It simply takes an understanding of the theories and basic principles" (Manion, 2005, p. 284), as well as the desire to develop these skills.
- *There is one kind of employee satisfaction.* Atchison (2003) discusses the pros and cons of "egocentric and other-centered satisfaction" and suggests that in the short run employees respond to specific rewards that they receive personally, but in the longer run they respond to quality performance of the team and the organization. Thus, they migrate from being self-centered to being other-centered in terms of job satisfaction—from a "me" to a "we" mentality.

MOTIVATIONAL STRATEGIES

The literature provides an array of strategies for managers to use in seeking to help motivate individuals. Some of these seem very obvious, while others represent the "tried and true" approaches to management. Still others represent innovations. No matter, they are worth enumerating here.

- *Expect the best.* People live up to the expectations they and others have of them. Henry Ford said it best: "Whether you think you can or you think you can't, you're right!'" (Manion, 2005, p. 292).
- *Reward the desired behavior.* Make sure that rewards are not given for undesirable behaviors and be sure to use many different types of rewards to achieve the desired outcomes (Manion, 2005, p. 295).
- *Create a "FUN (Focused, Unpredictable, and Novel) approach.* Atchison (2003, p. 21) suggests using money for a variety of creative employee rewards, such as giving $50 gift certificates to a shopping center in recognition of employees' exceeding expected patient outcomes.
- *Reward employees in ways that enhance performance and motivate them.* Don't waste money on traditional types of recognition. Though these are viewed as being nice, they don't motivate (Atchison, 2003). Money is better spent on true rewards for specific types of performance and outcomes.
- *Tailor rewards.* As mentioned in the previous section, Atchison (2003) steers managers away from standard types of rewards, such as giving the obligatory Thanksgiving turkey. Instead, he recommends

finding more creative ways to spend the organization's money and reward employees.

- *Focus on revitalizing employees.* Research shows that when employees are working on overloaded circuits motivation is diminished and productivity declines. This is particularly true in healthcare organizations. Hallowell (2005) suggests that managers can help to motivate employees by encouraging them to eat right, exercise regularly, take "real" vacations, get organized, and slow down.

- *Get subordinates to take responsibility for their own motivation.* This can be achieved by managers taking steps to deal with problem employees, to understand employees' needs, to determine what motivates their employees, to engage employees in the problem-solving process, and to really work hard at resolving, rather than ignoring, difficult employee problems (Nicholson, 2003).

- *Play to employees' strengths, promote high performance, and focus on how they learn.* This requires managers to know what their employees' strengths and weaknesses are, to find out what will be required to get specific employees to perform, and to understand how to capitalize on the ways those employees learn as an alternative method of encouraging and motivating them (Buckingham, 2005).

CONCLUSION

Motivation of employees is a tricky business. Managers often do not understand the concepts, principles, and myths about motivation well enough to put them in practice. Managers can improve their success rate by providing extrinsic rewards that will help their employees to be intrinsically motivated to become top performers.

DISCUSSION QUESTIONS

1. Compare and contrast needs-based theories of motivation. Which offers the most value to healthcare managers?

2. Discuss any limitations of the management approaches to motivation.

3. Which types of rewards are more important—intrinsic or extrinsic?

4. Does the importance of different types of rewards change over time as one progresses through one's career?

5. Which myth of motivation is the most important? Are there other myths that you can identify?

6. What motivational strategy would you apply with an employee who you think is capable of doing the work, but is underperforming?

7. What motivational strategy would you apply with a highly effective employee who you want to keep performing at a very high level?

REFERENCES

Adams, J. S. (1963, November). Towards an understanding of inequity. *Journal of Abnormal and Social Psychology, 67*(5), 422–436.

Alderfer, C. P. (1972). *Existence, relatedness and growth: human needs in organizational settings.* New York: Free Press.

Atchison, T. A. (2003, May/June). Exposing the myths of employee satisfaction. *Healthcare Executive, 17*(3), 20.

Buckingham, M. (2005, March). What great managers do. *Harvard Business Review, 3*(3), 70–79.

Hallowell, E. M. (2005, January). Overloaded circuits: why smart people underperform. *Harvard Business Review, 83*, 54–62.

Herzberg, F. (2003, January). One more time: how do you motivate employees? *Harvard Business Review, 81*, 86–96.

Locke, E. A., & Latham, G. P. (1990). *A theory of goal setting and task performance.* Englewood Cliffs, NJ: Prentice-Hall.

Manion, J. (2005). *From management to leadership.* San Francisco: Jossey-Bass.

Maslow, A. H. (1954). *Motivation and personality.* New York: Harper & Row.

McClelland, D. C. (1985). *Human motivation.* Glenview, IL: Scott, Foresman.

Morse, G. (2003, January). Why we misread motives. *Harvard Business Review, 81*(1), 18.

Nicholson, N. (2003, January). How to motivate your problem people. *Harvard Business Review, 81*(1), 57–65.

Ouchi, W. G. (1981). *Theory Z.* Reading, MA: Addison-Wesley Publishing Company.

Skinner, B. F. (1953). *Science and human behavior.* New York: Macmillan.

Vroom, V. H. (1964). *Work and motivation.* New York: Wiley.

CHAPTER 3

Organizational Behavior and Management Thinking

Sheila K. McGinnis

LEARNING OBJECTIVES

By the end of this chapter, the student will be able to:

- Explain what is meant by organizational behavior;
- State ten challenges of healthcare management;
- Define what is meant by cognition (or thinking) as it relates to behavior in organizations;
- Explain how perception and thinking influence behavior in the workplace;
- Describe the role of thinking in communication and problem solving in the workplace;
- Explain the role of thinking in organizational change and learning; and,
- Describe three ways a manager can use knowledge of thinking processes to improve communication between individuals, and within groups and organizations.

INTRODUCTION

Healthcare managers, like all managers in other industries, are responsible for effectively using the material, financial, information, and human resources of their organizations to deliver services. As you can see from the topics presented in this textbook, the manager's role requires a wide range of both technical and interpersonal skills. Leadership (Chapter 1), motivation (Chapter 2), managing healthcare professionals (Chapter 9), and teamwork (Chapter 11) are some of the most important interpersonal skills of a manager, examined at length in other chapters of this text. The purpose of this chapter is to provide a sample of how knowledge of human cognition (or thinking) provides valuable insight about communication skills and organizational behavior to help future healthcare managers understand human behavior at work. While this chapter will not make you an expert on organizational behavior or managerial thinking, it will help you appreciate how the science of organizational behavior and management thinking can be used to work with others in a way that leads to beneficial outcomes for both people and organizations.

The chapter begins with a brief background on the field of organizational behavior, describes several organizational behavior insights for health administration, and then offers an extended discussion and illustration of how the healthcare manager can use managerial thinking and organizational behavior to achieve important organizational goals.

THE FIELD OF ORGANIZATIONAL BEHAVIOR

Organizational behavior is a broad area of management that studies how people act in organizations. Managers can use theories and knowledge of organizational behavior to improve management practices for effectively working with and influencing employees to attain organization goals. The field of organizational behavior has evolved from the scientific study of management during the industrial era, administrative theories of the manager's role, principles of bureaucracy, and human relations studies of employees' needs (Scott, 1992). Organizational behavior is an interdisciplinary field that draws on the ideas and research of many disciplines that are concerned with human behavior and interaction. These include psychology, social psychology, industrial psychology, sociology, communications, and anthropology (Robbins, 2003). In this chapter, we will highlight ideas from cognitive psychology (the science of human thinking) and their extensions to organizational behavior.

ORGANIZATIONAL BEHAVIOR'S CONTRIBUTION TO MANAGEMENT

The most successful organizations make the best use of their employees' talents and energies (Heil, Bennis & Stephens, 2000; Huselid, 1995). Firms that effectively manage employees hold an advantage over their competitors. Pfeffer (1998) estimates that organizations can reap a 40% gain by managing people in ways that build commitment, involvement, learning, and organizational competence.

Because employees are key to an organization's success, how well the manager interacts and works with a variety of individuals is key to a manager's success. A manager who is skilled in organizational behavior will be able to work effectively with employees and colleagues across the organization, assisting and influencing them to support and achieve organization goals.

KEY TOPICS IN ORGANIZATIONAL BEHAVIOR

Organizational behavior is a broad field comprised of many subject areas. Work behaviors are typically examined at different levels—individual behavior, group behavior, and collective behavior across the organization—with different issues salient at each level. Studying individual behavior helps managers understand how perceptions, attitudes, and personality influence work behavior, motivation, and other important work outcomes, such as satisfaction, commitment, and learning. Examining interactions in the group setting provides insight into the challenges of leadership, teamwork, communication, decision making, power, and conflict. Studying organization-wide behavior (sometimes referred to as organization theory) helps explain how organizations structure work and power relationships, how they use systems for decision making and control, how an organization's culture affects behavior, how organizations learn, and how they adapt to changing competitive, economic, social, and political conditions.

ORGANIZATIONAL BEHAVIOR ISSUES IN HEALTH ORGANIZATIONS

Organizational behavior, whether in a healthcare or other type of organization, is concerned with behavior that occurs under the conditions posed by an organizational situation. While a specific organization setting may create unique challenges or certain sets of problems, the behaviors of interest are similar to those of individuals, groups, and often organizations in other settings or industries (Weick, 1969). Thus, healthcare organization behavior does not create unique management issues so much as certain issues are more prevalent in health care and occur along with other challenges (Shortell & Kaluzny, 2000).

Many of these challenges directly or indirectly affect what is expected of healthcare workers and how they behave in healthcare organizations. Health organizations are staffed with a highly professional workforce and impose exacting requirements on how work is organized and accomplished. The complex work has a high risk of serious or deadly error, which necessitates highly reliable systems of practice at all organization levels. Complex technical and medical systems demand sophisticated technical expertise, which requires a highly educated, efficient, and well-coordinated workforce. Professional workers, especially physicians, work with a great deal of autonomy and control over the technical and clinical aspects of care delivery. As a result, healthcare managers are responsible for facilitating the delivery of highly complex medical services that must be carefully coordinated by autonomous professionals over whom the manager has little direct authority—all within an industry system that is facing extreme financial and policy challenges.

Squeezed by rising costs and declining reimbursements, many health organizations struggle to survive financially. In the face of increased competition and consumer demands, the health delivery system is changing rapidly to create new services and adopt new technologies, often by forming new partnerships. The chronic health conditions that characterize an aging population demand more outpatient care, which dramatically changes the nature of care delivery. Concerns over patient safety and quality of care demands workers skilled in clinical information management, total quality management, and evidence-based practice, yet labor shortages abound and are predicted to increase.

The work of health care is carried out against the backdrop of these demands. Yet every day, the healthcare manager facilitates and orchestrates the accomplishment of organizational goals with an eye towards helping employees and colleagues successfully negotiate the complexities presented by the nature of healthcare work and the healthcare industry. To do this, the managers must be sure they themselves and those with whom they work continually find ways to effectively work together in a demanding industry. Organizational behavior skills help managers do this.

HOW THINKING INFLUENCES ORGANIZATIONAL BEHAVIOR

Organizational science explanations of human behavior increasingly draw upon human thinking, especially cognition and the creation of meaning. In the cognitive framework, behavior is inextricably tied to thinking. We cannot understand behavior without understanding the thoughts, assumptions, and attributes of a situation that precede behavior and its consequences.

Cognition refers to the mental processes involved in thinking, including attending to information, processing information, and ordering information to create meaning that is the basis for acting, learning, and other human activities. Cognitive science has taught us that information processing capacities and mental processes shape and govern one's perceptions, language, and, ultimately, one's behaviors. A focus on thinking highlights the importance of perceptions, assumptions, and social cues. It points out biases in information processing and creating common meaning during communication. Finally, it sets the stage for learning in that the human capacity to adapt is rooted in new ways of thinking and acting. Studies of thinking teach managers that humans have a limited capacity to process information, causing them to simplify and take shortcuts; that individuals' actions are largely determined by how they perceive the world; and that humans engage in an ongoing construction of their world by using stored information structures to guide their perception and interpretation of events and information (Fiske & Taylor, 1984).

In short, the lessons of cognition suggest that the foremost management task is to create common understanding among organization members. While thinking has long been implicit in understanding organization behavior, its importance grows in a knowledge economy that is driven by information (Huff, Huff & Barr, 2000). The effective healthcare manager works with organization members and constituents to make sense of their interactions and experiences and agree upon meaning so they can work together, make decisions, and take action. The rest of this chapter describes some cognitive principles commonly present in human interaction that often complicate organizational processes, and then discusses ways a manager can work to create a shared understanding that facilitates organizational effectiveness.

INDIVIDUAL PERCEPTION AND THINKING

Human understanding and the resulting organizational behavior are largely based upon how a person perceives and thinks about a situation (Elsbach, Barr, & Hargadon, 2005; Fiske & Taylor, 1984). **Perceptions** matter because how a person makes sense of a situation affects his or her attitudes, attributions, and behaviors. The process of perceiving involves noticing, selecting, and organizing information in order to respond. Information is naturally lost or distorted in this complex process, so the knowledge upon which a person's action is based may be incomplete or inaccurate. However, the actor assumes his or her knowledge is complete, and thus may act upon deficient information.

Experts have identified various habits of the mind that are based on the power of perceptions and patterns of thinking. Those with particular relevance for managers and organizations include perceptions, cognitive biases, Theory X and Theory Y, expectancies, expectancy theory, attribution theory, schemas, mental models, and sensemaking. Collectively, these principles demonstrate the power of thought, showing that how people view a situation has a strong effect on how they respond to and act upon that situation. They remind managers that much of organizational behavior is about each individual's "inner game," which is often not known by the individuals themselves nor revealed during interpersonal interactions. Thus, a valuable skill for managers is to elicit these thoughts in a way that organization members can work with them.

Perception

People vary greatly in what they notice and what draws their focused attention. Their attention processes will be influenced and filtered by their assumptions, values, knowledge, goals, past experiences, and other personal differences. As a result they will only take in part of the information they are presented with, and subsequently act upon partial information. In addition, the partial information that is taken in is subject to other mental processes that can create further distortions.

Cognitive Biases

As we have learned in recent decades, our human capacity to effectively process information is limited. So individuals compensate with judgment shortcuts (called **heuristics**) that simplify the decision process but create systematic biases affecting their judgments (Bazerman, 1998). These shortcuts make the complex processes of perceiving and judging vulnerable to the influence of assumptions and prior experiences that are readily recalled. A perceiver may notice and select only a subset of the information to which he is exposed because he is more apt to notice familiar cues or to arrange cues into meaningful groups based on his preconceptions and what he has learned from his own prior experiences and the experiences of others. For example, a mother can hear her child's voice in a noisy room and a star gazer finds it easier to locate a constellation once she knows the pattern to expect. Similarly, a physician who does not expect to see an exotic condition, like hanta virus, may fail to diagnose the problem because she is not attuned to the possibility.

Studies consistently document more than a dozen common biases, or systematic errors of perception and judgment, that, used inappropriately, diminish the quality of thinking by limiting the amount and richness of information processing. According to Das and Teng (1999) the four main categories of **cognitive biases** include 1) prior beliefs and assumptions that constrict one's capacity to absorb more information or prompt the use of preselected outcomes that narrow the range of options considered; 2) oversimplifying the problem definition or possible solutions, or relying on intuition, in a way that again limits the range of outcomes considered; 3) flawed assessments of the likelihood of occurrence; and 4) overestimating one's capacity to influence events (Korte, 2003).

The cognitive simplifications provided by judgment heuristics and biases do help the user streamline information processing. However, heuristics and biases are problematic when used inappropriately. The manager who can monitor and recognize situations with the potential for inappropriate biases and act to reduce biases and increase the appropriate use of information can significantly improve organizational decisions and actions (Bazerman, 1998).

Theory X and Theory Y

An early organizational psychologist, Douglas McGregor, described two very different ways of managing, termed **Theory X and Theory Y**. The two different approaches were based on very different underlying assumptions about human nature (McGregor, 1967). McGregor observed that early industrial management techniques were based on the negative beliefs that employees naturally dislike work and tend to avoid responsibility, so they must be compelled to perform (termed "Theory X"). He espoused a view based on the positive beliefs that employees are naturally motivated and committed, and that managers can fully tap employee talents by fostering employee growth, responsibility, and the development of their potential (termed "Theory Y"). One of the fundamental lessons from McGregor is that effective managers must "examine their deepest held beliefs about people and the nature of work" (Heil, Bennis, & Stephens, 2000, p. 15). Arguably the first step to managerial success begins with the manager's own philosophy of management—that is, the thoughts and assumptions that shape his or her own approach to management. Growing research support the merits of an intrinsically motivating (i.e., Theory Y) approach to engaging employees. Accordingly, managers must assess how well their own assumptions and behaviors and their organizations' policies and practices promote employee growth, development, engagement, and contribution (Heil, Bennis, & Stephens, 2000).

Expectancy

Perceptual expectations can create a situation in which "believing is seeing." That is, prior knowledge or experience tends to make us perceive what we expect to perceive. In addition, expectations or beliefs ("my boss won't like my idea") or situational cues ("organic chemistry is a difficult course") influence how we tend to act in certain situations and events (Bandura, 1977). In addition to individual expectations, expectations can also arise from social interactions between people. At an extreme, expectations about another's behavior can create a "self-fulfilling prophecy." For example, classroom teachers who expect students to perform a certain way may verbally and non-verbally transmit their expectations to students in a way that increases the likelihood that the expected effect will occur. Similarly, a manager who believes that a certain employee has an "attitude problem" may treat that person in a way that elicits the very behavior that is objectionable.

Expectancy Theory

The effect of expectancies is very robust, and also appears in the **expectancy theory** of individual work motivation (see Chapter 2). This is a cognitive theory of outcome expectancy in which an employee's motivation to put forth effort on the job depends on the expectations that the individual will be able to perform a task, and that successful performance will result in valued outcomes (Vroom, 1964). The manager who recognizes the role that employee and managerial expectations play in motivation can strengthen motivation by providing appropriate encouragement and assistance to help an employee succeed at a task, by identifying the employee's desired outcomes and rewarding appropriately, and by clearly conveying organizational goals and the manager's own performance expectations.

Attribution Theory

To attribute is to make an inference, or to explain what causes something. According to **attribution theory**, people naturally seek to explain the likely cause of another's behavior. Regardless of their accuracy, our perceptions will influence what we presume to be the cause of another's behavior. In general, the presumed cause of observed behavior will be attributed to either a person's disposition or personality, or else to the situation in which the behavior occurs. **Fundamental attribution error** is a cognitive bias in which an observer makes incorrect causal attributions. In fundamental attribution error, the observer erroneously attributes an actor's behavior to the actor's internal disposition, rather than external situation. For instance, if a stranger cuts in line ahead of you at the movies, you may conclude the action is intentional and decide the person is rude, even though it may have occurred because the entrance signs were not clear to the person who cut in line.

Managers are susceptible to fundamental attribution error when judging employee performance, blaming an employee for poor performance that may actually be caused by circumstances beyond the employee's control. For example, **attribution error** occurs when a manager decides an employee who performs a task poorly is lazy or incompetent, rather than recognizing the employee needs training, clear incentives, or improved work equipment. To avoid making an erroneous performance attribution requires the manager to fully understand both how the work context affects employee performance and how the employee perceives the work context and how it is affecting performance.

Schemas and Mental Models

Schemas are cornerstones of cognitive simplification. **Schemas** are mental representations of one's general knowledge and expectations about a concept, including the concept's attributes and relations among those attributes (Fiske & Taylor, 1984). Schemas direct how we perceive, classify, store, and act upon information received. They organize what we know and guide how we use our knowledge. In short, they help people make sense of the world. According to Fiske and Taylor, people develop schemas for many different concepts and situations. **Person schemas** characterize a certain person's traits and actions (my dad will loan me his car if I mow the lawn); **role schemas** define appropriate behaviors and expectations for a social category (grandmothers bake cookies, professors should grade fairly); and **event schemas** dictate one's expected "scripts" for how certain events should unfold (taking final exams, conducting a performance evaluation). Schemas are sophisticated mental devices that simplify information processing about people and situations. Because they are cognitive simplifications, they can also be incomplete, inaccurate, and difficult to change. Thus they provide another opportunity for distortion when organization members search for common understanding.

Thinking is an individual process. While an organization does not think, its capacity to take collective action depends upon the degree to which organization members share a common view or shared way of thinking about a situation. Organizational schemas and mental models can be viewed as a form of organizational thinking.

Common schemas can facilitate common understanding needed for collective action. When schemas are shared among organization members, they can define and guide organizational behaviors and actions. In healthcare organizations, members may hold schemas about strategies to attract and retain nurses, patients' roles in deciding about their treatment, or how to work with other healthcare organizations in the local market. These shared schemas enable organizational action consistent with the schemas, and may also hinder action that does not fit existing schemas.

Mental Models

Recent efforts to understand how organizations change and learn have led to the study of "mental models" in organizations. **Mental models** are "deeply held internal images of how the world works" (Senge, 1990, p 174). While expectancies and schemas are concerned with how we receive and store information, mental models are concerned with how we use that information in reasoning. Mental models are similar to expectancies and schemas in that they are abstract representations of reality that define expectations and interpretations. They are a guide to reasoning and they can also restrict how people think and act. Managers can change and improve organizations by discovering, sharing, challenging, and changing the schemas and mental models that guide how organization members think.

For example, a new longterm care center manager finds the facility's occupancy rate is too low, and the staff is convinced the center's location is undesirable. When the manager does a market analysis, he learns that client decisions are more influenced by available services rather than location. The staff's mental model that location drives client choice of facility was incorrect. When staff members revised their mental model to address range of services, the center's occupancy rate improved.

Sensemaking in Organizations

Perception and thinking are mainly concerned with how well one can accurately process and understand information and whether that understanding corresponds correctly to the information stimuli. A related problem is how people individually and collectively comprehend the meaning of ambiguous information or situations that are subject to several plausible interpretations. Ambiguous information is unclear and **equivocal**, in that it has multiple meanings and is open to several interpretations. Individuals frequently encounter ambiguous situations in organizations. Ambiguity becomes increasingly problematic as more individuals are involved, making it hard to find a common meaning on which to base action.

The term **sensemaking** refers to the process by which organizations arrive at a plausible interpretation of what an equivocal situation means (Weick, 1995). While sensemaking begins with the cognitive processes of individuals, involving multiple people (as in the organization setting) makes it a social process that also depends upon communication, interpersonal dynamics, and the give and take of dialogue and negotiation.

Studies on perception and thinking have given us new insight into mental habits. Sometimes these habits alter information processing, which can lead to miscommunications. Sensemaking calls attention to how organization members select information and communicate about alternative interpretations to arrive at an understanding that defines an equivocal situation and guides subsequent actions. Sensemaking is thus a fundamental component of many core organizational behaviors and processes, including communication, problem solving and decision making, coordination, conflict, and change. According to Weick, Sutcliff, and Obstfeld (2005), sensemaking has some important lessons for the manager. First, through the process of determining what is important in a situation, we define our environment and thus create our own opportunities and constraints—an organizational parallel to the self-fulfilling prophecy. Second, meaning is made retrospectively, in that the meaningful pattern we call understanding often emerges in hindsight as we process events with others. Third, sensemaking organizes information to create a plausible (if not necessarily accurate) understanding of a situation that is sufficient for organizational action and learning.

MANAGING AND LEARNING

As we have seen, perception and thinking among individuals are complex processes. Knowledge of biases, Theories X and Y, fundamental attribution error, mental models and sensemaking won't fix every situation encountered in an organization. However, these ideas point out that how people comprehend a situation can be very different from the actual facts of the situation, and will vary across individuals. The adage that perception is reality applies to organizations, and thinking and sensemaking principles can help the manager work with perceived realities. These ideas demonstrate that what one believes about a person or a situation, even if incomplete or inaccurate, will determine how one responds to that person or situation. The manager who is blind to assumptions and perceptions, both her own or others', will be working from an incomplete and inaccurate knowledge base.

A critical management task is to remedy the limits of human and organizational thinking and create common understanding among organization members, which is largely accomplished through conversation and discussion. The process of sharing assumptions and perceived realities makes them available to others, encourages individuals to refashion their own mental constructs, and promotes elaboration of common mental frameworks. In short, learning occurs and knowledge is created in the process of discussing and revising individual and organizational mental models (Easterby-Smith, Crossan, & Nicolini, 2000). In a knowledge economy, organizations with a superior ability to learn and adapt are expected to create new knowledge, master new behaviors, innovate, continually improve their work processes, outperform their competitors, and adapt to competitive pressures. The manager who can work with perceptions and mental models contributes to making a learning organization.

Current methods to foster learning and knowledge development in organizations often target ways to expand shared understanding, to improve shared mental models, and to engage in collective sensemaking. For example, Peter Senge (1990) outlines a set of five essential practices or "disciplines" that characterize the learning organization. His first two disciplines are systems thinking to discern the pattern of connections between elements of a system and a drive for individual proficiency that leads to personal mastery. Senge's last three disciplines help address the innate cognitive limits of individuals and groups. They include surfacing and challenging mental models, creating a common identity with a shared vision of the future, and team learning that uses dialog to remove assumptions and create shared meaning.

THINKING AND SENSEMAKING IN COMMUNICATION AND PROBLEM SOLVING

The bottom line of the organization and learning literature is that, instead of assuming meaning is clear, effective managers examine and test mental models and assumptions about the organizational world in order to increase shared understanding among members. Bias is inherent to human thinking, yet a manager can reduce bias through skillful collective communication and problem solving. One of the simplest ways to accomplish this is by sharing mental representations and beliefs with others through questioning, discussion, and debate (Heil, Bennis, & Stephens, 2000; Senge, 1990). Thus, communication and problem-solving skills are paramount to successfully working with thinking in organizations. However, as the ideas in this chapter suggest, successful communication and problem solving are less about following step-by-step procedures and more about creating clear common meaning.

Communication

Communication is "the creation or exchange of understanding between sender(s) and receiver(s)" (Shortell & Kaluzny, 2000, p. 224). Communication is one of the manager's most powerful tools and most important responsibilities because it can be used to create a shared, common focus. While communicating sounds easy, it is really much more than exchanging words and messages. Experts identify many barriers to communication. Communication failure may occur if the sender does not clearly convey the purpose or message, or provides too much information. The receiver may not correctly comprehend the message, may resist the message content or distort its meaning, or may not view the sender as credible. The communication setting also creates barriers, which can include relaying messages through an organizational chain of command, role or status differences between sender and receiver, or simply the logistical challenges of available time and media.

Some of the most potent communication barriers are the thoughts and perceptions of the sender and receiver. Successful communication only occurs when we overcome the myriad assumptions, biases and preconceptions brought to the conversation to achieve shared meaning. Shared understanding is the ultimate test of communication success (Shortell & Kaluzny, 2000).

Problem Solving

Perhaps the most important work of a manager is to assure that organizational problems are solved. A problem exists when the current and the desired state of affairs differ, and the manager solves the problem by finding a way to reach the desired state. Every day, healthcare organizations face problems related to treatment plans for patients, improving patient safety and quality of care, meeting patients' needs and expectations, determining the best mix of services to offer, and attracting and retaining the best workers. The successful manager is able to handle complex, ambiguous problems that are not clearly defined and for which opinions vary on the nature of the problem and possible solutions. This does not mean the manager always knows exactly what to do. Rather it means that the manager finds a way to engage others in finding an appropriate solution.

Problem solving involves two main phases, **problem identification** and **problem solution**, with various tasks occurring in each phase (Daft, 1992; Schein, 1988; Whetten & Cameron, 1998). The first phase involves recognizing and identifying the problem and its causes, setting goals, and generating options. The second phase involves assessing options, and choosing, implementing, and evaluating the chosen solution. While these problem-solving steps appear to be logical, actual problem solving and decision making in organizations often varies from this ideal process. Problem solving can be difficult because managers may have incomplete information or are unable to process all of the information related to the problem, goals and priorities may be unclear or in dispute, and results of alternatives may be uncertain.

CONCLUSION AND APPLICATIONS

This chapter offers a brief overview of organizational behavior in health care, and highlights how perceptions, thinking, mental models, and other thinking patterns play out in organizational life. The study of thinking processes indicates that human and organizational behavior is best understood as driven by people's perception of their world, rather than assuming they clearly comprehend all the facts of a complex world. The implication for managers is that fundamental organizational activities like communication, problem solving, and decision making depend less on following certain procedures and rely more upon the manager's efforts to bring employees together in defining a shared understanding that supports a focus on collective action.

As mentioned earlier, one of the best ways to address distortions and differences in thinking is by sharing mental models and understandings with others through questioning, discussion, and debate. The following scenarios provide the opportunity to examine these ideas more closely and work with them in practice.

ACTION INQUIRY: A FRAMEWORK FOR CHECKING ASSUMPTIONS

Torbert's (2004) Action Inquiry approach to organizational research fosters a type of dialogue that is an antidote to the assumptions and beliefs that limit thinking and learning, and serves to build shared understanding. Torbert's framework consists of four "forms of speech," or four steps to follow in the course of a conversation. Using these steps or forms of speech promotes awareness of self and awareness of others in a way that tests perceptions and assumptions. All four forms of speech are to be used sequentially during a conversation to steadily question (or inquire) how well practices (or action) support desired results:

- **Framing**—State the purpose and objectives for the current discussion, including any assumptions that need testing, to reveal the speaker's intentions and seek a common purpose;
- **Advocating**—State an opinion, perception, or feeling at an abstract level;
- **Illustrating**—Relate an anecdote or give an example that highlights the direction the speaker advocates; and,
- **Inquiring (and listening)**—Ask questions of listeners to learn their views and experiences regarding the speaker's explanation of the situation (as expressed by the speaker's prior framing, advocacy, and illustration statements).

Repeated questioning or inquiry using Torbert's four forms of speech will heighten awareness of the manager's own perspectives and practices, and also the perspectives and practices of other organization members. The purpose of this form of dialogue is to directly address assumptions and perceptions. The result is to increase personal and organizational effectiveness because this type of inquiry elicits and discusses people's understandings in a way that increases the parties' common understanding. Through the process of action inquiry, organization members can better create a common or collective viewpoint that provides a framework for collective organizational action.

APPLICATION EXERCISE 1: PRELUDE TO A MEDICAL ERROR

Mrs. Bee was lying in her bed after her morning physical therapy with Mr. Traction and felt like she couldn't breathe. "Is something bothering you, Mrs. Bee?" asked Nurse Karing. "I know you had a disagreement with your husband regarding rehabilitation last night," she said. Nurse Karing knew that Mrs. Bee had suffered a bad fall and that therapy was going to be difficult for her to handle. She had discussed the support issues that were important during stressful hospitalizations with Mrs. Bee's husband and he had appeared supportive. She felt that a disagreement wasn't the source of Mrs. Bee's discomfort.

Nurse Karing thought back to her previous night's visit with Mrs. Bee. Mrs. Bee had complained of terrible spasms within her left calf. Nurse Karing had proceeded to order a STAT venous doppler ultrasound to rule out thrombosis. She had also paged Dr. Cural to notify him that Mrs. Bee was having symptoms of thrombosis. Dr. Cural, upset that he was being bothered after a long day of work, had shouted into the phone, "I evaluated that patient this morning and nothing was wrong with her. I don't need incompetent nurses calling me at night to tell me that my patient is having leg cramps. Don't bother me again! And by the way, you had no right to order that test! Cancel it! (click)." The phone call had upset Nurse Karing, leaving her feeling humiliated and distracted. She had canceled the venous doppler test, as directed by Dr. Cural, thinking that he must have been right. Mrs. Bee was probably just having leg cramps from being sedentary during the day. And besides, she had thought, Dr. Cural always claimed to know his patients inside and out! Still, Nurse Karing had gone home that night feeling bothered by the incident and the lack of respect and communication displayed by her coworkers lately.

But today, Mrs. Bee was short of breath, pale, and had elevated blood pressure, and was losing consciousness. Nurse Karing ordered a STAT VQ scan to rule out a pulmonary embolus. Nurse Karing called for help. The nursing team and Dr. Krisis (from the ER) raced to the room to help stabilize Mrs. Bee. "Looks like we have another problem from one of the nursing floors," observed Dr. Krisis. "Someone must have not had time again to call the doctor yesterday to see if a venous doppler was necessary. Now she's really critical!" Nurse Karing ignored Dr. Krisis's comment and notified Dr. Cural. "Why didn't anybody call me to tell me that my

(*continued*)

patient was having problems? I am the physician! Can't you nurses do anything right? Don't you know that you need to focus on what symptoms Mrs. Bee is having. Get Mrs. Specimen up here to draw some blood. I want STAT ABGs now! Get ICU on the phone!"

At the same time, Mr. Friendly, the social worker, happened to be walking by. He stopped to speak to Dr. Cural and Nurse Karing. "Mrs. Bee's paperwork is all ready. Her insurance will allow her to go to a rehabilitation facility for one week of physical therapy. The MediCar will be here in 1 hour to pick her up." Nurse Karing was furious. She thought to herself, "It's time for administration to hear this one."

QUESTION A: Identify and discuss examples of preconceptions, assumptions, and mental models evident in this scenario. What are the consequences of the ways these health providers are thinking about the situation?

QUESTION B: Discuss some strategies each actor could use to deal with the preconceptions, assumptions, and mental models evident in this scenario. Roleplay the scenario using those strategies.

SOURCE: Scenario courtesy of Jennifer Krapfl, RN, MHA

APPLICATION EXERCISE 2: THE FINANCE DEPARTMENT AT ROSEVILLE COMMUNITY HOSPITAL

Kelly Munson, the new Finance Manager of Roseville Community Hospital, was reviewing a recent staff meeting in which the staff discussed reorganizing the Finance department. Louise Smith, who had been with the department for eight years, agreed that outdated computer systems compromised level of service to patients, but was unenthusiastic about making major changes. Frank Williams, who had applied for Kelly's job, but didn't get it, was unwilling to cooperate with the rest of the department. John Evans, who had recently completed his MHA degree, was eager to try new approaches that he learned in grad school. Kelly sighed, thinking how difficult it can be to help department members understand how their work fits together and to decide how to change operations to better serve patients and the hospital.

ACTIVITY A: Role-play a discussion between Louise, Frank, John, and Kelly as they discuss whether or not to reorganize the Finance department. Following the role-play, describe the assumptions and thought patterns that seemed to emerge in this scenario and discuss how they might be hindering the Finance department's ability to effectively solve this problem.

ACTIVITY B: Role-play a discussion between Louise, Frank, John, and Kelly on whether or not to reorganize the Finance department. Use the principles of Action Inquiry during the discussion to check each others' assumptions. Discuss how the conversation differs when you address underlying assumptions.

APPLICATION EXERCISE 3: REAL LIFE SCENARIO

Think of a recent situation in which you participated where it would have been helpful to address underlying assumptions. What was the situation, who was involved, what were their roles, what were they trying to accomplish, and what actually happened? What did you observe that leads you to believe assumptions played a role in this situation? What could you have done differently to change the situation? What will you do or say differently in similar situations in the future?

DISCUSSION QUESTIONS

1. Describe an incident from a past job where you would like to better understand how the organizational setting influenced employee behavior. What was the situation, and what happened? If you had been the manager in that situation, what would you have needed to understand to handle that situation?

2. Give examples of incidents from your past jobs where perceptions and cognition (or thinking) may have had a strong influence on employee behavior. What was the situation, who was involved, and how did they act? Describe the thinking patterns you observed.

3. Discuss the role of thinking in promoting organizational change and learning. In what ways could you as a manager use thinking to improve learning and change?

4. Discuss the role of thinking processes in organizational communication and problem solving. In what ways could you as a manager use thinking to improve communication and problem solving?

REFERENCES

Bandura, A. (1977). Self-efficacy: toward a unifying theory of behavioral change. *Psychological Review, 84,* 191–215.

Bazerman, M. (1998). *Judgment in managerial decision-making (4th ed.).* New York: Wiley & Sons.

Daft, R. L. (1992). *Organization theory and design.* St. Paul, MN: West Publishing Co.

Das T. K., & Teng, B. S. (1999). Cognitive biases and strategic decision processes: an integrative perspective. *Journal of Management Studies, 36*(6), 757–778.

Easterby-Smith, M., Crossan, M., & Nicolini, D. (2000). Organizational learning: debates past, present and future. *Journal of Management Studies, 37*(6), 783–795.

Elsbach, K. D., Barr, P. S., & Hargadon, A. B. (2005). Identifying situated cognition in organizations. *Organization Science, 16*(4), 422–433.

Fiske, S. T., & Taylor, S. E. (1984). *Social cognition.* New York: Random House.

Heil, G., Bennis, W., & Stephens, D. C. (2000). *Douglas McGregor, revisited.* New York: John Wiley & Sons.

Huff, A. S., Huff, J. O., & Barr, P. S. (2000). *When firms change direction.* Cambridge: Oxford University Press.

Huselid, M. A. (1995). The impact of human resources management practices on turnover, productivity, and corporate financial performance. *Academy of Management Journal, 38,* 645.

Korte, R. E. (2003). Biases in decision making and implications for human resource development. *Advances in Developing Human Resources, 5*(4), 440–457.

McGregor, D. (1967). *The professional manager.* New York: McGraw-Hill.

Pfeffer, J. (1998). *The human equation.* Cambridge, MA: Harvard Business School Press.

Robbins, S. P. (2003). *Essentials of organizational behavior.* Upper Saddle River, NJ: Prentice Hall.

Schein, E. H. (1988). *Process consultation.* Reading, MA: Addison-Wesley Publishing Company.

Scott, W. R. (1992). *Organizations: rational, natural, and open systems (3rd. ed.).* Englewood Cliffs, NJ: Prentice Hall.

Senge, P. M. (1990). *The fifth discipline.* New York: Currency-Doubleday.

Shortell, S. M., & Kaluzny, A. D. (2000). *Health care management (4th ed.)*. Albany, NY: Thomson Delmar Learning.

Torbert, B., & Associates (2004). *Action inquiry*. San Francisco: Berrett-Kohler.

Vroom, V. (1964). *Work and motivation*. New York: Wiley.

Weick, K. E. (1969). *The social psychology of organizing*. Reading, MA: Addison-Wesley.

Weick, K. E. (1995). *Sensemaking in organizations*. Thousand Oaks, CA: Sage Publications.

Weick, K. E., Sutcliff, K. M., & Obstfeld, D. (2005). Organizing and the process of sensemaking. *Organization Science, 16*(4), 409–420.

Whetten, D. A., & Cameron, K. S. (1998). *Developing management skills*. Reading, MA: Addison-Wesley.

CHAPTER 4

Strategic Planning
Susan Judd Casciani

LEARNING OBJECTIVES

By the end of this chapter, the student will be able to:

- Describe strategic planning and the strategic planning process;
- Identify healthcare market powers, trends, and potential impact on health services;
- Utilize a situational assessment or SWOT analysis;
- Define the links between market volume forecast, core customers, mission, vision, and values;
- Compare data collection methods and strategy tactical plans; and,
- Identify methods to monitor and control strategy execution.

INTRODUCTION

Every organization needs to be successful over the long term in order to survive. A factor critical to that success lies in how well an organization can plan for the future and tap market opportunities. Strategic planning is the process of identifying a desired future state for an organization and a means to achieve it. Through an ongoing analysis of the organization's operating environment, matched against its internal capabilities, an organization's leadership is able to identify strategies that will drive the organization from its present condition to that desired future state.

Strategic planning in health care has had a relatively short history. As recently as the 1970s, strategic planning in the healthcare industry mainly consisted of planning for new buildings and funding expanding services in response to population growth. With the introduction of the federal Prospective Payment System (PPS) in the 1980s, the field of healthcare strategic planning received a transforming jolt as organizations scrambled to compete in an increasingly demanding environment. The turbulent managed care era of the '80s and '90s only served to further fuel the growth of the field, as the cost of healthcare continually rose faster than the Gross Domestic Product (GDP) and competition among providers intensified. Today, hospitals and other healthcare organizations have come to embrace strategic planning as a valuable tool to evaluate alternative paths and help them prepare for the future. Healthcare managers at all levels need to understand the process of strategic planning, its purpose, benefits and challenges, and the key factors for its success.

PURPOSE AND IMPORTANCE OF STRATEGIC PLANNING

In any organization's operating environment there are forces, both controllable and uncontrollable, that will undoubtedly influence the future success of that organization. Only by identifying these forces and planning for ways to adapt to them can an organization achieve the greatest success. At one extreme, completely ignoring these forces can most certainly lead to organizational death. Although no one can predict the future, one can systematically think about it. Accordingly, the purpose of strategic planning is to identify market forces and how they may affect the organization, and determine an appropriate strategic direction to take that will counteract those forces, and/or tap their potential.

Strategic planning serves to focus the organization and also its resource allocation. At any given point in time, there are multiple, and often competing, initiatives and projects to be undertaken in an organization. By understanding the organization's operating environment and identifying a strategy to reach a desired future state, resources can be allocated appropriately and effectively.

THE PLANNING PROCESS

The **strategic planning process** consists mainly of two interrelated activities: the development of the strategic plan, and execution of the organization's strategy. The development of the plan usually spans a multi-year time horizon (3, 5, or 10 years, for example), and is updated annually. **Strategy execution**, on the other hand, is done on a continuous basis and is the critical factor in management of the organization's strategic intentions, optimally providing continual feedback for the development of any future plans.

Although strategic planning is a dynamic and not linear process, Figure 4-1 attempts to depict a logical progression of the steps undertaken to develop a strategic plan. As shown in Figure 4-1, the **Situational Assessment** provides a foundation for strategy development. This Assessment serves two important functions: to provide a snapshot of how the organization is currently interacting with the market in comparison to its internal capabilities and intended strategic direction, and to identify market opportunities and threats that the organization may want to address in future strategic efforts.

Through development of the Situational Assessment, strategy identification can begin. In this stage, the organization's leadership team uses the information and analyses provided in the Situational Assessment to identify specific strategies that may be worthy of pursuit, either to grow the organization or to protect current areas of strength. Once these strategies have been identified, they must be narrowed down to a manageable number through selection and prioritization, and tactical implementation plans must be created. With the strategic plan completed, operating, marketing, and other supporting plans are developed. Control and monitoring of the plan follows, and is most effectively done on an ongoing basis throughout the year. We will look at each of these stages of strategic planning in more detail; however it is important to keep in mind that strategic planning is not a linear process; the feedback loop depicted in Figure 4-1 shows the critical nature of planning being an ongoing, dynamic process.

SITUATIONAL ASSESSMENT

The Situational Assessment is often referred to as a **SWOT (Strengths, Weaknesses, Opportunities, Threats) Analysis,** as it aims to identify the internal strengths and weaknesses of an organization, along with market opportunities and threats. It includes three distinct but intricately related components: the **Market Assessment, the Mission, Vision,** and **Values** of the organization, and the **Internal Assessment.** The development of the Market Assessment may be the most complex and time-consuming section

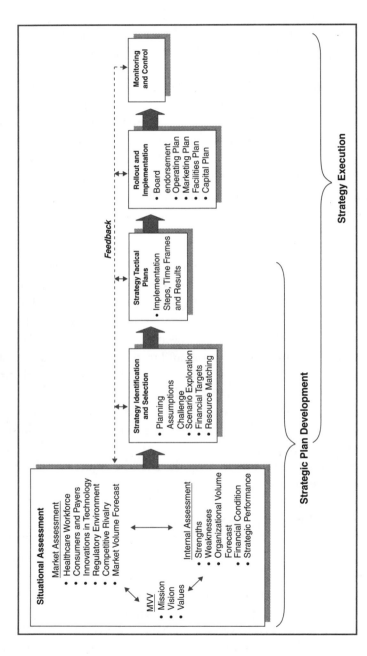

FIGURE 4-1 Strategic Planning Process

of the strategic plan in that, in this section, virtually all aspects of the market must be examined and analyzed to determine their future implications on the organization. Any of a number of market assessment models can be utilized for this analysis, but one of the most common is the **Five Forces Model** developed by Harvard University professor Michael Porter (1998). In this model, Porter identifies five market or industry forces that, when combined, determine the attractiveness of competing in a particular market. For health care, this model can be adapted to analyze the interactions between the **Power of the Healthcare Workforce,** the **Power of Consumers and Payers, Innovations in Technology,** the **Regulatory Environment,** and **Competitive Rivalry.**

The Power of the Healthcare Workforce can have significant strategic implications for any healthcare organization, as its employees act as the frontline caretakers in providing services. In the Market Assessment, an organization should look at the availability of all subsets of healthcare providers that are critical to its success. As an example, if obstetrics is a major clinical program of the organization, the organization should closely consider the future anticipated supply and demand of obstetricians in its market. Currently, with the significant increases in malpractice insurance targeted at obstetricians across the country, many OBs have elected to discontinue delivering babies and focus solely on gynecology, while others have opted to retire early. This has dramatically reduced the supply of obstetricians in many areas of the country, and forced some hospitals to hire their affiliated obstetrical staff in an effort to cover their malpractice insurance premiums and keep them practicing. Other hospitals have developed "laborists"—OBs who are hired solely to work in the hospital and deliver babies. These moves are examples of strategies that could be adopted by organizations to either maintain or grow their obstetrical services in response to market trends.

Another example of the power of the healthcare workforce is the potential ramifications of the current nursing and radiology personnel shortages. With a shortage of personnel, wage and hiring expenses increase, jeopardizing the ability to offer those specific services. A nursing shortage may affect a hospital's ability to add beds to meet growing demand. A shortage of radiology technicians may affect an organization's opportunity to offer new state-of-the-art technologies currently in demand. The influence of these and other healthcare personnel (and the organization's dependency on them) must be considered when developing future strategies.

At the other end of the spectrum are the ultimate purchasers of health care—consumers. The **Power of Consumers** is becoming a more significant market force, and one that has required a dramatic shift in the way the industry offers services. Today's consumers are demanding more and more from their healthcare providers on all levels (e.g. physicians, payers, hospitals, etc.), both in terms of the availability of specific service offerings and in the delivery of those services. For healthcare providers, this has required a shift from the traditional view, where the physician is the primary customer; to today's world, where the patient is the central focus of "customer" service. The potential impact of this shift needs to be considered when developing future strategies.

Consumers can influence the healthcare market in other ways as well. Different communities have different healthcare needs—one community may need increased access to primary care channels, while another may need better health education and screenings. By identifying specific community needs, healthcare organizations can better target their services and potential growth opportunities.

In concert with the Power of Consumers is the **Power of Payers**. Some markets have multiple payers of various sizes and strengths, while others have one or two major payers that dictate market payments. In either case, a healthcare organization that relies on these payers must stay abreast of their needs and demands and how each may affect future operations and strategies. A good example of this is a market with one or two powerful payers where the payers prefer a "late adopter" stance for new medical technologies. In other words, they prefer not to pay for new technologies until the technologies have been proven either medically effective, financially efficient, or both. This would be a significant threat to an organization that strives for a competitive advantage through being first-to-market with the adoption of new medical technologies. The Power of Payers may also create opportunities for an organization. An example would be the general preference of payers for less costly outpatient services. Healthcare organizations that specialize in these types of service offerings (e.g., ambulatory surgery centers, diagnostic/imaging centers) have capitalized on this payer influence in many areas of the country.

The third market power to be considered is **Innovations in Technology**. These innovations may represent the threat of substitute products, as new technologies often replace standard operations and services. A good example of this is the introduction of Picture Archive Communication

Systems (PACs). This filmless imaging system significantly reduces the need for storage space for films and readers and the staff to maintain those areas, as well as allows for remote electronic accessing of files, ultimately requiring a potentially smaller number of physicians necessary to interpret the images. Innovations in technology may also reduce the need for other types of clinical staff, as in the case of some surgical innovations (e.g., minimally invasive surgery, robotic technologies, drug advancements, etc.), and/or they may significantly increase the requirement of financial resources, as in the case of new radiology equipment (e.g., the 64-slice CT scanner, new fluoroscopy equipment, MRI machinery, etc.). As these and other new technologies become available, their potential impact on operations and systems needs to be considered in strategy development.

As the fourth market force, the **Regulatory Environment**—on all levels, federal, state, and local—needs to be monitored for its affects on strategy development as well. Congress continually enacts influential legislation, such as the 1986 Emergency Medical Treatment and Active Labor Act (EMTALA) and the 1996 Health Insurance Portability and Accountability Act (HIPAA), that are indicative of the current focus on mandatory error reporting and physician self-referrals that has significant and rippling effects on all participants in the healthcare industry. Further, the Centers for Medicare and Medicaid Services (CMS) take the lead in changes in healthcare payment formulas that are frequently followed by payers at local levels. Other far-reaching issues, such as liability reform and quality of care measures, may be dealt with on local, state, and federal levels as well. All of these actions can influence a particular healthcare organization's strategy, and need to be monitored and analyzed for their potential impacts.

Competitive Rivalry, the last market force to be considered, is probably given the most significant attention in most organizations' strategy development. Whether an organization operates in a near monopoly or an oligopoly, strategically savvy organizations always track their competitors' moves and suspected intentions. Although it is highly unlikely that you will gain access to the actual strategy of your competitors, much information on their strategic intent can be gleaned from their market activities. Information on their service volumes and market share, as well as news coverage and press releases, should be monitored. Ongoing discussions with the organization's own physicians, staff, and suppliers will likely also yield valuable competitive intelligence. Compiling and synthesizing this information to see a larger picture often leads to an indication of competitors' strategies. Once their strategic intent has been identified, market opportunities for and threats against one's own organization can be further addressed.

Market Volume Forecast

The final component of the Market Assessment is the **Market Volume Forecast**, the purpose of which is to initially develop a quantitative picture of the environment in which the organization will be operating in the future. The forecast is initiated by identifying the organization's service area—usually a zip code-defined area where 70–80% of its patients are drawn from—and determining the population use rates for your applicable service lines (e.g., cardiology, orthopedics, home care visits, CT scans, etc.). These data are usually collected for several historical time periods (e.g. the previous 3 years) and can then be forecasted out several more time periods simply by using a mathematical trend formula, resulting in a base forecast.

For a more realistic forecast, however, assumptions must be overlaid onto this base model. It is critical that the information and data gathered in the market assessment, including the competitor assessment, be incorporated into this forecast in the form of these assumptions. For example, are there new technologies on the horizon that will affect service volumes? Or is there a dearth of providers that may counteract predicted increasing utilization of a particular service for a period of time? Overlaying these assumptions onto the base forecast results in a future scenario for market volume, and any number of future scenarios can be created by adjusting the impacts of the planning assumptions. This is where strategic planning really becomes an art versus a science, and it is often difficult to quantitatively determine the extent to which market forces may affect future market volumes. To this end, there are several companies that provide assistance and/or models for quantifying market forces; a sampling of these companies is provided as additional resources at the end of this chapter.

Mission, Vision, Values

The information gleaned regarding the interaction of these five forces (Healthcare Workforce, Consumers and Payers, Innovations in Technology, Regulatory Environment, and Competitive Rivalry) in the market is matched against the organization's **Mission, Vision,** and **Value (MVV)** statements. As the driving purpose of the organization, the MVVs are re-verified as part of the strategic planning process to ensure they continue to be aligned with the organization's future market environment, and to help identify future desired strategic directions. The **Mission** of any organization is its enduring statement of purpose. It aims to identify what the organization does, whom it serves, and how it does it. For example, Radiologix, a radiology services company, "strives to be the premier provider of diagnostic imaging services through high-quality service to patients, referring physicians and mutually beneficial relationships with radiologists who provide expert interpretations of diagnostic images" (http://www.radiologix.com, Retrieved on August 29, 2006). On the other hand, a **Vision statement** strives to identify a specific future state of the organization, usually an inspiring goal for many years down the road. The vision of the American Hospital Association "[is] . . . of a society of healthy communities, where all individuals reach their highest potential for health" (http://www.aha.org, Retrieved on August 29, 2006). The **Values statement** should help define the organization's culture—what characteristics it wants employees to convey to customers. An example of one such value from Duke University Health System in North Carolina is: "We earn the trust our patients place in us by involving them in their healthcare planning and treatment and by exceeding their service expectations" (http://www.dukehealth.org/AboutDuke/Mission/mission_statement, Retrieved on August 29, 2006).

Although the mission statement is generally the most enduring of the three, each of these statements may be altered over time to adapt to the environment. As an example, the increasing influence of consumerism in healthcare drove many an organization to revise its vision and value statements to become more customer-service focused, which in turn (hopefully) helped to change the organization's culture. Reaffirming and/or adjusting these three statements in relation to market activity is a critical step in determining the desired future state of the organization.

Internal Assessment

The third component of the Situational Assessment, the **Internal Assessment**, is matched against both the Mission, Vision, and Values Statements and the Market Assessment to complete the situational snapshot. In conducting an internal assessment, an organization turns the analytical lens inward to examine areas of strength and weakness, as well as how it may build or sustain a competitive advantage in the market. Like the Market

Assessment, the Internal Assessment has both quantitative as well as qualitative components. The quantitative section of the internal assessment consists mainly of the organizational volume forecast and an assessment of the financial condition. The qualitative section focuses on past strategic performance, and leadership's interpretation of the organization's core capabilities (or lack thereof).

Organizational Volume Forecast

The **Organizational Volume Forecast** takes the base model forecast developed in the market assessment and applies historical market share information, therein highlighting some of an organization's strengths and weaknesses. By holding its market share growth trends constant in the future scenarios, an organization can formulate a preliminary idea of how well it would fare if it (and its competitors) were to stay its current course. Examining the forecast from the perspective of market share, contribution margin, and/or medical staff depth will also yield service lines of strength that may need to be protected, as well as service lines that could be developed further.

As with the development of the previous future scenarios however, it is important to apply assumptions to the forecasts. For example, will the organization plan to hold market share constant for a particular service, or will the organization hope to grow that market? Alternately, the organization may decide to discontinue a specific service, perhaps due to predicted declining reimbursements or lack of physicians. It is important to keep in mind that any alternative scenarios that are created will be used as input for the development of specific strategies in the next phase of the planning process, at which time their underlying planning assumptions should be debated extensively.

Financial Condition

As with the volume forecast, several years' worth of **key financial indicators** should be analyzed to highlight additional strengths and weaknesses of the organization. These may include indicators such as operating margin, net income, gross and net revenues, bond ratings, fund raising, key financial ratios, payer mix, pricing and/or rate setting arrangements. The organization's historical performance against budget is also helpful to analyze, and should yield further insight into strengths and weaknesses. Any financial forecasts that are available should also be included, as well as any routine or planned capital spending and/or facility improvement plans. It is critical to tie the financial reserves and needs of the organization to the strategic planning process to ensure the resulting strategies can and will be funded appropriately. Tying the financial information to the volume forecast also serves to provide budget targets for the upcoming year(s).

Strategic Performance

It is important to remember that, as mentioned earlier, strategic planning is a dynamic rather than a linear process and as such there should optimally be no distinct beginning or end. Thus, a review of the organization's past strategic performance should be included as part of future strategy development. This review can be as simple as an assessment of whether past strategies accomplished intended goals, or as multifaceted as an ad hoc leadership meeting to discuss roadblocks that led to failure or factors that drove success. Either way, this review can and should provide valuable information for future strategy development and implementation.

Leadership Input

In addition to the more quantitative strengths and weaknesses outlined through the volume forecast and financial condition review, there are subjective strengths and weaknesses that need to be identified for strategy development as well. Identifying these capabilities can be quite challenging, as planners usually have to rely on surveys of and/or interviews with the leadership of the organization to gather this information. This can be both time consuming and value laden, but this information will be critical input for the plan's overall success. With that said, Table 4-1 highlights some common methods of collecting this information, and the benefits and limitations of each.

The key to gathering the most value from the leadership input is to challenge leaders (e.g., executives, physicians, managers, etc.) to think within a strategic context, as opposed to the operational mode they are involved in on a day-to-day basis. Merely asking leaders to identify an organization's weaknesses, for example, can result in responses such as parking or a lack of marketing, whereas framing the question to identify challenges to the organization in growing service volumes may better yield answers such as an aging medical staff, lack of capacity, etc. It is important to incorporate these identified strengths and weaknesses into the Internal Assessment for further discussion.

TABLE 4-1 Data Collection Methods

	Pros	Cons
Interviews	▪ Opportunity to clarify responses ▪ Encourages free thinking ▪ Can ensure representative sample	▪ Time consuming ▪ Potential for interviewer bias ▪ Open answers difficult to analyze
Focus Groups	▪ Opportunity to clarify responses ▪ Allows for relatively large sample ▪ Can be economically efficient	▪ Potential for groupthink ▪ Open answers difficult to analyze
Surveys	▪ Effective way to obtain large sample ▪ Standardized answers allow for easier analysis ▪ No interviewer bias	▪ Can be expensive ▪ Lag time for responses ▪ Potential for low response rate

---

Strategy Identification and Selection

Throughout the development and analyses of the overall Situational Assessment, the building blocks for strategy identification begin to emerge. If the organization is at the start of the development of a multi-year plan, it will usually conduct a rather thorough Situational Assessment. However, if the organization has an identified long-term strategic direction, the Situational Assessment may selectively analyze only those areas that are relevant to the identified strategic direction. For example, if the organization has resolved to grow defined service lines, the assessment may focus more specifically on those areas of the market. Alternately, if the direction is diversification, the assessment may focus more on areas related to the organization's current strengths, whether they are service line or internal capability related. Regardless of the depth of the Situational Assessment, it serves as input for the next step in the process, **Strategy Identification** and **Selection.**

With the backdrop of the Situational Assessment, strategy identification begins by analyzing and challenging the planning assumptions, further exploring any future scenarios developed earlier, and incorporating any desired financial targets as determined by leadership. From this analysis, several potential strategic directions for the organization may emerge. The strategic direction is the goal that the organization desires to accomplish within the planning timeframe. Generally, as each direction may have different probabilities for success and require different levels of resource investment, the specific direction that will ultimately be chosen will often depend on an organization's tolerance for risk.

Once a strategic direction is chosen, specific desired outcomes should be targeted and strategies identified to accomplish it. As an example, if an organization concludes it will differentiate itself through its orthopedic services (strategic direction), the desired outcome may be to lead the market in orthopedic service volumes within two years. To accomplish this, the organization may identify strategies to increase its surgeon base, add rehabilitation services, or develop a center of excellence program. A strategy is a carefully designed plan to accomplish the desired outcomes.

Even the largest and most fiscally sound organization cannot successfully implement all the strategies it can conceive of, nor should it try to. A successful strategic plan is focused and, just as importantly, executable; too many strategies may render the plan ineffective simply because there is too much to do. Strategy is all about making choices. A clear and focused strategy will guide decision making, prioritize resource allocation and keep the organization on its desired course; in choosing which strategies to pursue, an organization is also choosing which strategies not to pursue. At this stage in the planning process, the organization's leadership must determine its ability to successfully execute the strategies it has identified.

Factors to consider in making this determination include the degree to which the strategy has the ability to help the organization meet its financial targets. Alternately, does the organization have the financial resources to fund the strategy appropriately in terms of operating and capital expense? Additionally, does the organization have the internal capabilities to successfully execute the strategy—does it have, or can it acquire, the necessary human resources? Is the strategy transformational enough to bring about the desired change? Equally important, is there a champion to take ownership of the strategy's success? By going through the exercise of matching potential strategies to financial and other targets, and matching implementation requirements to resource availability, strategy selection is accomplished (see Table 4-2).

STRATEGY TACTICAL PLANS

The final step in the actual development of the strategic plan is the creation of specific tactical plans for each strategy, which are necessary for translating the plan into action.

TABLE 4-2 Successful Strategies

Successful strategies:

- Are focused on the desired future state
- Align internal capabilities with market opportunities and threats
- Provide or sustain a competitive advantage for the organization
- Are funded and resourced long term

Tactical plans answer the who, what, when, where, and how questions of strategy implementation. Table 4-3 shows an example of a basic template for a tactical plan that, when completed, will help drive implementation of the strategy.

ROLLOUT AND IMPLEMENTATION

With the development of the tactical plans, the strategic plan is complete. The plan is then presented to the Board of Directors for approval and endorsement, and is then rolled out across the organization. **Rollout** of the plan has two main steps: first, the plan is communicated at all levels of the organization; only by communicating the strategy to all necessary stakeholders can an organization gain the support necessary for successful execution of the strategy.

Second, supporting plans such as the financial and budgeting plans, operating plan, marketing plan, capital plan, and master facilities plan are developed or updated with the intent and strategies developed in the strategic plan. Having all of the organization's supporting plans tied to the

---

TABLE 4-3 Tactical Plan Template

Goal	Key Actions	Target Completion Date	Resources Required	Dependencies	Revenue Projection	Success Metric

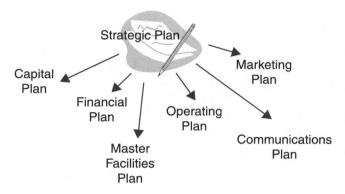

FIGURE 4-2 Supporting Plans

strategic plan is a critical factor in reinforcing its strategic direction. Figure 4-2 depicts some of the supporting plans that may be drawn from the strategic plan.

MONITORING AND CONTROL

Monitoring and control of the strategic plan is most often accomplished through the use of an **organizational dashboard,** or **scorecard.** A dashboard is a visual reference used to monitor an organization's performance against targets over time. Its simplistic design should allow for quick assessment of areas that may need adjustment, similar to an automobile dashboard. Dashboards can depict strategic, operational and/or financial indicators, depending on the organization's needs, but care must be taken to highlight a manageable number of indicators or the dashboard will lose its functionality. Figure 4-3 depicts an example of a dashboard, although many other templates abound in the industry.

Depending on the organization's needs, and depending on the types of indicators management identifies, the dashboard should be monitored regularly (e.g. monthly or quarterly). At a minimum, as soon as an indicator highlights a variance from the desired target, managers must address the variance with tactics that correct or alter the results, but optimally, the dashboard should serve to facilitate management discussion regarding execution of the strategy. To best ensure success of the strategic plan, dashboard indicators are aligned with operational plans and their associated identified goals.

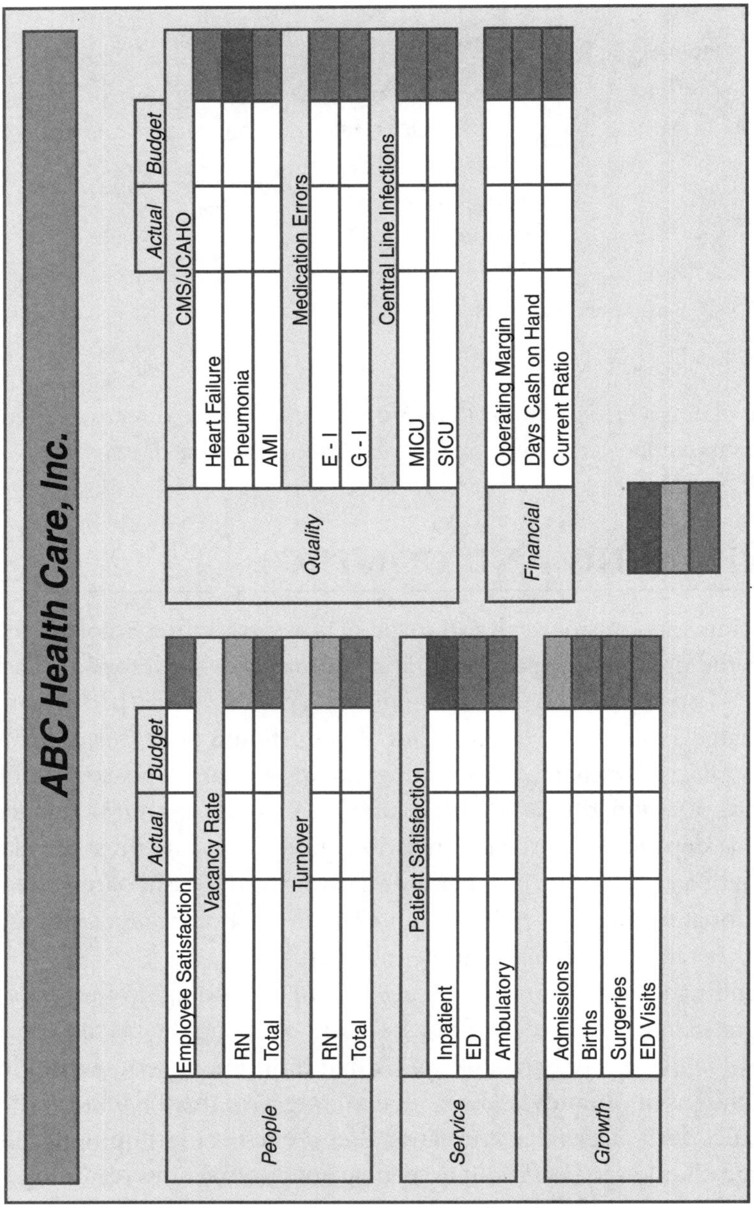

FIGURE 4-3 Dashboard

STRATEGY EXECUTION

Although the development of the actual strategic plan occurs in a logical progression, other than perhaps the creation of the Situational Assessment, every stage of the plan's development should be viewed as part of its execution. **Strategy execution** is crucial for organizational success and cannot be overstated in terms of importance. Unfortunately, this is often an element of strategic planning that many organizations overlook. With the flurry of activity and intensity that usually surrounds the development of the strategic plan itself, there can be a collective sigh of relief following board approval of the plan, and leadership may be relieved to be able to return to their "real work" and the day-to-day operations. Yet successful organizations know that execution is much more important than the plan.

Execution, however, isn't easy and there are many roadblocks on the path to success. For example, it has been said that "culture eats strategy for lunch," and even that may be an understatement. If an organization's stakeholders are not ready for the strategy, it will not be executed by even the most tenacious of leaders. With the heightened influence of consumerism, many healthcare organizations attempted strategies early on to shift the organization from a more physician-centric to a patient-centric focus, aiming to gain a competitive advantage on this emerging market trend. However, many of these same organizations were faced with a strong undercurrent of resistance from an internal culture that was not prepared for this new paradigm, and the strategy failed. This example demonstrates the need for strategy execution to start early in the planning process, enabling the organization to either better prepare itself for implementation of the strategy or to table the strategy until the organization is ready to implement it successfully.

Other barriers to successful strategy execution include a lack of strategic focus. Often during the plan development phase, leadership will inevitably develop more strategies than it can successfully execute. If this list is not pared down to a reasonable number, or if the few strategies that are planned do not align appropriately, execution attempts will be futile. Additionally, as mentioned earlier, if the strategies are not appropriately funded and resourced they cannot be executed, or if they result in competing priorities, the organization will likely be unsuccessful. All of these barriers can be overcome, however, in part by focusing on execution at the earliest stages of strategy development.

Strategy execution is also most successful with a combination of strong leadership and organizational buy-in. Although leadership will need to have flexibility to adjust strategies as market conditions warrant, they must also have the consistency over time to stay the course. Too often, strategies have failed because an organization has fallen to the temptation of new priorities, or has simply neglected to resource the strategy over multiple years or time periods. Strategy is not a quick fix nor does it promise immediate turnaround; strong leadership is needed to maintain a long-term focus. In addition, organizational buy-in at all levels is critical. As demonstrated earlier in the example regarding culture, strategy cannot be implemented solely in the top layers of an organization. All stakeholders must be aware of and buy into the desired future state and the path that leads them there in order to ensure the momentum necessary to achieve results. Optimally, a successfully conducted strategic planning process will generate strategy champions at all levels of the organization.

Participants

All organizations generally involve key leadership in the strategic planning process, but the extent to which other stakeholders are involved varies considerably. There is no one best answer as to who should be involved in the planning process and how as each organization and culture is different, but one caveat generally always holds true: the more stakeholders that are aware of and own the strategy, the greater the chance of success. That said, the strategic planning process should involve representatives from the Board of Trustees, upper and middle management, the medical staff, general staff, and community leaders throughout the process, as much as is feasible. When the plan is completed, it should be communicated to all stakeholders as discussed earlier.

STRATEGIC PLANNING AND EXECUTION— THE ROLE OF THE HEALTHCARE MANAGER

A good portion of this chapter has been dedicated to discussion of the content of the strategic plan, and with good reason—healthcare managers need to understand the types of information and intelligence gathered and analyzed for plan development, and how that information is interpreted and acted upon. However, it has often been said that the plan is worthless, but planning is priceless; the value of strategic planning lies not in the plan itself, but in the planning process. Properly conducted, the strategic planning process will challenge management to robustly confront the brutal facts of its market and the organization, to persistently test planning assumptions, and to continually refine the organization's execution skills.

Healthcare managers at all levels have the responsibility to continually monitor their environment—both internal and external—and assess and act upon the possible implications of any trends or events that are of note. They have the responsibility to understand their local market on an ongoing basis and to know their organization's strategic direction and intent. They are responsible for identifying ways to support the organization's strategy, and for ensuring that their subordinates have the knowledge and understanding of the strategy in order to do the same. Strategic planning may be driven by the planning or business development function of an organization, but it is the responsibility of leadership at all levels to help execute and manage the organization's strategy.

CONCLUSION

Effective strategic planning is a critical element in the success of today's healthcare organizations. Through understanding its competitive and other market environments, an organization can best identify a desired future state and a means to achieve it, but as discussed, the true value of strategic planning lies in the process, and less in the resulting plan. In a recent study, Begun and Kaissi (2005) investigated the perceived value of strategic planning to leaders in 20 healthcare organizations. Consistent with the information presented in this chapter, the authors found that leadership stressed the dynamic versus static nature of planning, and the importance of execution of the strategic plan. Strategic planning will likely continue to be a valued function in healthcare organizations in the future, and management at all levels needs to understand the process and its purpose, and its role in development and execution of the successful strategy.

DISCUSSION QUESTIONS

1. What are some of the healthcare market trends you can identify in your market? How might they affect your job as a manager, and how would you react to/prepare for them?

2. In what ways can you, as a manager, contribute to the management and execution of your organization's strategy?

3. Discuss how strategic planning is a dynamic, versus linear, process. Why is this important?

4. What is the purpose of the Situational Assessment, and how is it best used in the planning process?

REFERENCES

Begun, J. & Kaissi, A. (2005). An exploratory study of healthcare strategic planning in two metropolitan areas. *Journal of Healthcare Management, 50*(4), 264–274.

Porter, M. (1998). *On competition.* Cambridge, MA: Harvard Business School Publishing.

Additional Readings

Bossidy, L., & Charan, R. (2004). Execution: the discipline of getting things done. *AFP Exchange, 24*(1), 26–30.

Brandenburger, A., & Nalebuff, B. (1995). The right game: use game theory to shape strategy. *Harvard Business Review, 73*(4), 57–71.

Collins, J. (2001). *Good to great: why some companies make the leap . . . and others don't.* New York: Harper Business.

Collis, D., & Montgomery, C. (1995). Competing on resources: strategy in the 1990's. *Harvard Business Review, 73*(4), 118–129.

Ginter, P., Swayne, L., & Duncan, W. J. (2002). *Strategic management of healthcare organizations (4th ed.).* Malden, MA: Blackwell Publishers, Inc.

Jennings, M. (Ed.). (2000). *Health care strategy for uncertain times.* San Francisco, CA: Jossey-Bass.

Kaplan, R., & Norton, D. (1996). *The balanced scorecard: translating strategy into action.* Cambridge, MA: Harvard Business School Publishing.

Kaplan, R., & Norton, D. (2005). The balanced scorecard: measures that drive performance. *Harvard Business Review, 83*(7), 172.

Prahalad, C. K., & Ramaswamy, V. (2004). *The future of competition: co-creating unique value with customers.* Cambridge, MA: Harvard Business School Publishing.

Senge, P., Kleiner, A., Roberts, C., Ross, R. B., Roth, G., & Smith, B. J. (1994). *The fifth discipline fieldbook: strategies and tools for building a learning organization.* New York: Doubleday.

Zuckerman, A. (2005). Creating competitive advantage: product development. *Healthcare Financial Management, 59*(6), 110–113.

Additional Websites to Explore

Sg2	www.sg2.com
Solucient	www.solucient.com
Data Bay Resources	www.databayresources.com
The Advisory Board Company	www.advisoryboardcompany.com

CHAPTER 5

Performance Improvement in Health Care: The Quest to Achieve Quality

Grant T. Savage
Eric S. Williams

LEARNING OBJECTIVES

By the end of this chapter the student will be able to:

- Define healthcare quality from a variety of stakeholder perspectives;
- Discuss the importance of quality to a healthcare system;
- Trace the evolution of quality thinking, from quality assurance to continuous quality improvement to systems improvement;
- Describe the leading models of quality improvement;
- Define and apply key quality concepts; and,
- Describe and discuss four future challenges.

INTRODUCTION

Cost, access, and quality form the health policy triumvirate. Quality, as a key policy consideration, gained significant public focus in the United States with two recent publications by the Institute of Medicine (IOM):

To Err is Human (Kohn, Corrigan, & Donaldson, 2000) and *Crossing the Quality Chasm* (Institute of Medicine, 2001). *Too Err is Human* is the IOM report that first brought public attention to the issue of medical errors, concluding that between 44,000 and 98,000 people die every year from these errors. It also diagnosed the quality problem as not one of poorly performing people, but of people struggling to perform within a system riddled with opportunities for mistakes—known as latent errors—waiting to happen. The second IOM report, *Crossing the Quality Chasm*, outlines a number of goals for improving the quality and performance of the United States healthcare system, as well as some of the methods for achieving those goals.

This chapter builds on these two significant reports. The first two sections describe several of the more common definitions of quality and present the case for the importance of quality as the ultimate measure of performance for healthcare organizations. The third section examines the historical evolution of quality thinking in health care, from initial conceptions of quality assurance in the 19th century to the adoption of continuous quality improvement in the 1980s and 1990s. The fourth section presents the leading models of quality currently used in health care, while the fifth section expands on some of the key quality concepts that underlie many of the quality models discussed in the text. The sixth section traces the emergence of system improvement and system thinking during the turn of the 21st century, while the final section presents a number of quality and performance challenges that appear on the horizon for patients, policy makers, and providers.

DEFINING QUALITY IN HEALTH CARE

Healthcare quality may be defined in various ways, with differing implications for healthcare providers, patients, third-party payers, policy makers, and other stakeholders. In what follows, we examine the leading definitions and some of their implications for stakeholders. The National Academies' Institute of Medicine (IOM) provides the most widely accepted definition of healthcare quality as the "degree to which health services for individuals or populations increase the likelihood of desired health outcomes and are consistent with the current professional knowledge" (Institute of Medicine, 1990). This definition highlights several aspects of quality. First, high quality health services should achieve desired health outcomes for individuals, matching their preferences for variety. Second, they should achieve desired health outcomes for populations, matching the societal preferences of policy makers and third-party payers for efficiency. And, third, they should adhere to professional standards and scientific evidence, consistent with the clinical focus and preferences of healthcare providers for effectiveness.

Another way to view quality is as the result of a system with interdependent parts that must work together to achieve outcomes such as those noted above. Avedis Donabedian, a physician who was a leading advocate for improving healthcare quality during the last half of the 20th century, introduced the idea that quality could be viewed from a system perspective as structure, processes, and outcomes (Donabedian, 1966). The structural elements of quality involve the material and human resources of an organization and the facility itself. Simply put, this is the quality of the setting and the people, whether in a hospital, physician's office, nursing home, or hospice. Processes are the actual activities of patient care and all the ancillary activities attending the interaction between patients and providers. Outcomes are the resulting health status of the patients. As a physician, Donabedian championed the development of "best practices" to achieve better care (Cooper, 1999), linking structures, processes, and outcomes with a feedback loop. Moreover, he defined quality as having at least four components (Donabedian, 1986):

1. The technical management of health and illness
2. The management of the interpersonal relationship between the providers of care and their clients
3. The amenities of care
4. The ethical principles that govern the conduct of affairs in general and the healthcare enterprise in particular.

The four parts of this definition highlight the need to incorporate multiple stakeholder perspectives to understand healthcare quality. On one hand, the technical management of health focuses on the clinical performance of healthcare providers; on the other hand, the management of interpersonal relationships underscores the co-production of care by both providers and patients. In other words, at the patient-provider encounter level, health service quality is driven both by clinical and non-clinical processes (Marley, Collier, & Goldstein, 2004). The "amenities of care" speak to patients' interest in pursuing individual well-being (or variety);

the "ethical principles" speak to providers' interests in furthering societal and organizational well-being (or effectiveness).

A related and more focused view of quality represents two fundamental questions about any clinical service, procedure, or activity occurring in a healthcare setting: 1) "Are the right things done?" and 2) "Are things done right?" The first question assesses the effectiveness of clinical care; the second considers the efficiency of care services. Importantly, the performance of healthcare organizations depends on their effectiveness and their efficiency. Moreover, both effectiveness and efficiency are discussed in the IOM's *Crossing the Quality Chasm* as two of six specific aims for quality improvement. Effectiveness is defined as "providing services based on scientific knowledge to all who could benefit and refraining from providing services to those not likely to benefit (avoiding underuse and overuse)"; efficiency is defined as "avoiding waste, in particular waste of equipment, supplies, ideas, and energy" (Institute of Medicine, 2001).

WHY IS QUALITY IMPORTANT?

One of the key issues in healthcare quality and performance is the appropriate use of scarce resources to improve the health of both individuals and the entire population. Problems in this domain can take three forms: underuse, overuse, and misuse. Chassin (1997) defines these terms as follows:

> [**Underuse** is] the failure to provide a service whose benefit is greater than its risk. **Overuse** occurs when a health service is provided when its risks outweigh its benefits. **Misuse** occurs when the right service is provided badly and an avoidable complication reduces the benefit the patient receives.

Underuse is a problem since clinical research has produced a large number of proven, effective treatments that are not widely used. For example, beta blockers are effective in preventing heart attacks among patients who previously have had a heart attack. A study in the late 1990s found that only 21% of eligible elderly patients were prescribed beta blockers upon release after their first heart attack (Soumerai, McLaughlin, Spiegelman, Hertzmark, Thibault, & Goldman, 1997). More recent studies suggest that the underuse of beta blockers, not only in the United States but also in other parts of the world, may occur because of hospital- and clinician-based prescribing patterns (Fonarow, 2005; Nicholls, McElduff, Dobson, Jamrozik, Hobbs, & Leitch, 2001).

Overuse is also a quality problem, as certain treatments are provided despite evidence that the treatment is ineffective or, even, dangerous. Gonzales, Steiner, and Sande (1997) document the overuse of antibiotics among their sample of adults. They found that antibiotics were prescribed 51% of the time for common colds, 52% for upper respiratory infections, and 75% for bronchitis. Such prescriptions are written even though these maladies are caused by viruses, not bacteria. Further, the indiscriminant use of antibiotics has fed the rise of multi-drug resistant strains of bacteria (Steinberg, 2000).

Misuse caught the public's attention with the publication of the first IOM report on patient safety, *To Err is Human* (Kohn, Corrigan, & Donaldson, 2000), which examined the high rate of medical errors in hospitals, noting that between 44,000 and 98,000 hospitalized patients die each year from preventable adverse events and a further 1,000,000 are injured. Moreover, the IOM estimated that the costs to the U.S. economy totaled between $37.6 to $50 billion dollars each year in 1999. Importantly, these figures only represent inpatient, hospital-based services. Recent studies estimate that 3.5% to 6% of outpatients will experience moderate to serious adverse drug events. Solberg and his colleagues used four years of claims data to identify potential drug-drug interactions that alter the effectiveness or toxicity of one or more drugs (Solberg, Hurley, Roberts, Nelson, Frost, Crain, Gunter, & Young, 2004). They found that about 3.5% of those prescribed drugs are at risk in any given year for moderate to severe drug-drug interactions. Using a different methodology of chart auditing and patient surveys, Gandhi and his colleagues reported that 6% of outpatients experienced adverse drug events that were either serious and preventable or ameliorable (Gandhi, Weingart, Borus, Seger, Peterson, Burdick, Seger, Shu, Federico, Leape, & Bates, 2003).

The *Dartmouth Atlas of Health Care* (see http://www.dartmouthatlas.org/) illustrates the prevalence of healthcare service underuse, overuse, and misuse in the United States. The atlas, created by John Wennberg and his associates, captures and displays wide variations in medical practice that cannot be explained by illness severity or patient preference. The pattern of these variations is "often idiosyncratic and unscientific, and local medical opinion and local supply of resources are more important than science in determining how medical care is delivered" (Wennberg, 2002). For example, Boston and New Haven are demographically similar, geographically close, and might be expected to be fairly similar in their utilization of surgical services. However, residents of New Haven were "more than twice as likely to receive coronary bypass surgery and 50% more likely to undergo hysterectomy" than Bostonians. In addition, Bostonians "were two times more likely to undergo carotid artery surgery and 50% more likely to have their hip joints replaced than the residents of New Haven" (Wennberg, 2002).

A BRIEF HISTORY OF QUALITY AND PERFORMANCE IMPROVEMENT

While healthcare policy makers in the United States and other industrialized countries have recently focused their attention on quality, both patients and the providers of health services have valued it for countless millennia. For example, the Codex Hammurabi (circa 1700 BC) imposes several forms of punishment—including death—to physicians and nurses providing poor quality care (Spiegel & Springer, 1997). Similarly, the Hippocratic Oath (circa 400 BC) admonishes physicians to keep patients from "harm or injustice" (von Staden, 1996). Modern versions of the oath continue to be adhered to by physicians and to be incorporated into medical training (Smith, 1996), evolving during the past century into a professional code of ethics (Davis, 2003). Even though the concern about healthcare quality has a long history, its connection to performance improvement is much more recent, arising during the second half of the 19th century and continuing today. The modern history of quality and performance improvement in healthcare services can be divided into three relatively distinct eras: Quality Assurance (QA), Continuous Quality Improvement (CQI), and Systems Improvement (SI). We are now immersed in this latter era, but the techniques and practices of QA and CQI remain and are the basis for improving the system of health care in the United States and around the world.

QUALITY ASSURANCE

The beginnings of the quality assurance era can be traced to the mid-19th century, about the same time as the scientific understanding of germ-induced illness was gaining support in Europe. For most healthcare practitioners, quality assurance is associated with the observations and reforms made by Florence Nightingale during the Crimean War of 1854. During her service as a nurse, she noted a correlation between poor hospital sanitation and an alarming rate of fatalities among wounded soldiers. Acting on this observation, she developed hospital sanitation and hygiene standards during the war that sharply decreased mortality and morbidity rates. Nightingale promoted such basic precautions as washing hands, cleaning surgical tools, providing fresh bed linens, and ensuring hospital wards were clean. During the remainder of the 19th century, she devoted her life to a reform movement that significantly upgraded the practices of sanitation and hygiene in hospitals, while also significantly improving the training of nurses and expanding their role in health care (Henry, Woods, & Nagelkerk, 1990).

THE END RESULT SYSTEM AND THE FLEXNER REPORT

Building upon Nightingale's precepts, Ernest Codman, a Harvard Medical School surgeon, advocated that hospitals should examine whether the services provided to patients were beneficial and address the reasons for failure. His "End Result System" was introduced in 1910, and articulated three core principles of quality assurance: 1) examining quality measures to determine if problems are patient-, system-, or clinician-related; 2) assessing the frequency and prevalence of quality deficiencies; and 3) evaluating and correcting deficiencies so that they do not reoccur (Cooper, 1999). By 1917, the End Result System was acknowledged as critical to ensuring quality health care, and it became the basis for the Hospitalization Standardization Program of the American College of Surgeons. This program established "minimum standards" that focused on the quality of care within hospitals, including the 1) organizing of hospital medical staffs; 2) restricting of medical staff membership to well-trained, competent, and licensed physicians; 3) framing of policies and procedures to ensure regular staff meetings and clinical reviews; 4) recording of medical histories, physical exams, and laboratory tests; and 5) developing diagnostic and treatment facilities under physician oversight (Luce, Bindman, & Lee, 1994). When the American College of Surgeons began on-site inspections of hospitals in 1918, only 89 of 692 hospitals surveyed met minimum standards; by 1950, more than 3,200 hospitals were approved under the Hospitalization Standardization Program (JCAHO, 2006).

About the same time as Codman set forth his ideas, a committee headed by Abraham Flexner was investigating the quality of medical education in

North America for the Carnegie Foundation. His committee's report, *Medical Education in the United States and Canada*, was published in 1910 (Flexner, 1972, c1910). The report strongly criticized proprietary medical schools, including homeopathic and osteopathic approaches, and faulted their poor apprenticeship system. To improve medical education, the committee endorsed biomedical studies in biology, chemistry, and physics that were integrated with rigorous clinical training. The Flexner report revolutionized medical education, supplanting many other forms of physician education with the biomedical model, and integrating it with supervised clinical training. Both Codman and Flexner advanced the science of medical practice, laying the groundwork for future health professionals' acceptance and participation in quality assurance activities.

THE JOINT COMMISSION

In 1951, the American College of Physicians, the American Hospital Association, the American Medical Association, the Canadian Medical Association, and the American College of Surgeons created the Joint Commission on the Accreditation of Hospitals (JCAH). The Joint Commission was formed as a not-for-profit organization to provide voluntary accreditation to hospitals. The American College of Surgeons' Hospital Standardization Program—inspired by Codman's End Result System—was adopted as JCAH's accreditation tool, and the ACS officially transferred this program to the Joint Commission in 1952, and began surveying hospitals in 1953 (JCAHO, 2006). Although the Canadian Medical Association withdrew from the Joint Commission in 1959 in order to establish a Canadian accrediting body, the American Dental Association became a corporate member in 1979 (Viswanathan & Salmon, 2000).

With the passage of legislation authorizing Medicare and Medicaid in 1965, the Joint Commission grew in importance. The legislation contained a provision that JCAH accredited hospitals were deemed to be in compliance with most of the Medicare Conditions of Participation for Hospitals and, thus, could participate in the Medicare and Medicaid programs (JCAHO, 2006; Sprague, 2005). On one hand, this provision made the accreditation process much more compelling to hospital administrators. On the other hand, it meant a change in focus for the Joint Commission's quality assurance approach, from ensuring that minimum standards were followed by hospitals to one based on optimal achievable standards (Luce, Bindman, & Lee 1994). It also marked the beginning of the expansion of the Joint Commission's scope of accreditation. In 1966 it began accrediting long-term facilities; psychiatric facilities, substance abuse programs, and community mental health programs in 1970; ambulatory healthcare facilities in 1975; and hospice organizations in 1983. Thus, it was not surprising that in 1987, the Joint Commission changed its formal name to the Joint Commission on Accreditation of Healthcare Organizations (JCAHO) to reflect its expanded scope of activities beyond hospital accreditation (JCAHO, 2002).

QA ESSENTIALS

As the Joint Commission expanded its scope and activities from the 1950s to the 1980s, the End Result System evolved into Quality Assurance (QA). Essentially, QA involves the development of standards, and the measurement of individual, group, or organizational performance against such standards. In terms of Donabedian's structure-process-outcome framework (Donabedian, 1966), most QA standards focus on structural variables, with some recognition of process and outcome variables. Indeed, until the 1990s, the Joint Commission tended to focus on structural standards, such as assuring that a hospital's physicians were board certified, its nurses licensed, and other key employees had appropriate certifications (Gilpatrick, 1999). It also assured that a hospital had the appropriate numbers and quality of items (e.g., beds, surgical equipment) and appropriate policies and procedures.

Critical to the operation of these standards is the function of tracking and trending. Tracking begins with the identification and monitoring of indicators that reflect standards of care. Benchmarking is often used to identify clinical indicators and "best practices" associated with each. For instance, beginning in 2002, the JCAHO has required hospitals to measure quality of care indicators for the following illnesses: acute myocardial infarction, heart failure, pneumonia, and pregnancy. Care indicators associated with each of these illnesses were identified through an intensive process of reviewing clinical studies and conferring with expert panels of physicians. Field tests of the indicators resulted in four sets of validated measures (Williams, Schmaltz, Morton, Koss, & Loeb, 2005). A few examples of quality of care measures for acute myocardial infarction (heart attack) include aspirin and beta-blocker within 24 hours of admission and smoking-cessation counseling. Indicators such as these are then monitored at repeated intervals, requiring extensive data collection by trained individuals familiar with the measurement process. Gathering data for many clinical process indicators now requires that hospital or medical group personnel abstract data from patient charts. However, the increased use of electronic medical records should eventually automate this process, while prompting physicians to employ best practices (Delpierre, Cuzin, Fillaux, Alvarez, Massip, & Lang, 2004; Rubenfeld, 2004).

QA ASSUMPTIONS AND ACTIONS

From a QA perspective, once sufficient data is gathered, there are two possible outcomes. The first is that the healthcare provider meets or exceeds the standard. When this outcome occurs, no action needs to take place. However, if a provider does not meet the standard for a measure, then the responsible party for QA—a medical director, quality assurance department, or regulatory agency—must take action. The book, *Forgive and Remember: Managing Medical Failure* (Bosk, 1979), portrays the surgical culture of personal accountability upon which QA is grounded, and underscores QA's core assumption that people are responsible for most medical errors. Hence, the responsible party will identify those individuals, groups, or organizations causing the poor performance. Those associated with the quality deficiency will then face one of several responses, depending on the severity of the deficiency. They may be required to attend educational or retraining sessions, provided with technical assistance, and/or be disciplined. For individual providers, disciplinary actions may lead to the revocation of their licenses to practice; for organizations, certification or operating licenses may be rescinded.

At the same time that the Joint Commission was refining the practices associated with QA, the federal government was committed to assuring the quality of services provided to Medicare and Medicaid recipients. Moreover, both the Joint Commission and the Health Care Financing Administration (HCFA)—now known as the Centers for Medicare and Medicaid Services (CMS)—gradually moved away from QA to CQI approaches for improving healthcare quality. How and why these changes took place is discussed next.

FROM PEER REVIEW TO QUALITY IMPROVEMENT ORGANIZATIONS

The introduction of Medicare and Medicaid in 1965 dramatically changed the role and responsibilities of the federal government in the United States. Because Medicare and Medicaid were providing health insurance to a substantial portion of the population, Congress demanded assurance that public funds were being spent for both medically necessary and quality services and items. Initially, Congress authorized the Experimental Medical Care Review Organizations (EMCRO) in 1971. The EMCRO reviewed inpatient and ambulatory services for appropriateness and quality of care, establishing the model for the Professional Standards Review Organizations (PSRO) that would soon follow (Bhatia, Blackstock, Nelson, & Ng, 2000).

PROFESSIONAL STANDARDS REVIEW ORGANIZATIONS (PSROs) PROGRAMS

The U.S. Congress amended the Social Security Act in 1972, establishing the PSROs to review services and items reimbursed through Medicare. Specifically, the PSROs had three responsibilities: 1) assure the quality of services; 2) respond to beneficiary complaints; and 3) protect the Medicare trust funds from fraud and abuse (Jencks, 2004). The PSROs were physician-run organizations with authority to grant or deny payments for Medicare and Medicaid services; some PSROs were funded through grants, others were financed via cooperative agreements, and some directly contracted with the federal government (Bhatia et al., 2000). Regardless of their funding and governance structures, the PSROs typically engaged in retrospective utilization review, auditing medical records and charts to ensure that Medicare and Medicaid patients received care that met recognized standards. Even though by 1981 PSROs were established in 187 of the 195 designated regions of the United States, they often were perceived as focused primarily on denying payments and restricting medical practice and were resisted by the American Medical Association, state medical societies, and many state government agencies (Luce, Bindman, & Lee, 1994). The localized structure of the PSROs, the differing funding and governance arrangements for the PSROs, and the resulting wide variations in care standards and their evaluation undoubtedly contributed to medical providers' disdain for this program (Bhatia et al., 2000).

PEER REVIEW ORGANIZATION (PRO) PROGRAM

At the same time that the PSRO program was floundering, Congress was deeply concerned about containing the inflationary costs of Medicare while sustaining enrollees' access to quality services. The PSROs were dissolved by the Peer Review Improvement Act of 1982, to be replaced by the utilization and quality control peer review organization (PRO) program. The urgency to establish PROs was further propelled by the Deficit Reduction Act of 1984, which mandated Medicare to establish and implement a prospective payment system (PPS). PPS represented a radical change in the way Medicare reimbursed hospitals for patient care, replacing service fees based on reasonable or prevailing charges with fixed fees for each case involving a patient, from admission through discharge (Luce et al., 1994). The fee paid per case by PPS depended on the resources needed for treating patients within various diagnosis-related groups (DRGs). PPS provided clear incentives for hospitals to reduce the length of stay for patients or the kinds and amounts of services provided to patients (Bhatia et al., 2000). This change in funding and incentives also gradually changed the focus of quality review organizations from primarily seeking to reduce overuse to seeking to improve the overall quality of health services.

Hence, beginning in 1984, HCFA requested proposals to contract with PROs for utilization and quality control across 54 regions in the United States and its territories (later reduced to 53 regions). During the first three contract periods (1984–1986; 1986–1989; 1989–1993) the PROs engaged mostly in retrospective utilization reviews (Bhatia et al., 2000). Specifically, the PROs were responsible for reviewing a random group of patients, assessing their DRG classifications, reviewing readmissions, reducing unnecessary hospital admissions and operations, and lowering death and complication rates. These reviews used six generic screens: 1) adequacy of discharge planning; 2) medical stability at discharge; 3) unexpected deaths; 4) nosocomial infections; 5) unscheduled returns to surgery; and 6) trauma suffered in the hospital (Luce et al., 1994).

QUALITY IMPROVEMENT ORGANIZATION (QIO) PROGRAM

By the late 1980s, the value of retrospective case reviews and traditional QA were being questioned both within the healthcare industry and by policy makers. At the request of Congress, HCFA sponsored a study by the Institute of Medicine on quality assurance for Medicare (Lohr, 1990b). The IOM study concluded that many health services did not meet standards and that retrospective case review was an unreliable method for judging the quality of services. The IOM report recommended a major shift in QA strategy toward quality improvement, urging both the PROs and JCAHO to assess clinical outcomes (Lohr, 1990a).

To address these concerns, HCFA began engaging in several quality improvement initiatives during the early 1990s. These initiatives focused on a small number of explicit, evidence-based measures of quality for inpatient care. At the same time that HCFA was piloting quality improvement initiatives with PROs, it gradually expanded the range of partners, from hospitals and physician offices to nursing homes and home health agencies (Bhatia et al., 2000). These changes in the PROs scope, intent, and activities have transformed the PRO from a confrontational agency primarily engaging in retrospective utilization review to a cooperative agency engaging in quality improvement with a wide variety of healthcare organizations (Bradley et al., 2005; Hertz & Fabrizio, 2005; "Quality Directors Give QIOs High Marks in New Study," 2005). As a result, a new designation was coined for the PROs by the newly renamed Centers for Medicare and Medicaid Services (CMS): the organizations are now called Quality Improvement Organizations (QIOs).

As the preceding discussion illustrates, both the Joint Commission and the QIOs have moved from primarily engaging in quality assurance to partnering with all forms of health service delivery organizations. Indeed, both the Joint Commission and the QIOs now champion continuous quality improvement (CQI) efforts. The next section defines and provides multiple examples of CQI principles.

CONTINUOUS QUALITY IMPROVEMENT

During the 1970s, oil shortages compelled many people in the United States to purchase fuel efficient and inexpensive cars. Although U.S. automobile manufacturers tried to produce such cars, only the Japanese were manufacturing fuel efficient yet inexpensive automobiles that were reliable and durable. The quality of these small Japanese vehicles greatly surpassed those manufactured in the United States. Newspapers, magazines, and television news asked the question, "Can America Compete with Japan?" This rapid shift in the marketplace created a new awareness among U.S. industrial leaders that quality mattered.

To address the quality deficit, automobile and other manufacturers in the United States sought the help of quality improvement experts. The contributions assured that total quality management (TQM)—referred to as continuous quality improvement (CQI) in health care—became the new paradigm for quality improvement within the United States during the 1980s and 1990s. These quality gurus and advocates included Walter A. Shewhart, W. Edwards Deming, Joseph M. Juran, and Malcolm Baldrige. They shared a common interest in improving the quality of production in manufacturing and other industries, and their extraordinary lives were intertwined both by industry experience and interest.

During the mid-1920s, Walter A. Shewhart, a physicist at Bell Laboratories, was asked to study the variations in Western Electric's production processes and formulate a means to assure that products met specifications. Rather than inspecting each product for defects, Shewhart's practical perspective led him to try to control the source of quality variation in the production process. This led him to differentiate between "common cause" and "special cause" variations. He knew that "common cause" variations in the production process—due to natural variations in raw materials, minor electrical voltage fluctuations, etc.—often were impractical to control. However, "special cause" variations—due to operator behaviors, incorrectly calibrated machinery, the substituting of different types of raw materials, etc.—could be controlled (Kolesar, 1993). His book, *Economic Control of Quality of Manufactured Product* (Shewhart, 1931), articulated these principles of statistical process control (SPC) for reducing quality variation in production processes. With editorial assistance from his protégé, W. Edwards Deming, Shewhart also wrote a monograph on quality control, *Statistical Method from the Viewpoint of Quality Control*, which introduced the Plan-Do-Check-Act (PDCA) cycle model for improving production processes (Shewhart, 1939).

Known also as the Shewhart cycle in the United States, the PDCA cycle was popularized by W. Edward Deming and it is called the Deming cycle in Japan. A statistician, Deming further developed the principles underlying TQM/CQI while working with the Japanese to reconstruct their industries after World War II. His approach with the Japanese was to help them fundamentally change work processes. Deming developed a management philosophy that encouraged worker participation in process change, focused on data-based decision making, and embraced a standardized approach to quality improvement. This management philosophy was eventually codified into 14 points (see Table 5-1).

Joseph M. Juran was a contemporary and colleague of Deming's. Born in Braila, Romania in 1904, Juran immigrated to the United States with his family in 1912, and began working at the age of 9. He earned a bachelors degree in engineering, but also excelled in mathematics and statistics.

TABLE 5-1 Deming's 14 Points

1. Create and publish to all employees a statement of the aims and purpose of the company or organization. The management must demonstrate constantly their commitment to this statement.
2. Learn the new philosophy, top management and everybody.
3. Understand the purpose of inspection, for improvement of processes and reduction of cost.
4. End the practice of awarding business on the basis of price tag alone.
5. Improve constantly and forever the system of production and service.
6. Institute training.
7. Teach and institute leadership.
8. Drive out fear. Create trust. Create a climate of innovation.
9. Optimize toward the aims and purposes of the company the efforts of teams, groups, and staff areas.
10. Eliminate exhortation for the workforce.
11a. Eliminate numerical quotas for production. Instead, learn and institute methods for improvement.
11b. Eliminate management by objective. Instead, learn the capabilities of processes and how to improve them.
12. Remove barriers that rob people of pride of workmanship.
13. Encourage education and self-improvement for everyone.
14. Take action to accomplish this transformation.

Upon graduating, he was hired as an engineer at Western Electric's Hawthorne Works in 1925. He was one of the first engineers trained by Shewhart to apply the principles of SPC. While at Western Electric, Juran championed the Pareto principle from economics, focusing attention and resources on those important quality problems that are attributable to a small number of factors (e.g., the 80/20 rule). During WWII, Juran worked as assistant to the administrator of the Foreign Economic Administration under the Office for Emergency Management. In this role, he oversaw the logistics for providing materials and supplies to allied governments and troops on both fronts. Building on this experience, another of Juran's important contributions was the "Juran Trilogy" of quality planning, quality control, and quality improvement. All of these notions were first codified in the 1951 publication of the *Quality Control Handbook* (Juran, Gryna, & Bingham, 1974); his work now is carried on by the Juran Institute (see http://www.juran.com/).

Malcolm Baldrige, Secretary of Commerce under President Reagan, died in office as a result of a rodeo accident on July 25, 1987. "Mac" Baldrige was born in Nebraska. During the course of his life he worked as a ranch hand; was a professional team roper on the rodeo circuit; served in combat during WWII as an infantry captain in the Pacific; graduated from Yale University; worked as a foundry hand in an iron company, eventually becoming its president; and was the chairman and CEO of Scovill, Inc. before serving as commerce secretary. A strong advocate of free trade and a proponent of efficiency and effectiveness in government, Baldrige is credited with transforming Scovill from a financially-troubled brass mill to a successful manufacturer of consumer products, housing, and other goods (see http://www.quality.nist.gov/Biography.htm). In his honor, the Malcolm Baldrige National Quality Award was created in 1988 for companies that display excellent performance across seven dimensions. These dimensions of quality have been continually refined and expanded from their original manufacturing base to include healthcare organizations. The Baldrige Award models excellence using a structure-process-outcomes framework.

THE CONCEPT OF CQI IN HEALTH CARE

Now that we have discussed some of the important contributors to continuous quality improvement, let's examine the concept and application of CQI in health care. The concept of continuous quality improvement can be defined as an organizational process, in which employee teams identify and address problems in their work processes. When applied across the organization, CQI creates a continuous flow of process improvements that meet or exceed customer—or patient—expectations. Inherent within this definition are five dimensions of CQI: 1) process focus, 2) customer focus, 3) data-based decision making, 4) employee empowerment, 5) organization-wide scope.

CQI focuses on the process part of Donabedian's quality conception as key to developing high quality health care. Specifically, CQI promotes the view that understanding and addressing the factors that create variation in an administrative or clinical process (e.g., long wait times, high rehospitalization rates) will produce superior patient care quality and organizational performance. Further, quality improvement should not be a one-time activity; rather it should be a normal activity, resulting in a continual flow of improvements.

Underpinning this approach are the concepts and tools of statistical process control (SPC), which Shewhart developed. For example, a manager of an ambulatory clinic has tracked an increase in complaints about patient wait time from quarterly patient satisfaction surveys. For the next month, the wait time for each patient is collected and the daily average is graphed. At the same time, data is collected about why waiting time increases, and the clinic manager finds that the "special cause" variation is driven by 1) the number of medically complex, time-consuming patients each day; 2) the training needs of a new LPN and receptionist; and 3) the over scheduling of new patients. Armed with these findings, the manager is able to work with the clinical and administrative staff to address these concerns to reduce both the variability and the average wait time.

The second element in CQI is the focus on the customer. The organization must make every effort to "delight the customer." CQI defines "customer" in broad terms. Normally, patients are thought of as the main customers in health care. CQI's view is that any person or organization that is on the downstream end of a process is a customer. For example, a doctor ordering a MRI can be considered a customer because she receives the service of the radiology department. Thus, CQI takes the position that each process has a variety of both internal and external customers. The customer focus is best exemplified in the widespread use of patient satisfaction surveys by hospitals and physician groups.

The third element in CQI is an emphasis on using data to make all quality improvement decisions. The foundation of SPC, as discussed earlier, rests on the collection, analysis, and use of data to improve processes and monitor the success of process interventions. The use of carefully collected data reduces both uncertainty and the dependence on uninformed impressions or biases for improving an organizational process. It also provides good evidence to convince skeptics that a process problem exists. Returning to our earlier example, the collected data on waiting times enabled not only the clinic manager to understand the "special cause" factors that were creating them, but also helped physicians, nurses, and front desk and other staff understand the sources of the problem.

The fourth element of CQI is employee empowerment. This empowerment is manifested by the widespread use of quality improvement teams. The typical CQI team will consist of hourly employees whose day-to-day work gives them a unique perspective and detailed knowledge of patient care processes. Another important individual for a CQI team is the facilitator, who typically provides training on CQI tools and philosophy. Members of the CQI team are not only empowered to improve their work environment, but can also become an advocate for change, overcoming resistance among other employees. In our prior example, the clinic manager worked with both clinical employees (e.g., RNs, LPNs, and the nurse supervisor) and administrative employees (e.g., receptionists, admission and billing clerks, and their supervisor) to decrease the wait times and improve patients' satisfaction with the clinic.

The final element in CQI is its strategic use across the organization, accomplished through the coordinated and continuous improvement of various operational processes. Such coordination requires a broader management philosophy for improving the organization, similar in scope and intent to the system improvement notions discussed later in this chapter. Specifically, for CQI to be effective at the organization level, three elements must be in place: executive leadership, a strategic orientation, and a commitment to cultural change.

The first element is executive leadership. Without the support of the top managers, any attempt to apply CQI principles across the healthcare organization will be likely to fail. Overcoming organizational inertia, the natural resistance to change among departmental managers and work-unit supervisors, requires an overarching organizational commitment to CQI. The second element is a strategic orientation. CQI principles must be incorporated into the strategic plans and goals of the healthcare organization. If CQI is not a budget item with clear goals that are aligned with the strategic direction of the organization, organization-wide CQI initiatives are doomed to fail. The final element is cultural change. CQI emphasizes a culture in which quality is a central value shared across the entire organization and permeating all organizational and individual activities.

APPLYING CQI

In order to make specific quality improvements, the Shewhart/Deming cycle of PDCA is generally used in manufacturing and other industries. However, during the early 1980s, the Hospital Corporation of American (HCA) modified the PDCA cycle to create the FOCUS-PDCA framework, which has become the most commonly used quality improvement framework in the healthcare industry. FOCUS stands for Find, Organize, Clarify, Understand, and Select. The addition of FOCUS clarifies the steps that need to be done prior to the implementation of any process change. The changes in the process will then be guided by the PDCA cycle.

Find means simply to find a process to improve. Problems may be identified by employees, managers, or customers. Problem identification may be helped by brainstorming about the performance problems facing a work unit or department. Once this list is complete, the next step is selecting the problem on which to focus. Problems that cause "high pain" should be chosen. Keep in mind that CQI projects are time and personnel intensive. In order to be worthwhile and be approved by management, some statement about return on investment is necessary.

Organize means to organize a team. A good CQI team has three elements. First, the team is composed of people directly involved in the process. This ensures that team members will have intimate knowledge of the process to be improved. It also has the side benefit of reducing resistance to change. Second, the team must represent the range of professional and occupational groups involved in a process. If certain stakeholders are left out of a CQI project, then the knowledge base of the project is incomplete. Moreover, any solutions developed may be resisted by those stakeholders not represented on the team. The final element is the presence of a resource person who is responsible for providing necessary CQI training and facilitating the group's activities. Without this person, the team is very likely to be ill-prepared and fail to accomplish its mandate.

Clarify is commonly done by flowcharting the process. Once a team is organized and trained, then it must turn to clarifying the process. Flowcharting documents the sequence of activities that take place in a process. Creating a usable flowchart often takes a number of meetings, particularly if there is substantial variation in how the process is performed, which may have been the reason it was selected in the first place. Flowcharting also raises the issue about the scope of the project. It is at this point that teams need to assess if the scope of their project is too big or too small.

Understand is a three-part process of identifying measures, collecting data, and analyzing it. Once there is a usable flowchart, then the team can turn to understanding the process. The first part is identifying existing or developing new quality measures; the second is collecting the data, which provide insight about how well the process is performed. Sometimes quality measures are already collected and they just need to be accessed (e.g., manual medical chart audits, patient satisfaction scores). Other times, measures need to be developed and data collected (e.g., wait times). In either case, it is important that the methods and measures used to collect data are valid and reliable. Once data has been collected, the third step, analysis, can take place. Analysis involves documenting the variation as measured and uncovering the causes of the variation. As discussed in more detail later, a wide variety of tools for uncovering causes of process variation can be used.

Select is determining the quality improvement process to implement. After the process is mapped and the process problem and its causes understood, a process improvement plan can be selected. Studying the key causes of the problem uncovered in the analysis should inspire a number of alternative plans for improving the process. The team should develop criteria for deciding which plan to use. Such criteria might involve time, costs, feasibility, and potential for employee, managerial, or customer resistance. After each alternative is weighed on the criteria, the team should be able to make a rational selection of an improvement plan.

After the selection of the quality improvement plan, the CQI team moves to the PDCA cycle. This transition is important because PDCA represents a cyclical set of actions that take place until a process improvement is deemed to have met its goals. **Planning** converts the idea proposed for process improvement into a specific set of actions. During this planning, the questions of who, what, and how should be addressed. The "Who?" question pertains to that specific group or people who will pilot test the process improvement. The "What?" question asks about the specific actions of the planned intervention, and the "How?" question addresses the step-by-step operations for implementing the intervention. Another important question is that of measurement. During the understanding part of the framework, at least one, and preferably several, measures are identified and used. In the planning stage, goals for each measure need to be developed. Often these are derived from benchmarks, which may also be used during the **Understand** part of the FOCUS-PDCA framework. The "How?" question is answered by developing a detailed set of actions to be taken in reworking and improving the process.

Once the plan is complete, then it needs to be implemented. During this stage, data are collected and implementation issues are resolved. After a suitable pilot period, the data are compared with the goals to determine if the effort is successful. Also, this is where lessons on implementation and insights into the teams' own functioning may be discussed.

The final stage of the cycle is the **A** for **Act** to hold the gains. If the goals are not met, the cycle returns to the plan step and a new process improvement idea is selected. Alternatively, if the goals are met, then the cycle terminates. However, important work often needs to be done to make sure that the improvement becomes permanent. If the improvement was pilot tested in one group (e.g., a nursing ward within a hospital), then it might be spread to other wards. Among the activities that need to be done are training personnel in the new process, revising policies, automating data collection, and educating stakeholders to reduce resistance to change.

OTHER LEADING QUALITY IMPROVEMENT MODELS

In addition to the methods discussed under CQI, there are three additional methods of quality improvement that bear brief mention, including **Six Sigma**, **reengineering**, and **ISO 9000**.

Six Sigma

Six Sigma is an extension of Joseph Juran's approach to quality improvement, and was developed by Motorola and popularized by Jack Welch at General Electric. It has been defined as a "Data-driven quality methodology that seeks to eliminate variation from a process" (Scalise, 2001). Six

Sigma employs a structured process called **DMAIC**, which stands for *Define, Measure, Analyze, Improve,* and *Control.* **Define** includes delimiting the scope of work, determining due dates, and mapping the future state of the process, including improvements. **Measure** encompasses both the creation of measures or metrics, as well as their application to determine how well a process is performing. **Analyze** further breaks down the understanding of the process, and often includes flowcharting the process. **Improve** specifies the steps that will be taken to meet the goals outlined during the define step. **Control** is about ensuring that the improvements are permanent rather than temporary.

While DMAIC guides the actual improvement project, Six Sigma also features major training and human resource components. Because of these components, many large hospital and health systems have begun adopting Six Sigma as a way to change the organization and establish a culture of quality. Such change begins with a CEO who supports the method; without top level management support, efforts like this generally founder. A champion is a senior executive (generally VP level or above) who has full-time responsibility for quality improvement efforts. Further into the organization are three levels of "belts." At the top are Master Black Belts, full-time employees who provide technical leadership and training to those running QI projects. Black Belts direct multiple projects, and Green Belts are those who lead specific projects.

Business Process Reengineering

Reengineering is another quality improvement method that has gained favor in recent years. It was popularized by the book, *Reengineering the Corporation* (Hammer & Champy, 1993). Its development was born from managers' frustration with the slow pace of other quality improvement methods. Specifically, it advocates the "radical redesign of business processes for dramatic improvement." Rather then improving existing processes, it relies on a clean sheet approach to quality improvement. It focuses on the complete end-to-end set of activities that provide value for customers. This approach has great value when it is used to rapidly pilot change within an organization and to create business options (Lillrank & Holopainen, 1998). On one hand, experience has demonstrated that large scale reengineering projects have a high risk of failure, largely because of the resistance to radical change within most organizations ("The Trouble with Re-engineering," 1995). On the other hand, large public sector health organizations, such as the Veterans Health Administration in the United States (Jha, Perlin, Kizer, & Dudley, 2003), have achieved remarkable results through reengineering. And its use is supported by the National Health System in the United Kingdom (McAdam & Corrigan, 2001).

ISO 9000

The International Organization for Standardization (ISO) is a not-for-profit organization, which provides a framework for developing voluntary technical and management system standards for international business. ISO unites a network of national standards institutes in 156 countries (see http://www.iso.org/iso/en/aboutiso/introduction/index.html). ISO's goal is to provide a world-wide consensus for the standardization of processes and services for all industries, thus benefiting consumers, businesses, and governments. ISO 9000 was proposed in 1987 and improved in 1994 to provide a non-prescriptive management system quality standard for non-technical business functions. Similar to Deming's TQM principles, ISO 9000 certification is grounded on eight principles (http://www.iso.org/iso/en/iso9000-14000/understand/qmp.html): 1) customer focus, 2) leadership, 3) involvement of people, 4) process approach, 5) system approach to management, 6) continual improvement, 7) factual approach to decision making, and 8) mutually beneficial supplier relationships. Healthcare organizations seeking ISO 9000 certification pursue the International Workshop Agreement 1:2005 standards for quality management systems, which provide guidelines for process improvements in health services (http://www.iso.ch/iso/en/CatalogueDetailPage.Catalogue Detail?CSNUMBER=41768&ICS1=11&ICS2=20&ICS3=&scopelist CATALOGUE). The healthcare organizations then demonstrate that their quality management processes meet international standards through a quality audit conducted by various ISO 9000 certification bodies.

KEY QUALITY IMPROVEMENT CONCEPTS

Across the many ways of thinking about quality and ways to improve quality, there is a common set of four key concepts: measurement, process variation, statistical process control, and quality improvement tools.

Measurement

The most basic concept in quality improvement is that of measurement and the metrics associated with it. **Measurement** is the translation of observable events into quantitative terms, while metrics are the means actually used to record phenomenon. All quality improvement efforts require numerical data because "you can't manage what you can't measure." In this way, quality improvement is driven by data-based evidence rather than subjective judgments or opinions.

Good measurement begins with the rigorous definition of the concept to be measured. It then requires the use of a measurement methodology that yields **reliable** (i.e., consistent) and **valid** (i.e., accurate) measures of the concept. Rigorous definition means that the concept to be measured (e.g., wait times) needs to be defined in very specific terms. This definition should be written and include the unit of measure. For example, wait times could be defined as the time interval between the arrival of a patient at the office and the time they are first seen by the doctor. The unit of measure is time, but the start and end points are important for assessing the reliability and validity of the measure.

Once a good definition of the concept is developed, one challenge is to measure it reliably. If every recorded wait time starts with the arrival of the patient and ends with the patient's first encounter with the doctor, then the measure should be consistent, or reliable. **Measure reliability** means that if a measure is taken at several points over time or by various people, that the measure will generally be consistent (that is, not vary too much). For example, if a person takes his/her temperature each morning, it should be close to 98.6°F each time assuming that she or he is not ill. If it substantially deviates from that temperature, then that person is either ill or the thermometer is broken and not giving consistent readings. Another example of reliability is that of reliability among people. If two nurses in a practice are measuring wait times but use different definitions of waiting, then their measurement of waiting time will not be consistent (e.g., reliable) because the two nurses are measuring the same concept, but in different ways.

Another challenge is to ensure that the measure of the concept is valid. Its validity depends on the accuracy of the measure. If two nurses use the same stopwatch to record waiting times, so long as the clock itself is accurate and the nurses adhere to the same definition of waiting, the wait times should be accurate. In other words, **validity** is the extent to which the measure used actually measures the concept. As with reliability, having a rigorous definition and method of data collection will yield a valid measure.

Process Variation and Statistical Process Control (SPC)

Process variation is the range of values that some quality metric can take as a result of different causes within the process. As Shewhart noted, these causes can take two forms: **special** and **common cause variation** (Shewhart, 1931). **Special cause variation** is due to unusual, infrequent, or unique events that cause the quality metric to deviate from its average by a statistically significant degree. **Common cause variation** is due to the usual or natural causes of variation within a process. Following Shewhart, quality improvement now involves 1) detecting and eliminating special cause variation in a process; and 2) detecting and reducing, whenever feasible, common cause variation within a process.

Statistical Process Control (SPC) is a method by which process variation is measured, tracked, and controlled with the goal of improving the quality of the process. SPC is a branch of statistics that involves time series analysis with graphic data display. The advantage of this method is that it often yields insight into the data in a way that is intuitive for most decision makers. In essence, it relies on the notion that "a picture is worth a thousand words" for its import. Quality data from a particular process are graphed across time. At some point when there is enough data, a mean and standard deviation for the data are calculated and a control chart constructed. The construction begins with the graphing of data across time. It continues with the calculation of upper and lower control limits. Think of these limits as similar to the tolerances for machined parts. Complex machinery, like aircraft, requires parts that are manufactured to very tight tolerances so that they will fit together well. The larger the tolerance, the greater the likelihood that a part will not fit the way it is supposed to fit. These limits show the range of variation where the process is thought to be "in control." Typically these limits are set at plus and minus three standard deviations. With these control limits in place, the data can be interpreted and times when the process was "out of control" investigated and remedied.

QUALITY IMPROVEMENT TOOLS

In addition to the use of control charts, there are a number of other tools that are commonly used in quality improvement activities. They can be divided into three categories: data collection, process mapping, and process analysis.

Data Collection Tools

The check sheet is a simple data collection form in which the occurrence of some event or behavior is tallied. At the end of the data collection period, they are added up. The best check sheets are those that are simple and have well-defined categories of what constitutes a particular event or behavior. For example, a doctor's office staff wanted to find out the reasons why patients showed up late. They brainstormed about the reasons and after carefully defining each reason, they developed a check sheet. The check sheet was pilot tested, and several new reasons were added while other reasons were refined. The check sheet was then employed during a month-long data collection period. They found that transportation problems and babysitting problems jointly accounted for 63% of the late shows.

Another example is the use of chart abstractions or chart audits. In this process, a check sheet is used to collect information from a patient's medical record. Most of the time this is a manual process that involves an individual looking at the medical record, finding the requested information, and recording it on a check sheet. The use of electronic medical records may take some or all of the labor out of this process, as pertinent medical information can be collected more easily or, better yet, a complete report produced at the click of a mouse.

Geographic mapping is a pictorial check sheet in which an event or problem is plotted on a map. This is often used in epidemiological studies to plot where victims of certain diseases live, work, play, etc. For example, a public health agency was trying to isolate and contain an outbreak of a virulent form of influenza. The agency plotted the places where the infected individuals' lived, worked, and/or went to school. Using that plot, they were able to focus their efforts on a specific area where the disease occurred most often.

A more focused application of geographic mapping is the workflow diagram. Simply put, this reflects the movements of people, materials, documents, or information in a process. Plotting these movements on the floor plan of a building or around a paper document can present a very vivid picture of the inefficiency of a process. With the advancement of information technology, increasingly sophisticated geographic mapping and tracking programs have become available, making this complex task easier to do.

Mapping Processes

Flowcharting is the main way that processes are mapped. A flowchart is nothing more than a picture of the sequence of steps in a process. Different actions within a process are denoted by different geometric shapes. A basic flowchart just outlines the major steps in a process. A detailed flowchart is often more useful in quality improvement. Developing such a flowchart requires substantial investigation of each aspect of the process to be charted. Determining the appropriate level of detail should be driven by the flowchart's use within the quality improvement process. A top down flowchart is often used for providing an overview of large or complex processes. It shows the major steps in the process and lists below each major step the sub-steps. The development flowchart adds another dimension to the flowchart. Often it is useful for tracking the flow of information between people. That is, the development flowchart shows the steps of the process carried out by each person, unit, or group involved in a process. Since hand-offs are often where errors may occur, this flowchart provides a target for data collection efforts.

Analyzing Processes

The cause-and-effect diagram helps to identify and organize the possible cause for a problem in a structured format. It is commonly referred to as a **fishbone diagram** for its resemblance to a fish. It is also called an **Ishikawa diagram**, in honor of Kaoru Ishikawa who developed it. The diagram begins with the problem under investigation described in a box at the right of the diagram. The fish's spine is represented by a long arrow pointing to the box. The major possible causes of the problem are arrayed as large ribs along the spine. These are broad categories of causes to which smaller ribs are attached that identify more specific causes of the problem.

A **Pareto chart** is a simple frequency chart. The frequency of each problem, reason, etc. is listed on the X-axis and the number or percent of occurrences is listed on the Y-axis. This analysis is most useful in identifying the major problems in a process and their frequency of occurrence. Another version of the frequency chart is the **histogram**, which shows the range and frequency of values for a measure. When complete, it shows the complete distribution of some variable. This is often useful in basic data analysis.

As mentioned earlier, CQI has its greatest impact if it becomes a part of the strategic mission of a healthcare organization. When that occurs, it is then possible to look beyond the boundaries of the organization and to consider ways in which the healthcare system at the local, regional, and national levels could be improved. The next section addresses why system improvement is important and outlines some of the initiatives within the United States for improving the healthcare system

SYSTEM THINKING AND HEALTHCARE QUALITY IMPROVEMENT

Within the healthcare industry, the paradigmatic shift between CQI and system improvement became fully visible with the publication of the 1999 IOM report, *To Err is Human*. Most important to the evolution of thinking about system improvement was the 2001 report, *Crossing the Quality Chasm*, which laid out an agenda for the creation of a 21st century healthcare system in the United States. The report identified six aims for health care, specifying that it should be:

- Safe—avoiding injuries to patients from care that is intended to help them;
- Effective—providing services based on scientific knowledge to all who could benefit and refraining from providing services to those not likely to benefit (e.g., avoidance of overuse and underuse);
- Patient-Centered—providing care that is respectful of and responsive to individual patient preferences, needs, and values and ensuring that patient values guide all clinical decisions;
- Timely—reducing waits and sometimes harmful delays for both those who receive and those who give care;
- Efficient—avoiding waste, including use of equipment, supplies, ideas, and energy; and,
- Equitable—providing care that does not vary in quality because of personal characteristics such as gender, ethnicity, geographic location, and socioeconomic status (IOM, 2001)

System Thinking and Active vs. Latent Errors

Taken together, the two IOM reports introduced both to the public and to many healthcare professionals a new way of thinking about quality, namely system thinking. Specifically, the authors of the IOM reports viewed many medical errors as latent and occurring in complex, tightly-linked organizations. **Latent errors** are those types of errors "whose adverse consequences may lie dormant within the system for a long time, only becoming evident when they combine with other factors to break the system's defenses" (Reason, 1990). They are likely to be spawned by "those whose activities are removed in both time and space from the direct control interface." The effects of **active errors**, on the other hand, are likely to be felt immediately and are likely to be committed by service providers directly interacting with the patient. Note that active errors are also the types of errors that are typically the ones detected by QA.

For example, consider an operating room nurse faced with setting up three different infusion pumps for the administration of anesthesia, as well as an oxygen pump. For the anesthesia to be administered without error, each pump must be set up correctly. Active errors could include overdosing the patient with an anesthetic or providing too little oxygen during surgery, either of which would potentially produce deadly harm to the patient. One potential latent error lies in having three different types of infusion pumps, each with their own set up procedure, and often with strikingly different means for turning on and off critical valves. Or the infusion pumps may have similar valves, but these may be different from those used for the oxygen pump. Moreover, dosages for different medications administered through the infusion pumps may be confused with one another, introducing other latent errors. Lastly, another latent error may be inadequate or incomplete training for the OR nurses on how to set up and operate the three different types of infusion pumps in conjunction with the oxygen.

While QA techniques probably would detect this latter problem and address it, all the other latent errors would most likely not be detected and appropriately addressed. However, we know CQI techniques are capable of detecting the other latent errors and helping to produce solutions to eliminate them. The system improvement perspective takes the knowledge gained from both QA and CQI in this example; moreover, it would focus both on (a) enabling all other hospital operating rooms to detect these latent errors and (b) diffusing the best practices for eliminating these errors.

System Interactiveness and Coupling

Beyond active and latent errors, two other important concepts are system **interactiveness** and **coupling**, which are discussed in Normal Accident Theory (Perrow, 1984).

System Interactiveness

Interactiveness is the level and type of interaction among system components; such interactions can be characterized as either linear or complex. Linear interactions follow a sequential logic: A interacts with B to produce C; C interacts with D to produce E; and so forth. Complex interactions, on the other hand, have "branching paths, feedback loops, jumps from one linear sequence to another because of proximity. The connections are not only adjacent, serial ones, but can multiply as other parts of units or subsystems are reached." Think for a moment about the following example: A interacts with B and C to produce D; E interacts with A, C, and D to produce F; while G and E interact with F to produce H. Now use the following to make this abstract formula more concrete: A = patient; B = admissions staff; C = nurse; D = medical complaint/history; E = attending physician; F = medical exam; G = consulting physician; H = diagnosis. As this example illustrates, even a routine visit to a family doctor often involves complex interactions. For many patients, however, obtaining a diagnosis is only the first part of an increasingly complex journey through the health system.

System Coupling

Coupling is the amount of time, distance, or slack between two elements in a system. Loosely coupled systems have more time or slack between system elements than a tightly coupled system. As the prior example illustrated, even a doctor's office contains a number of complex interactions. Complexity increases by several magnitudes in an acute care hospital, which is composed of many interacting sub-systems of care, often with tight coupling among several of the sub-systems. For example, a patient admitted into the emergency department typically will need laboratory tests and x-rays, each of which are produced by separate departments (subsystems) within the hospital. The patient's diagnosis and treatment by an

ER physician depends on these ancillary services not only being conducted correctly, but also being produced quickly and in conjunction with each other. In other words, the emergency department, imaging department, and laboratory are tightly coupled sub-systems.

HEALTH CARE AS HIGH HAZARD INDUSTRY

Because of the tightly coupled, complex interactions within healthcare organizations, Gaba (2000) argues that health care is a high hazard industry, like nuclear power or airlines. The likelihood of an adverse outcome (e.g., a medical error, long wait time, etc.) occurring increases both as a system gets more complex, and as the system's interactions become more tightly coupled. In a system characterized by complex interactions many latent errors may occur; add tightly coupled interactions between system elements, and it becomes difficult to detect and correct such errors. Consider the example of the patient admitted to the ER. Given an inaccurate or mislabeled test result or mislabeled or misread x-ray, the patient's diagnosis and treatment may be tragically wrong—although based on clinically correct decision making. Determining what went wrong, why it happened, and how to prevent its reoccurrence, requires more than simply optimizing performance by separately applying CQI techniques at the sub-system levels of the laboratory, the imaging department, or the emergency department. Instead, CQI techniques must be applied to the emergency care micro-system that encompasses each of the sub-systems. In other words, system thinking about quality improvement shifts the focus to the system encompassing the tightly coupled sub-systems. Again, the goals of system improvement are twofold: 1) to detect and eliminate latent errors in complex organizations by using CQI across the organization; and 2) to diffuse the best practices for doing so both within and across healthcare organizations. The various ways that system improvement in the United States are being attempted are discussed next.

APPROACHES TO SYSTEM IMPROVEMENT

System improvement moves quality from an issue of concern for a department or work unit, and makes it a concern for the entire organization, its network of partners, and the market and governmental institutions supporting the healthcare sector. Quality thus viewed is a property of the entire system of health care, which has to be addressed at four levels of increasing degrees of abstraction: the patient, the micro-system of care, the healthcare organization, and the healthcare environment (Berwick, 2002). The environment includes not only the network of healthcare organizations providing services, but also the incentives and restrictions they face from training, market, governmental, and accrediting institutions. The example of the patient admitted to the ER focuses on not only the patient, but also the micro-system of care. If we extend the example to include the patient's admission to the critical care unit in the hospital, discharge to a nursing home for rehabilitation, followed by home health care and ambulatory rehabilitation visits, it becomes clear that each healthcare organization involved has a responsibility to improve the quality of care for the patient. The most difficult aspect within not only the United States but also within other countries' health systems, is ensuring that there is continuity of care as a patient is transferred from one healthcare setting to another (Plochg & Klazinga, 2002; Schoen, Osborn, Hoynh, Doty, Zapert, Peugh, & Davis, 2005). Improving the quality of both healthcare practices and the continuity of care at the system level requires both governmental and industry-wide involvement and oversight.

Federal Government Initiatives

Since the 2001 publication of *Crossing the Quality Chasm*, there has been increasing activity to improve healthcare systems in the United States, involving not only governmental agencies, but also large employers, accrediting agencies, trade and professional organizations, and nonprofit organizations. The federal government's efforts to improve system quality are fivefold (Schoenbaum, Audet, & Davis, 2003):

1. The Agency for Healthcare Research and Quality (AHRQ; see http://www.ahrq.gov/) manages an active research program in quality of care and patient safety, including the Center for Quality Improvement and Patient Safety;

2. The National Quality Forum (NQF; see http://www.qualityforum .org/) is a public-private partnership working on improving quality performance measures;

3. The Patient Safety Task Force (see http://www.ahrq.gov/qual/task force/psfactst.htm) is a multi-agency research program on the quality of care and patient safety that links the AHRQ, the Centers for

Disease Control and Prevention, the CMS, and the Food and Drug Administration;

4. The Veterans Health Administration's (VHA) Quality Enhancement Research Initiative (see http://www.hsrd.research.va.gov/queri/) translates research findings and promotes innovations to improve systems of patient care (McQueen, Mittman, & Demakis, 2004); and,

5. Medicare's quality assurance program contracts with the Quality Improvement Organizations (QIOs), whose efforts to improve quality were previously discussed (see http://www.cms.hhs.gov/Quality ImprovementOrgs/).

Employer-Sponsored Initiatives

Large corporations have also become involved in improving health system quality, most notably through the Leapfrog Group, made up of more than 170 companies and corporations (see www.leapfroggroup.org/). Through partnerships with health insurance companies, medical associations, and nonprofit foundations, the Leapfrog Group has actively promoted the use of rewards and incentives for hospitals and physicians that provide high quality health services. Indeed, many of the current pay-for-performance projects either involve the Leapfrog Group or are modeled upon its efforts.

The National Business Coalition on Health (NBCH) is a national, not-for-profit organization; its members include about 90 business coalitions in 33 states, representing over 7,000 employers and about 34 million employees and their dependents (see http://www.nbch.org/more.cfm). As a coalition of coalitions, the NBCH helps member coalitions seek community health reform through value-based healthcare purchasing. Such purchasing is based both on measuring the quality and efficiency of providers and health plans and on creating incentives for rewarding providers who provide high-value care.

Accrediting Agency Initiatives

Both the Joint Commission (JCAHO; see http://www.jcaho.org/pms/ index.htm) and the National Committee for Quality Assurance (NCQA; see http://www.ncqa.org/index.htm) are important contributors to system improvement in health care. During the late 1980s and early 1990s, the Joint Commission attempted to integrate performance measurement into the accreditation process through the **Indicator Measurement System**

(IMSystem). When it became clear that system improvement would require multi-faceted collaborations, the Joint Commission launched the ORYX® initiative in 1997. This initiative is open to multiple external measurement systems developed by the QIOs, NQF, CMS, AHRQ, and other organizations, and involves a wide range of activities with two overarching objectives: "1) the continuing expansion and coordination of nationally standardized core measurement capabilities and 2) increasing the use of measure data for quality improvement, benchmarking, accountability, decision making, accreditation, and research" (JCAHO; see http://www.jcaho.org/pms/reference+materials/future+goals+and+objectives.htm).

The NCQA originally began in the early 1990s as an accrediting agency for health maintenance organizations (HMOs). However, it soon assumed responsibility for reporting on HMO performance to employers and government agencies with the Health Plan Data and Information Set (HEDIS). Now it accredits not only HMOs but also preferred provider organizations (PPOs) and managed behavioral healthcare organizations (MBHOs); moreover, it has deeming authority for Medicare Advantage plans (Medicare Part C). Available to consumers, employers, and government agencies, NCQA's Health Plan Report Card (http://hprc.ncqa.org/menu.asp) assesses participating health plans throughout the United States, benchmarking them on such measures as access and services, the quality of the providers, and ability to maintain health, improve health, and help those with chronic illnesses.

Other Initiatives

A leading advocate of system-wide quality improvement, not only in the United States but worldwide, is the Institute for Healthcare Improvement (IHI; see www.ihi.org/IHI/). Founded by Donald M. Berwick, MD, the IHI is a nonprofit organization that provides training and resources for improving healthcare systems, as well as numerous programs to improve patient safety and care. It often partners with the Robert Wood Johnson Foundation (RWJF; see www.rwjf.org/index.jsp), a nonprofit philanthropy devoted to improving the health and health care of all Americans. The RWJ Foundation has been particularly focused on reducing ethnic and racial disparities in health and healthcare services, as well as pay-for-performance projects.

A leading advocate of pay-for-performance initiatives in the private sector, Bridges to Excellence (BTE; see http://www.bridgestoexcellence.org/

bte/index.htm) is a multi-state, multi-employer coalition developed by employers, physicians, health services researchers, and other experts. Its mission is to reward quality care that is safe, timely, effective, efficient, equitable, and patient-centered. Partners include HealthGrades, the Leapfrog Group, Medstat, Michael Pine and Associates, NBCH, NCQA, and WebMD; BTE is also supported by a grant from the RWJ Foundation.

Lastly, the Hospital Quality Alliance (HQA) was founded by the American Hospital Association (http://www.aha.org/aha/key_issues/qualityalliance/index.html), the Federation of American Hospitals (http://www.fah.org/issues/quality_initiative/), and the Association of American Medical Colleges (http://www.aamc.org/quality/hospitalalliance/start.htm). A national public-private collaboration, the HQA encourages hospitals to voluntarily collect and report hospital quality performance information. As we discuss later, the HQA makes important information about hospital performance accessible to the public, helping to inform and invigorate efforts to improve quality. CMS and the Joint Commission participate in the HQA, along with the AHA, the FAH, the AAMC, the American Medical Association, the American Nurses Association, the National Association of Children's Hospitals and Related Organizations, American Association of Retired People, the American Federation of Labor and Council of Industrial Organizations, the Consumer-Purchaser Disclosure Project, the AHRQ, the NQF, and the U.S. Chamber of Commerce.

These various initiatives have had a positive impact on improving healthcare quality in the United States and elsewhere, but much still remains to be done. A latter section in this chapter discusses the quality and performance challenges facing healthcare organizations, especially in the United States.

A good place to start when considering the quality and performance challenges facing healthcare organizations and institutions is an assessment of what has been done. To that end, the Commonwealth Fund recently published an Issue Brief entitled, *Medical Errors: Five Years after the IOM Report* (Bleich, 2005).

ASSESSING HEALTHCARE SYSTEM IMPROVEMENT

In its report, *Crossing the Quality Chasm* (Institute of Medicine, 2001), the IOM recommended a fourfold strategy for improving system quality:

1. Establish a Center for Patient Safety within the Agency for Healthcare Research and Quality (AHRQ);
2. Develop a nationwide mandatory error-reporting system for adverse events that cause death and serious harm, as well as voluntary error-reporting systems for events that cause minimal harm;
3. Raise explicit performance standards for patient safety and enforce them through licensing, certification, and accreditation; and
4. Implement safety systems and best practices at the delivery level in healthcare organizations.

As noted in the previous section, many of these recommendations are being carried out. AHRQ's Center for Quality Improvement and Patient Safety has helped address the first recommendation, as has its other efforts to support research and disseminate best practices on patient safety. Also, JCAHO and NCQA have begun fulfilling the third recommendation by requiring healthcare organizations and health plans, respectively, to meet and improve patient safety standards. Moreover, CMS, BTE, JCAHO, the Leapfrog Group, QIOs, and the IHI are collaborating to improve safety systems and disseminate best practices among healthcare organizations, helping to address the fourth recommendation.

The second recommendation, to develop mandatory and voluntary error-reporting systems, has been much harder to initiate. As of 2005, mandatory reporting was required in only 22 states (Bleich, 2005), and there is a great deal of variation in what is reported and the transparency of this reporting to the public (McQueen, Mittman, & Demakis, 2004). Moreover, there is considerable opposition to voluntary reporting systems from hospital administrators and from physicians, largely because of the threat of malpractice litigation (Andrus, Villasenor, Kettelle, Roth, Sweeney, & Matolo, 2003; Weissman, Annas, Epstein, Schneider, Clarridge, Kirle, Gotsanis, Feibelmann, & Ridley, 2005).

HEALTHCARE SYSTEM
IMPROVEMENT CHALLENGES

The difficulty that the United States has encountered in implementing the IOM's error-reporting recommendation underscores not only this but also other performance and quality improvement challenges. These challenges occur not only because of legal constraints (Pawlson & O'Kane, 2004), but also because of the uncertainty in diagnosing and providing medical treatments (Lillrank & Liukko, 2004), deficits in the information technology infrastructure in the health system (Ortiz, Meyer, & Burstin, 2002; Schoenbaum et al., 2003), and the economic incentives within the healthcare financing system (McNeil, 2001). We discuss each of these four challenges to conclude this chapter.

Reforming Medical Malpractice

Medical malpractice litigation exists in part to deter carelessness (i.e., negligence) on the part of medical providers; it does so by allowing patients to be compensated for harm and suffering (Wood, 1998). The evidence for the effectiveness of medical malpractice litigation in deterring poor quality is meager. Not only does it do little to improve healthcare quality (Pawlson & O'Kane, 2004), but it also does much to decrease healthcare quality in two ways. First, the so-called defensive practice of medicine increases the overuse of unnecessary medical services, especially diagnostic tests and imaging services (Rubin & Mendelson, 1994). Both physicians and hospitals are likely to order more, rather than less, testing to avoid legal liability for a misdiagnosis or failure to provide treatment, even if the testing or treatment may have limited benefit. Second, inflated medical malpractice awards have periodically brought about crises in malpractice insurance costs. When malpractice insurance becomes unaffordable, this induces many physicians to restrict or leave the practice of medicine and contributes to the scarcity of needed medical services, such as obstetrics (Amon & Winn, 2004).

Understandably, physicians and hospitals are particularly sensitive to the disincentives that medical malpractice litigation poses for reporting medical errors. For example, without immunity from medical malpractice prosecution, physicians are reluctant to report medical errors (Andrus, Villasenor, Kettelle, Roth, Sweeney, & Matolo, 2003). Reforming medical malpractice legislation at the national level to provide immunity to physicians reporting medical errors would be one way to address this issue. Another would be to encourage medical error reporting through incentives from the companies issuing medical malpractice insurance (Pawlson & O'Kane, 2004).

Others argue that the system of malpractice litigation should be moved from the courts to third-party arbitration and that the National Practitioner Data Bank should be more transparent, to allow for data mining and quality improvement efforts (Lehrman, 2003). Still others argue that the standard of care on which malpractice is judged should be empirically determined, encouraging the use of practice guidelines and protecting physicians who follow them (Hall & Green, 2004). A more refined argument along this vein is that malpractice cases should distinguish among three categories of care: effective care, preference-sensitive care, and supply-sensitive care (Wennberg & Peters, 2004).

Effective care has established clinical evidence that it is the most beneficial treatment or diagnostic test for a particular illness. For such care, a legal standard should be that all of those in need should receive the treatment. **Preference-sensitive care**, in contrast, occurs when various treatments or tests are available for a specific illness, each with different risks and benefits. The law should adopt a standard of informed patient choice for the treatment that best advances patient preferences. Lastly, **supply-sensitive care** occurs when less intensive care can be substituted for more intensive care with essentially equivalent outcomes, and applies particularly to those with chronic illnesses. For such care, providers should be protected under the "respectable minority" doctrine if they adopt conservative patterns of practice (Wennberg & Peters, 2004).

Accounting for Medical Uncertainty

The distinctions among effective, preference-sensitive, and supply-sensitive care point to different aspects of medical uncertainty facing both providers and patients. As we have emphasized, CQI and other quality improvement approaches are effective to the extent that they reduce process variation in the provision of health care. Care processes that can be circumscribed sufficiently to be found effective—what Wennberg and his colleagues call effective care (Wennberg, 2005; Wennberg & Peters, 2004) and others label evidence-based medicine (McNeil, 2001)—have little uncertainty. Lillrank and his colleagues note that effective care assumes that standard operating procedures for a care process can be developed for (a) assessing a patient, (b) specifying decision rules for generating an appropriate treatment, and (c) implementing a treatment to eliminate or alleviate the patient's illness (Lillrank, 2002, 2003; Lillrank & Liukko, 2004). In other words, given a patient with a particular condition, specific medical personnel examine and diagnose the patient; determine the appropriate treatment based on existing knowledge and decision rules; and deploy certain facilities, equipment, and medical supplies to treat the patient and to produce an expected outcome. CQI helps to create standard operating procedures so that each aspect of the care process is repeated the same way each time a patient with a particular condition is seen. For instance, the process of examining a patient with an apparent cold, diagnosing a viral upper respiratory infection, and prescribing decongestants and antihistamines, as well as adequate fluids and rest, are steps that should and can be repeated from one patient to another without error by a primary care physician or nurse practitioner.

However, most healthcare processes are not standard. Many healthcare processes have more than one type of input and two or more types of alternative outputs. Lillrank and his colleagues (Lillrank, 2002, 2003; Lillrank & Liukko, 2004) call these *routine* types of care processes. For example, one patient with type II diabetes may have hypertension and glaucoma, while another type II diabetes patient may be obese and have impaired circulation. While the dominant disease state is the same and similar health outcomes may be sought for both patients, the treatment for each patient will differ because of their co-morbidities. With the diabetes type II patient with co-morbidity, a single standard operating procedure is not appropriate. Rather, the physician—and the patient—must make choices across different procedures for treating each of the diseases.

Hence, routine healthcare processes are more likely to encompass what Wennberg and his colleagues (Wennberg, 2005; Wennberg & Peters, 2004) call preference-sensitive care. On one hand, some obese patients may be willing and able to use both exercise and diet to control diabetes type II, if the physician can prescribe appropriate medication and devices to improve blood circulation and prevent leg cramps. On the other hand, other obese patients may seek gastric bypass surgery, while still others may seek only nutrition and dietary counseling along with support groups. Whether physicians can accommodate these different patient preferences is also influenced by supply-sensitive care. In a community with a large number of bariatric surgeons and few registered dieticians, patients face a greater likelihood that they will be asked to consider the high-risk treatment alternative of gastric bypass surgery. In contrast, if the community has a high degree of managed care penetration by health maintenance organizations (HMOs), physical therapy and dietary counseling may be the predominant services available.

Lastly, some healthcare processes are non-routine. In many such instances, the inputs provided by the patients' symptoms are unclear and not easily diagnosed (Lillrank, 2002, 2003; Lillrank & Liukko, 2004). In other instances, given a confirmed diagnosis, the efficacy of various treatments for the disease may be uncertain, with no clear understanding of the possible outcomes (McNeil, 2001). In the first case, an iterative process of testing and excluding various diseases that manifest similar symptoms is necessary. In the second case, a similar iterative process of trying various treatments is required. In both cases, physicians' interpretive and information seeking capabilities account for much of the variation in the care process. Here, especially, preference-sensitive and supply-sensitive care processes come into play. Some patients may demand highly invasive and risky diagnostic tests or treatments, while other patients prefer low risk, non-invasive testing or treatments. Moreover, some physicians may recommend invasive diagnostics and treatments rather than non-invasive tests and treatments, particularly if such tests and treatments are readily accessible. Again, patients' access to healthcare organizations and the restrictions placed on such access by their health insurance, especially in the United States, will have a great deal of influence on when and whether patients receive more or less invasive tests and treatments.

Significantly, the quality problems facing standard, routine, and non-routine healthcare processes differ as follows (Lillrank & Liukko, 2004, p. 43):

Non-compliance with a standard process produces a deviation from the target.

Inappropriate selection from known alternatives in a routine process produces an error.

Improper assessment of input [*or an output*] in a non-routine process produces a failure.

To address these different types of quality problems, healthcare managers and health professionals must use appropriate methods. Standard healthcare processes can see significant quality improvement through CQI and other quality system approaches. The quality of non-routine healthcare processes, in contrast, will be improved by the clinical experience and intuition of the health providers. Here, healthcare organizations benefit from a strong quality culture—developed by health professionals' clinical training and reinforced by organizational and institutional values, such as those espoused by QA proponents. Routine healthcare processes, of course, lie between these two extremes and benefit both from CQI and a strong QA culture. Recall the difficulties healthcare providers have in ensuring that there is continuity of care as a patient is transferred from one healthcare setting to another. On one hand, the uncertainty involved in medical care often is reduced as patients move from primary to secondary to tertiary care settings, as non-routine processes in physician offices become the routine, albeit, complex and tightly-coupled processes performed in diagnostic clinics, surgical centers, and hospitals. On the other hand, the method of sharing medical or health records between healthcare providers across these different settings often creates new quality problems. The inadequacies of the health information technology (HIT) infrastructure linking healthcare facilities and providers are discussed next.

DEVELOPING A NATIONAL INFORMATION TECHNOLOGY INFRASTRUCTURE

Currently, most healthcare providers rely on faxing or couriering paper patient records from one healthcare setting to another. Incomplete, missing, or poorly organized information within these health records may cause problems ranging from duplicative diagnostic tests, to delays in diagnosis and treatment, to adverse drug-drug interactions, to surgery on the wrong limb or the wrong patient. "If the state of the US medical technology is one of our great treasures, then the state of US HIT is one of our great disgraces" (Kleinke, 2005, p. 1247). Despite HIT investments by insurers and large hospitals, only the two largest integrated healthcare systems in the United States—the Veterans Health Administration and Kaiser Permanente, a California-based HMO—have the HIT infrastructure that allows patients' electronic health records to be accessed by providers throughout those organizations. This situation represents a massive market failure, and has led to multiple calls for intervention by the federal government (Halvorson, 2005; Kleinke, 2005; Middleton, 2005; Shortliffe, 2005). As a result, the U.S. federal government has set a target of 2014 for establishing a national information technology infrastructure for health care.

> [S]uch a system would dramatically improve the quality of patient care and reduce the nation's healthcare costs by:
>
> - Making the patient's up-to-date medical record instantly available whenever and wherever it is needed and authorized;
> - Avoiding costly duplicate tests and unnecessary hospitalizations;

- Providing health professionals with the best and latest treatment options for the patient's needs;
- Helping eliminate medical errors;
- Streamlining the reporting of public health information for early detection and response to disease outbreaks and potential bioterrorism;
- Creating opportunities to gather non-identifiable information about health outcomes for research to identify the most effective treatment options;
- Providing better, more current medical records at lower costs; and,
- Protecting privacy (HHS, 2004).

To fulfill the above goals, a national information technology infrastructure for health care must overcome certain barriers. These barriers include ensuring that (a) electronic health records (EHRs) use a shared medical terminology and standard codes; (b) different EHR systems are interoperable, allowing the sharing of information; (c) shared EHR information is secure; (d) legal barriers to collaboration on EHR systems are removed; and (e) the costs for implementing EHRs in physician offices and other small healthcare organizations are offset (Yasnoff, Humphreys, Overhage, Detmer, Brennan, Morris, Middleton, Bates, & Fanning, 2004). The latter costs occur because there is a significant EHR adoption gap between large and small healthcare organizations; a negative business case for EHRs in physician practices, small clinics, and ambulatory centers; and limited access to HIT expertise and implementation support within these settings (Bates, 2005; HHS, 2005).

To overcome these barriers, the President of the United States issued an executive order in 2004 authorizing the establishment of the Office of the National Coordinator for Health Information Technology within the Department of Health and Human Services (HHS; see http://www.white house.gov/news/releases/2004/04/20040427-4.html). The National Coordinator, David Brailer, MD, PhD, has broad responsibility to establish a national health information technology infrastructure that will inform and interconnect clinicians, personalize care, and improve the population health of the United States (http://www.hhs.gov/healthit/goals.html). As indicated in the sidebar, the Office of the National Coordinator for Health Information Technology has initiated five projects.

1. Working with the Commission on Systemic Interoperability, authorized by the 2003 Medicare Modernization Act to make recommendations for establishing a national health information technology

infrastructure; its report, *Ending the Document Game: Connecting and Transforming Your Healthcare through Information Technology*, issued in October, 2005, has 12 recommendations (http://www.hhs.gov/healthit/comsystinter.html);

2. Overseeing the Consolidated Health Informatics Initiative (CHI) to establish health information interoperability standards for sharing EHRs and other health data among all federal agencies and departments (http://www.hhs.gov/healthit/chi.html);

3. Establishing the American Health Information Community, a federally-chartered commission, tasked with making "recommendations to HHS on how to make health records digital and interoperable, and assure that the privacy and security of those records are protected" (http://www.hhs.gov/healthit/ahic.html);

4. Awarding contracts to three different public-private groups in October, 2005, for accelerating adoption of HIT (http://www.hhs.gov/news/press/2005pres/20051006a.html), and to four consortia of healthcare and HIT organizations in November, 2005, for developing prototypes for a Nationwide Health Information Network architecture (http://www.hhs.gov/news/press/2005pres/20051110.html); and,

5. Proposing regulatory changes to allow exceptions to the Stark and anti-kickback laws, thus enabling hospitals and other healthcare organizations to furnish hardware, software, and training services to physicians for interoperable e-prescribing and EHR systems (http://www.hhs.gov/healthit/e-prescribing.html).

While a fully operational national health information technology infrastructure is needed to improve the quality of health care in the United States, the widespread adoption of EHRs, e-prescribing, and other HIT also requires aligning the economic incentives between providers and payers (Poon, Jha, Christino, Honour, Fernandopulle, Middleton, Newhouse, Leape, Bates, Blumenthal, & Kaushal 2006).

Aligning Economic Incentives

One of the dilemmas facing any healthcare financing system is ensuring that payments to healthcare providers reward them for services and outcomes that improve the health of patients. In other words, healthcare providers should provide effective care for standard cases where the diagnosis or treatments are evidence-based, preference-sensitive care for other routine and non-routine cases, and minimize or eliminate supply-sensitive care. On one hand, fee-for-service financing systems are prone to overuse of services because providers induce their own demand for services (Rice & Labelle, 1989), i.e., generate supply-sensitive care (Wennberg, 2005). On the other hand, capitated financing systems, where physicians are salaried or providers are paid prospectively per patient, are prone to underuse of effective and, especially, preference-sensitive services (Blomqvist & Leger, 2005; Iversen, 2004; Lien, Ma, & McGuire, 2004).

As mentioned previously, the Leapfrog Group, Bridges to Excellence, and Medicare are experimenting with **pay-for-performance (PFP)** programs in hospitals, physician group practices, skilled nursing facilities, and home health agencies (Beich, Scanlon, Ulbrecht, Ford, & Ibrahim, 2006; Bokhour et al., 2006; Chassin, 2006; Galvin, 2006; Grossbart, 2006; Hackbarth, 2006; Levin-Scherz, DeVita, & Timbie, 2006; Nahra, Reiter, Hirth, Shermer, & Wheeler, 2006). Ideally, as an incentive program, PFP should use evidence-based performance measures to reward healthcare providers for improving both patient safety and the quality of health care, while avoiding the rationing of care services simply to reduce costs (Baumann & Dellert, 2006). The latter concern is particularly important to physicians, many of whom are skeptical and some of whom are opposed to PFP programs as yet another means to reduce physician autonomy and income (Bodenheimer, May, Berenson, & Coughlan, 2005; Steiger, 2005; Weber, 2005).

The three most notable PFP initiatives in the United States include the Leapfrog Group's Hospital Rewards Program (see https://leapfrog.medstat.com/hrp/index.asp); the Bridges to Excellence PFP programs that reward physicians who improve cardiac and diabetes care outcomes and use HIT to improve patient care (see http://www.bridgestoexcellence.org/bte/physicians/home.htm); and the federal government. Medicare is pursuing ten PFP initiatives and demonstration projects as part of its overall Quality Initiative that was launched in 2001 (CMS, 2005c; Kuhn, 2005).

1. The *Hospital Quality Initiative* is a voluntary reporting by hospitals of 20 quality measures vetted by the CMS, HQA, JCAHO, NQF

and the QIOs. There is a strong incentive for hospitals to report this information because the Medicare Modernization Act of 2003 authorizes CMS to reduce annual payments by 0.4% if the 10 quality measures are not submitted (CMS, 2005b). The results of these measures are reported in the website, *Hospital Compare* (www .hospitalcompare.hhs.gov).

2. In partnership with Premier Inc., a nationwide organization of not-for-profit hospitals, CMS launched the *Premier Hospital Quality Incentive Demonstration* in March, 2003 and announced the first year results in November, 2005 ("Pay for Performance Works Says CMS," 2006). PFP is explicit in this demonstration; CMS increases Medicare patient payments for the participating top performing hospitals (http:// new.cms.hhs.gov/HospitalQualityInits/35_HospitalPremier.asp).

3. The *Physician Group Practice Demonstration*, authorized by the Medicare, Medicaid, and SCHIP Benefits and Improvement Act of 2000, is a 3-year PFP project that targets large group practices with at least 200 physicians. It began in April, 2005 with 10 participating physician group practices located in 10 different states (CMS, 2005e). Each of the group practices will be rewarded for coordinating the care of chronically ill and high cost beneficiaries in an efficient and effective manner. The "groups will have incentives to use electronic records and other care management strategies that, based on clinical evidence and patient data, improve patient outcomes and lower total medical costs" (CMS, 2005e).

4. The *Medicare Care Management Performance Demonstration* is modeled on the Bridges to Excellence framework. It is a 3-year pay-for-performance demonstration with physicians to promote the adoption and use of HIT to improve the quality of patient care for chronically ill Medicare patients. Doctors who meet or exceed performance standards established by CMS in clinical delivery systems and patient outcomes will receive bonus payments. In contrast to the *Physician Group Practice Demonstration*, this demonstration focuses on small and medium-sized physician practices (CMS, 2005c).

5. The *Medicare Health Care Quality Demonstration* projects, authorized by Section 646 of the 2003 Medicare Modernization Act, have a 5-year mandate to encourage a variety of quality improvements, including improving patient safety, reducing variations in utilization

via evidence-based care and practice guidelines, encouraging shared decision making, and using culturally and ethnically appropriate care (CMS, 2005c). Physician groups, integrated delivery systems, and regional healthcare consortia are eligible for the 8–12 demonstration projects, with proposals due in two phases during 2006 (CMS, 2005d).

6. The *Chronic Care Improvement Program* pilot tests a population-based model of disease management. Participating organizations are paid a monthly per beneficiary fee for managing a population of chronically ill Medicare patients with advanced congestive heart failure and/or complex diabetes. Nine sites have been selected: Humana in South and Central Florida; XLHealth in Tennessee; Aetna in Illinois; LifeMasters in Oklahoma; McKesson in Mississippi; CIGNA in Georgia; Health Dialog in Pennsylvania; American Healthways in Washington, DC and Maryland; and Visiting Nurse Service of NY and United Healthcare in Queens and Brooklyn, New York (CMS, 2005c).

7. The *ESRD Disease Management Demonstration* tests the effectiveness of disease management models to increase quality of care for end stage renal disease (ESRD) patients. Five percent of the payment will be linked to ESRD-related quality measures. Three organizations are participating in this multi-state project: DaVita, Fresenius Medical Care North America, and Evercare of Georgia (CMS, 2005a).

8. The *Disease Management Demonstration for Severely Chronically Ill Medicare Beneficiaries* tests whether disease management and prescription drug coverage improves health outcomes and reduces costs for beneficiaries with illnesses such as congestive heart failure, diabetes, or coronary artery disease. Three disease management organizations are participating: XLHealth in Texas; CorSolutions in Louisiana; and HeartPartners in California and Arizona. They receive a monthly payment for every beneficiary they enroll to provide disease management services and a comprehensive drug benefit, and must guarantee that there will be a net reduction in Medicare expenditures as a result of their services (CMS, 2005c).

9. *Disease Management Demonstration for Chronically Ill Duel-Eligible Beneficiaries* focuses on dually (Medicare & Medicaid) eligible beneficiaries in Florida who suffer from advanced-stage congestive heart failure, diabetes, or coronary heart disease. The demonstration com-

bines the resources of the state's Medicaid pharmacy benefit with a disease management activity funded by Medicare to coordinate the services of both programs and achieve improved quality with lower total program costs. LifeMasters, the demonstration organization, is being paid a fixed monthly amount per beneficiary and is at risk for 100% of its fees if performance targets are not met. Savings above the targeted amount will be shared equally between CMS and LifeMasters (CMS, 2005c).

10. *Care Management for High Cost Beneficiaries* targets beneficiaries who are both high-cost and high-risk. The payment methodology will be similar to that implemented in the Chronic Care Improvement Program, with participating providers required to meet relevant clinical quality standards, as well as to guarantee savings to the Medicare program (CMS, 2005c).

While the effectiveness of PFP initiatives is still being scrutinized by health services researchers and policy makers, preliminary evidence shows some support for the effectiveness of PFP programs in hospitals and within disease management programs (Beich, Scanlon, Ulbrecht, Ford, & Ibrahim, 2006; Grossbart, 2006; Levin-Scherz, DeVita, & Timbie, 2006; Nahra, Reiter, Hirth, Shermer, & Wheeler, 2006). Experts caution that these early studies all exhibit some flaws in their research designs, are positively biased because the sample of providers volunteered to be part of the PFP programs, and that generalizing the results to other settings and to non-volunteer providers may not be warranted (Chassin, 2006; Galvin, 2006). Nonetheless, both the Medicare Payment Advisory Commission (MedPac) and CMS believe that the effectiveness of PFP programs is sufficient to ask Congress to link Medicare payments to quality (Hackbarth, 2006; "Pay For Performance Works," 2006).

CONCLUSION

Healthcare quality may be defined in various ways, with differing implications for healthcare providers, patients, third-party payers, policy makers, and other stakeholders. High quality health services are co-produced by both providers and patients. On one hand, such care should achieve the desired health outcomes for individuals, matching their preferences for various types of outcomes. On the other hand, health services should adhere to professional standards and scientific evidence, consistent with the clinical focus and preferences of healthcare providers for effectiveness. Moreover, such services should achieve desired health outcomes for populations, matching the societal preferences of policy makers and third-party payers for efficiency.

Quality is important in health care because there are limited resources to improve the health of both individuals and the population as a whole. High quality healthcare services avoid the inappropriate use of resources that occur when services are underused, overused, or misused. The overuse of health services not only increases the overall costs of care, but also exposes patients to undue risks. In contrast, the underuse of health services leads to unacceptable levels of morbidity and mortality within a population. Lastly, misuse of health services directly harms patients and wastes resources. Both ethical and economic concerns are raised by each of these quality problems. Modern attempts to guarantee healthcare quality have ranged from quality assurance to continuous quality improvement to system improvement.

The United States is engaged in multiple governmental initiatives and public-private partnerships to improve the quality of the healthcare system that include the Agency for Healthcare Research and Quality, the National Quality Forum, the Patient Safety Task Force, the VHA's Quality Enhancement Research Initiative, and the QIOs that contract with Medicare. Most employer-sponsored initiatives originate with either the Leapfrog Group or the National Business Coalition on Health; accrediting agency initiatives are associated with the Joint Commission and the National Committee for Quality Assurance. Other notable quality improvement initiatives have been produced by the Institute for Healthcare Improvement, the Robert Wood Johnson Foundation, the Bridges to Excellence coalition, and the Hospital Quality Alliance.

Taken together these efforts have addressed many of the goals for improving the quality of health care as presented in the IOM's report, *Crossing the Quality Chasm*. Nonetheless, in the United States four significant challenges remain: 1) reforming medical malpractice; 2) accounting for and reducing medical uncertainty; 3) developing a national information technology infrastructure; and 4) aligning economic incentives. Meeting these challenges will take both talent and persistence. As the next generation of healthcare managers emerges, healthcare quality and performance improvement will be important factors for judging the competencies of those managers. In other words, understanding and appropriately applying the concepts of QA, CQI, and system improvement will be essential for healthcare managers.

DISCUSSION QUESTIONS

1. Why is quality of care a concern in the United States and around the world?
2. How can quality of care be measured from a patient's perspective? A healthcare provider's perspective? A purchaser's perspective?
3. In what ways has the concern for quality of care changed in the last 150 years—from the time of Florence Nightingale to that of Donald Berwick?
4. What are the pros and cons of different methods for improving the delivery of care within the healthcare organizations?
5. What barriers do healthcare providers and organizations face when attempting to improve care?

REFERENCES

Amon, E., & Winn, H. N. (2004). Review of the professional medical liability insurance crisis: lessons from Missouri. *American Journal of Obstetrics and Gynecology, 190*(6), 1534–1538; discussion 1538–1540.

Andrus, C. H., Villasenor, E. G., Kettelle, J. B., Roth, R., Sweeney, A. M., & Matolo, N. M. (2003). "To Err Is Human": uniformly reporting medical errors and near misses, a naive, costly, and misdirected goal. *Journal of the American College of Surgery, 196*(6), 911–918.

Bates, D. W. (2005). Physicians and ambulatory electronic health records. *Health Affairs, 24*(5), 1180–1189.

Baumann, M. H., & Dellert, E. (2006). Performance measures and pay for performance. *Chest, 129*(1), 188–191.

Beich, J., Scanlon, D. P., Ulbrecht, J., Ford, E. W., & Ibrahim, I. A. (2006). The role of disease management in pay-for-performance programs for improving the care of chronically ill patients. *Medical Care Research and Review, 63*(1_suppl), 96S–116.

Berwick, D. M. (2002). A user's manual for the IOM's 'Quality Chasm' report. *Health Affairs, 21*(3), 80–90.

Bhatia, A. J., Blackstock, S., Nelson, R., & Ng, T. S. (2000). Evolution of quality review programs for Medicare: quality assurance to quality improvement. *Health Care Financing Review, 22*(1), 69–74.

Bleich, S. (2005). *Medical errors: five years after the IOM report* (Issue Brief). New York: Commonwealth Fund.

Blomqvist, A., & Leger, P. T. (2005). Information asymmetry, insurance, and the decision to hospitalize. *Journal of Health Economics, 24*(4), 775–793.

Bodenheimer, T., May, J. H., Berenson, R. A., & Coughlan, J. (2005). Can money buy quality? Physician response to pay for performance. *Issue Brief Center for Studying Health System Change*(102), 1–4.

Bokhour, B. G., Burgess, J. F., Jr., Hook, J. M., White, B., Berlowitz, D., Guldin, M. R., et al. (2006). Incentive implementation in physician practices: a qualitative study of practice executive perspectives on pay for performance. *Medical Care Research and Review, 63*(1_suppl), 73S–95.

Bosk, C. L. (1979). *Forgive and remember: managing medical failure*. Chicago: University of Chicago Press.

Bradley, E. H., Carlson, M. D., Gallo, W. T., Scinto, J., Campbell, M. K., & Krumholz, H. M. (2005). From adversary to partner: have quality improvement organizations made the transition? *Health Services Research, 40*(2), 459–476.

Chassin, M. R. (1997). Assessing strategies for quality improvement. *Health Affairs, 16*(3), 151–161.

Chassin, M. R. (2006). Does paying for performance improve the quality of health care? *Medical Care Research and Review, 63*(1_suppl), 122S–125.

CMS. (2005a, September 15). *Details for ESRD Disease Management Demonstration.* Retrieved March 1, 2006, from http://new.cms.hhs.gov/DemoProjectsEvalRpts/MD/itemdetail.asp?filterType=none&filterByDID=-99&sortByDID=3&sortOrder=ascending&itemID=CMS024167

CMS. (2005b, December). *Hospital quality initiative: overview.* Retrieved March 1, 2006, from http://www.cms.hhs.gov/HospitalQualityInits/downloads/HospitalOverview200512.pdf

CMS. (2005c, January 31). *Medicare "pay for performance (P4P)" initiatives.* Retrieved March 1, 2006, from http://new.cms.hhs.gov/apps/media/press/release.asp?Counter=1343

CMS. (2005d). *Medicare health care quality demonstration programs fact sheet.* Retrieved March 1, 2006, from http://www.cms.hhs.gov/DemoProjectsEvalRpts/downloads/MMA646_FactSheet.pdf

CMS. (2005e, January 31). *Medicare physician group practice demonstration fact sheet.* Retrieved March 1, 2006, from http://new.cms.hhs.gov/DemoProjectsEvalRpts/downloads/PGP_Fact_Sheet.pdf

Cooper, M. R. (1999). Quality assurance and improvement. In L. F. Wolper (Ed.), *Health care administration: planning, implementing, and managing organized delivery systems (3rd ed.*, pp. 545–573). Gaithersburg, MD: Aspen Publishers, Inc.

Davis, M. (2003). What can we learn by looking for the first code of professional ethics? *Theoretical Medicine and Bioethics, 24*(5), 433–454.

Delpierre, C., Cuzin, L., Fillaux, J., Alvarez, M., Massip, P., & Lang, T. (2004). A systematic review of computer-based patient record systems and quality of care: more randomized clinical trials or a broader approach? *International Journal for Quality in Health Care, 16*(5), 407–416.

Donabedian, A. (1966). Evaluating the quality of medical care. *Milbank Memorial Fund Quarterly, 44*(3), Suppl:166–206.

Donabedian, A. (1986). Quality assurance in our health care system. *Quality Assurance, 1*(1), 6–12.

Flexner, A. (1972, c1910). *Medical education in the United States and Canada: a report to the Carnegie Foundation for the Advancement of Teaching.* New York: Arno Press.

Fonarow, G. C. (2005). Practical considerations of beta-blockade in the management of the post-myocardial infarction patient. *Am Heart J, 149*(6), 984–993.

Gaba, D. (2000). Structural and organizational issues in patient safety: A comparison of health care to other high-hazard industries. *California Management Review, 43*(1), 83–100.

Galvin, R. S. (2006). Evaluating the performance of pay for performance. *Medical Care Research and Review, 63*(1_suppl), 126S–130.

Gandhi, T. K, Weingart, S. N, Borus, J., Seger, A. C., Peterson, J., Burdick, E., et al. (2003). Adverse drug events in ambulatory care. *New England Journal of Medicine, 348*(16), 1556.

Gilpatrick, E. (1999). *Quality improvement projects in health care: problem solving in the workplace.* Thousand Oaks, CA: Sage Publications.

Gonzales, R., Steiner, J. F., & Sande, M. A. (1997). Antibiotic prescribing for adults with colds, upper respiratory tract infections and bronchitis by ambulatory care physicians. *Journal of the American Medical Association, 278*, 901–904.

Grossbart, S. R. (2006). What's the return? Assessing the effect of "pay-for-performance" initiatives on the quality of care delivery. *Medical Care Research and Review, 63*(1_suppl), 29S–48.

Hackbarth, G. (2006). Commentary. *Medical Care Research and Review, 63*(1_suppl), 117S–121.

Hall, M. A., & Green, M. D. (2004). Malpractice litigation reform: empirical approaches to establishing the legal standard of care. *Journal of Medical Practice Management, 19*(5), 279–282.

Halvorson, G. C. (2005). Wiring health care. *Health Affairs, 24*(5), 1266–1268.

Hammer, M., & Champy, J. (1993). *Reengineering the corporation: a manifesto for business revolution.* New York: Harper Business.

Henry, B., Woods, S., & Nagelkerk, J. (1990). Nightingale's perspective of nursing administration. *Nursing & Health Care, 11*(4), 201–206.

Hertz, K. T., & Fabrizio, N. (2005). The many faces of QIOs, and what their latest incarnation means for your practice. *MGMA Connexion, 5*(7), 41, 42–45.

HHS. (2004, May 6). *Harnessing information technology to improve health care.* Retrieved January 15, 2006, from http://www.hhs.gov/news/press/2004pres/20040427a.html

HHS. (2005, May 23). *Barriers to adoption.* Retrieved February 20, 2006, from http://www.hhs.gov/healthit/barrierAdpt.html

Institute of Medicine. (1990). *Medicare: A strategy for quality assurance.* Washington, DC: National Academy Press.

Institute of Medicine. (2001). *Crossing the quality chasm: a new health system for the 21st Century.* Washington, DC: National Academy Press.

Iversen, T. (2004). The effects of a patient shortage on general practitioners' future income and list of patients. *Journal of Health Economics, 23*(4), 673–694.

JCAHO. (2006). *A Journey Through the History of the Joint Commission.* Retrieved August 28, 2006, from http://www.jointcommission.org/AboutUs/joint_commission_history.htm

Jencks, S. F. (2004). *The QIO program: legal foundation, recent history and current directions.* Retrieved December 12, 2005, from http://www.medqic.org/dcs/Blob Server?blobcol=urldata&blobheader=application%2Fpdf&blobkey=id&blobtable=MungoBlobs&blobwhere=1106669436962

Jha, A. K., Perlin, J. B., Kizer, K. W., & Dudley, R. A. (2003). Effect of the transformation of the Veterans Affairs health care system on the quality of care. *New England Journal of Medicine, 348*(22), 2218–2227.

Juran, J. M., Gryna, F. M., & R. S. Bingham, J. (Eds.). (1974). *Quality control handbook (3rd ed.).* New York: McGraw-Hill.

Kleinke, J. D. (2005). Dot-gov: market failure and the creation of a national health information technology system. *Health Affairs, 24*(5), 1246–1262.

Kohn, J. T., Corrigan, J. M., & Donaldson, M. S. (Eds.). (2000). *To err is human: building a safer health care system.* Washington, DC: Institute of Medicine.

Kolesar, P. J. (1993). The relevance of research on statistical process control to the total quality movement. *Journal of Engineering and Technology Management, 10*(4), 317–338.

Kuhn, H. (2005, March 16). *Pay for performance initiatives.* Retrieved February 28, 2006, from http://www.hhs.gov/asl/testify/t050315a.html

Lehrman, T. D. (2003). Reconsidering medical malpractice reform: the case for arbitration and transparency in non-emergent contexts. *Journal of Health Law, 36*(3), 475–506.

Levin-Scherz, J., DeVita, N., & Timbie, J. (2006). Impact of pay-for-performance contracts and network registry on diabetes and asthma HEDIS(R)Measures in an integrated delivery network. *Medical Care Research and Review, 63*(1_suppl), 14S–28.

Lien, H. M., Albert, Ma C. T., & McGuire, T. G. (2004). Provider-client interactions and quantity of health care use. *Journal of Health Economics, 23*(6), 1261–1283.

Lillrank, P. (2002). The broom and nonroutine processes: a metaphor for understanding variability in organizations. *Knowledge and Process Management, 9*(3), 143–148].

Lillrank, P. (2003). The quality of standard, routine and nonroutine processes. *Organization Studies, 24*(2), 215.

Lillrank, P., & Holopainen, S. (1998). Reengineering for business option value. *Journal of Organizational Change Management, 11*(3), 246.

Lillrank, P., & Liukko, M. (2004). Standard, routine and non-routine processes in health care. *International Journal of Health Care Quality Assurance Incorporating Leadership in Health Services, 17*(1), 39–46.

Lohr, K. (1990a). IOM study urges a major shift in QA strategy. *QA Review, 2*(5), 1, 7–8.

Lohr, K. (Ed.). (1990b). *Medicare: a strategy for quality assurance.* Washington, DC: National Academy Press.

Luce, J. M., Bindman, A. B., & Lee, P. R. (1994). A brief history of health care quality assessment and improvement in the United States. *West J Med, 160*(3), 263–268.

Marley, K. A., Collier, D. A., & Goldstein, S. M. (2004). The role of clinical and process quality in achieving patient satisfaction in hospitals. *Decision Sciences, 35*(3), 349–369.

McAdam, R., & Corrigan, M. (2001). Re-engineering in public sector health care: A telecommunications case study. *International Journal of Health Care Quality Assurance, 14*(5), 218–227.

McNeil, B. J. (2001). Hidden barriers to improvement in the quality of care. *New England Journal of Medicine, 345*(22), 1612–1620.

McQueen, L., Mittman, B. S., & Demakis, J. G. (2004). Overview of the Veterans Health Administration (VHA) Quality Enhancement Research Initiative (QUERI). *Journal of the American Medical Informatics Association, 11*(5), 339–343.

Middleton, B. (2005). Achieving U.S. health information technology adoption: the need for a third hand. *Health Affairs, 24*(5), 1269–1272.

Nahra, T. A., Reiter, K. L., Hirth, R. A., Shermer, J. E., & Wheeler, J. R. C. (2006). Cost-effectiveness of hospital pay-for-performance incentives. *Medical Care Research and Review, 63*(1_suppl), 49S–72.

Nicholls, S. J., McElduff, P., Dobson, A. J., Jamrozik, K. D., Hobbs, M. S. T., & Leitch, J. W. (2001). Underuse of beta-blockers following myocardial infarction: a tale of two cities. *Internal Medicine Journal, 31*(7), 391–396.

Ortiz, E., Meyer, G., & Burstin, H. (2002). Clinical informatics and patient safety at the Agency for Healthcare Research and Quality. *Journal of the American Medical Informatics Association, 9*(90061), S2–7.

Pawlson, L. G., & O'Kane, M. E. (2004). Malpractice prevention, patient safety, and quality of care: a critical linkage. *American Journal of Managed Care, 10*(4), 281–284.

Pay for performance works, says CMS . . . (2006). *Healthcare Financial Management, 60*(1), 17–18.

Perrow, C. (1984). *Normal accidents: Living with high-risk technologies.* New York: Basic Books.

Plochg, T., & Klazinga, N. S. (2002). Community-based integrated care: myth or must? *International Journal for Quality in Health Care, 14*(2), 91–101.

Poon, E. G., Jha, A. K., Christino, M., Honour, M. M., Fernandopulle, R., Middleton, B., et al. (2006). Assessing the level of healthcare information technology adoption in the United States: a snapshot. *BMC Medical Informatics and Decision Making, 6,* 1. Available from http://www.biomedcentral.com/1472-6947/6/1

Quality directors give QIOs high marks in new study. (2005). *Healthcare Benchmarks and Quality Improvement, 12*(6), 68–69.

Reason, J. (1990). *Human Error*. Cambridge, UK: Cambridge University Press.

Rice, T. H., & Labelle, R. J. (1989). Do physicians induce demand for medical services? *Journal of Health Politics, Policy and Law, 14*(3), 587–600.

Rubenfeld, G. D. (2004). Using computerized medical databases to measure and to improve the quality of intensive care. *Journal of Critical Care, 19*(4), 248–256.

Rubin, R. J., & Mendelson, D. N. (1994). How much does defensive medicine cost? *Journal of American Health Policy, 4*(4), 7–15.

Scalise, D. (2001). Six Sigma: The Quest for Quality. *Hospitals and Health Networks, 75*(12), 41–45.

Schoen, C., Osborn, R., Huynh, P. T., Doty, M., Zapert, K., Peugh, J., et al. (2005). Taking the pulse of health care systems: experiences of patients with health problems in six countries. *Health Affairs*, w5, 509–525.

Schoenbaum, S. C., Audet, A. M., & Davis, K. (2003). Obtaining greater value from health care: the roles of the U.S. government. *Health Affairs, 22*(6), 183–190.

Shewhart, W. A. (1931). *Economic control of quality of manufactured product*. New York: Van Nostrand.

Shewhart, W. A. (1939). *Statistical method from the viewpoint of quality control*. Washington, DC: The Graduate School of the Department of Agriculture.

Shortliffe, E. H. (2005). Strategic action in health information technology: why the obvious has taken so long. Today the United States is poised to achieve what has been sought and anticipated for at least three decades. *Health Affairs, 24*(5), 1222–1233.

Smith, D. C. (1996). The Hippocratic Oath and Modern Medicine. *Journal of the History of Medicine and Allied Sciences, 51*(4), 484–500.

Solberg, L. I., Hurley, J. S., Roberts, M. H., Nelson, W. W., Frost, F. J., Crain, A. L., et al. (2004). Measuring patient safety in ambulatory care: potential for identifying medical group drug-drug interaction rates using claims data. *American Journal of Managed Care, 10*(11 Pt 1), 753–759.

Soumerai, S. B., McLaughlin, T. J., Spiegelman, D., Hertzmark, E., Thibault, G., & Goldman, L. (1997). Adverse outcomes of underuse of beta-blockers in elderly survivors of acute myocardial infarction. *Journal of the American Medical Association, 277*(2), 115–121.

Spiegel, A. D., & Springer, C. R. (1997). Babylonian medicine, managed care and codex hammurabi, circa 1700 b.c. *Journal of Community Health, 22*(1), 69–89.

Sprague, L. (2005). Hospital oversight in Medicare: accreditation and deeming authority. *NHPF Issue Brief, 2005* (802), 1–15.

Steiger, B. (2005). Poll finds physicians very wary of pay-for-performance programs. *Physician Executive, 31*(6), 6–11.

Steinberg, I. (2000). Clinical choices of antibiotics: Judging judicious use. *The American Journal of Managed Care, 6*(23 Supplement), s1178–s1188.

The trouble with re-engineering. (1995). *Management Decision, 33*(3), 39–40.

Viswanathan, H. N., & Salmon, J. W. (2000). Accrediting organizations and quality improvement. *American Journal of Managed Care, 6*(10), 1117–1130.

von Staden, H. (1996). "In a pure and holy way": personal and professional conduct in the Hippocratic Oath? *Journal of the History of Medicine and Allied Sciences, 51*(4), 404–437.

Weber, D. O. (2005). The dark side of P4P. *Physician Executive, 31*(6), 20–25.

Weissman, J. S., Annas, C. L., Epstein, A. M., Schneider, E. C., Clarridge, B., Kirle, et al. (2005). Error reporting and disclosure systems: views from hospital leaders. *Journal of the American Medical Association, 293*(11), 1359–1366.

Wennberg, J. E. (2002). Unwarrented variation in healthcare delivery: Implications for academic medical centres. *British Medical Journal, 325*, 961–964.

Wennberg, J. E. (2005). *Variation in use of Medicare services among regions and selected academic medical centers: is more better?* (No. 874). New York: The Commonwealth Fund.

Wennberg, J. E., & Peters, P. G., Jr. (2004). Unwarranted variations in the quality of health care: can the law help medicine provide a remedy/remedies? *Specialty Law Digest: Health Care Law*(305), 9–25.

Williams, S. C., Schmaltz, S. P., Morton, D. J., Koss, R. G., & Loeb, J. M. (2005). Quality of care in U.S. hospitals as reflected by standardized measures, 2002–2004. *New England Journal of Medicine, 353*(3), 255–264.

Wood, C. (1998). The misplace of litigation in medical practice. *Australian & New Zealand Journal of Obstetrics & Gynaecology, 38*(4), 365–376.

Yasnoff, W. A., Humphreys, B. L., Overhage, J. M., Detmer, D. E., Brennan, P. F., Morris, R. W., et al. (2004). A consensus action agenda for achieving the national health information infrastructure. *Journal of the American Medical Informatics Association, 11*(4), 332–338.

Information Technology
Carla Wiggins

LEARNING OBJECTIVES

By the end of this chapter the student will be able to describe:

- The history and evolution of health information technology;
- Types of health information, including internal and external data;
- Health information users;
- Health information technology and applications, including electronic medical records, computerized physician order entry, bar coding, and Telehealth;
- The role of the healthcare manager in health information management;
- The impact of regulation, laws, and policies regarding confidentiality of patient information; and,
- The challenges faced by healthcare organizations in adopting new technology.

INTRODUCTION

Few topics have more potential to change health care delivery, quality, and efficiency than information technology (IT). IT impacts every area, function, caregiver, organization, and patient in this, the largest industry in the United States. The United States is the most advanced country in the world when it comes to clinical technology. Yet, health care is far behind most other U.S. industries when it comes to the use of integrated information systems to enhance the efficiency, accuracy, quality, and the security of the information that is its vital lifeblood.

HISTORICAL OVERVIEW

Computers were first used in health care as financial management tools. The introduction of Medicare and Medicaid in the 1960s resulted in a rapid expansion of patients and services. Health providers and health organizations were quickly overwhelmed by the volume of work that was necessary to accurately keep track of services, billing, and payments using strictly paper methods. Hospitals in particular recognized the need for automated billing. Thus, the first computer systems commonly used in the management of health organizations were automated versions of the paper billing process. Automated patient billing had the added benefit of increasing the accuracy of organizations' records, and of their cost, expense, and insurance reimbursement reports. Hospitals hired data processing staff, usually under the supervision of the Chief Financial Officer (CFO), and developed "home grown" financial data processing systems that ran on state-of-the-art computer equipment of the time—large mainframe computers. This mainframe computer was housed in its own large, temperature-controlled room and required a relatively large staff to maintain, program, and produce the reports requested by administration.

Healthcare computing evolved in the 1970s with the introduction of minicomputers. Minicomputers no longer required their own temperature-controlled rooms; rather, they were approximately the size of a small refrigerator and could process large amounts of data reasonably quickly. A number of large computer companies such as Digital Equipment Corporation (DEC) and Meditech began selling "turn-key" systems for hospitals and physician offices. A turn-key system is just as its name implies; the system is loaded into the minicomputer and simply turned on. The sellers of turn-key systems sold maintenance and package upgrade contracts to complement the basic systems in addition to 24-hour, 7-day-per-week access to help lines and technical support. Because processes, systems, reports, and databases were built directly into the software, the organization's data processing department no longer needed to write and implement its own programs. The data processors, still under the supervision of the CFO, became users, as opposed to creators, of the turn-key systems, only writing small, fine-tuning programs and accessing the system to produce the information and reports requested by management. However, even these activities were discouraged, as the guarantees, maintenance, and upgrade contracts were often made void by an organization's attempt to change or interfere with the system's built-in programs.

At the same time that turn-key systems were emerging on the administration side of health care, there was an increase in "free standing" clinical systems for laboratory, radiology, and pharmacy functions. These systems were self-contained, turn-key systems dedicated to very specific clinical applications. They ran on their own minicomputers and had no connection, interaction, or communication with other computer systems in the facility.

Turn-key systems allowed individual users to have access to the computer via desktop terminals. These were "dumb" terminals, simple input and output work stations that did not have the ability to actually compute. The turn-key systems came with built-in applications and programs to produce and execute most regularly requested functions and reports. Information requests could be entered at a dumb terminal and then sent to the main computer. Here it was either **batched**, i.e., held and processed later in a group, or if the minicomputer had adequate capacity, processed in "real time." The output was sent back to the dumb terminal for the user to collect and use.

The 1980s and 1990s saw quantum leaps in computer technology and computer applications. Minicomputers were replaced with microcomputers, more commonly called personal computers or PCs. PCs, unlike dumb terminals, had the ability to compute and manipulate data without relying on the main computer. PCs could be linked together or linked to a minicomputer forming Local Area Networks (LANs) and intranets, i.e., networks within an organization, to increase their computing power, data capacity, and the users' access to information. PCs were an important step forward in healthcare computing as they made computing accessible and affordable not only to hospitals and large organizations, but also to small group practices and physician offices. In addition, they provided access to health information on the Internet for anyone seeking health information. The number of vendors of health systems expanded rapidly, both in the areas of overarching, enterprise-wide systems and small, very specific routines or dedicated systems.

From this point forward, health organizations began to recognize the importance of information systems as a vital tool in the delivery of high quality care. Many health organizations chose to move the information management function, taking it from the supervision of the CFO and moving it into its own department under the supervision of the Chief Information Officer (CIO). Quality of care, along with issues of efficiency, information security, and system interoperability, moved to the forefront and remain the foci of health computing today.

HEALTH INFORMATION AND ITS USERS

Health care is an incredibly transaction-intense industry. Every patient contact, care experience, and outcome must be documented in an accurate and timely way. If patient care is not documented, from an accreditation and financial point of view, it didn't happen. Accrediting bodies, such as the Joint Commission on Accreditation of Healthcare Organizations (JCAHO) review documentation to assess compliance with standards of care for quality assurance. If a hospital is not accredited by JCAHO or another appropriate accreditor, it cannot receive Medicare or Medicaid payments. Therefore, good record-keeping is critical to ensure both quality of care and payment for care. Patient information is messy, complex and complicated. Methods of organizing multifaceted patient information require teamwork and the ability to track patient encounters from the time the patient is admitted until the time the patient is discharged. Patient information is found not only in the medical record, but also in administrative systems and in the dedicated clinical systems discussed above. Wager, Lee, & Glaser (2005) present the following framework for health information:

Internal Data/Information

Patient Encounter:

- *Patient Specific*—clinical, demographic, and administrative information that is specific to an individual patient and from which a specific patient might be identified.
- *Aggregate*—information about groups of patients such as disease indexes, outcomes data, statistical reports, cost reports, and trend analyses.
- *Comparative*—a combination of internal and external data and information to help the organization evaluate its performance.
- *General Operations*—information needed for the running and managing of the organization, such as accounting, financial planning, personnel, and facility data.

External Data/Information

- *Comparative*—data from other organizations, industries, or countries used for benchmarking and self analysis.
- *Expert/Knowledge-based*—information provided by experts who are not part of the organization. This information, often found in professional journals and databases, is used by both clinical and administrative personnel for planning and decision making (Wager, Lee, & Glaser, 2005, p 5–7).

The users of health information are as diverse as the information itself. Physicians and clinical professionals are not the only users who need access to health information. Other users of health information include administration, support services (such as admission and discharge), and the business office. Patients also need information about their medical situations as well as their financial responsibilities. Non-hospital providers such as pharmacies, therapists, off-site imaging providers, free standing emergency and urgent care services, dentists, and mental health providers need information to care for patients. Accrediting organizations such as The Joint Commission for the Accreditation of Health Organizations (JCAHO) and The Centers for Medicare and Medicaid Services (CMS) require health information and reports. Local, state, and federal governments, state and local health districts, the legal system, and third-party insurers require information. This list is not exhaustive, yet it is clear that not every user of health information requires the same information, the same depth of information, nor should have the same level of access to information. It is one of the great challenges in today's health industry to be able to provide exactly the right information—not too much and not too little—in a timely, accurate, and user-friendly format to all legitimate health information users.

The challenge of providing appropriate information to all users is magnified when health information resides in many places, in many formats, and in numerous, non-interfacing systems within the organization. For example, what does it mean to ask for a copy of one's medical record? The medical record is considered the vital core of patient clinical information and it is imperative to know what it is and where it is at all times. Health organizations and providers have a legal obligation to control and protect their patients' health information. In nearly all hospitals, the main component of the medical record is the paper file located in the Medical Record or Health Information Management department. However, patient information may also be housed on computers in imaging, pathology (slides, x-ray, or digital images), pharmacy (records of medications and the administration of medications while in the facility), and administration (demographic information, insurance protocols, formularies, etc.). Many hospitals and physician offices are in some interim stage of implementing **electronic medical records (EMR) systems**, making the exact location of the medical record even more confusing.

HEALTH INFORMATION TECHNOLOGY AND APPLICATIONS

EMR is not simply an automated form of the paper record. In the most ideal situation, EMR is an active and fluid tool that incorporates far more than patient notes. EMR can provide caregivers with immediate access to decision support, expert knowledge, care prompts, reminders, alerts, connectivity to the Internet, e-mail, and other real-time tools. It is wireless and portable. In addition, it can automatically record charges, post them to patient bills and enter the use of materials into the organization's inventory control system.

While the paper medical record has traditionally been seen as the "gold standard," there are many inherent problems with the paper record that EMR resolves:

- illegible writing;
- incomplete, inaccurate, or late documentation and/or notes;
- the physical record only being in one place at any given time;
- the limited access available to off-site providers;
- the fact that storage space for paper files often requires entire rooms and/or buildings;
- the passive, non-interactive nature of the paper record; and,
- the difficulty in collecting and aggregating information across patients, providers, and the organization.

EMR is a powerful tool that not only enhances the caregiver's ability to deliver and document care, it also provides easy and accessible aggregate and comparison data. For example, a physician who would like to discuss a patient's diagnosis could click on a link and obtain data on how common this diagnosis is in her or his practice, discover the most common treatment within the practice and/or within the region or nation, and find the most recent research on the patient's diagnosis, treatment, and outcome probabilities.

Despite the positive attributes of EMR, organizations and users have been slow to purchase, implement, and use it. Even though a fully implemented EMR provides improved efficiency, productivity, quality of care, health outcomes, patient satisfaction, and cost reductions, the expense of purchasing the system and the non-monetary implementation costs such as organization-wide training, a slow learning curve, culture changes, and power issues have affected health organizations' decisions to adopt EMR. It is important to recognize that EMR is much more than just an automated version of the paper record. EMR represents a change in the way healthcare organizations do business. In particular, the entire patient-provider encounter is likely to be drastically changed by the use of a fully implemented EMR. Caregivers record their notes at point of care and it may be disconcerting to them to see real-time alerts, warnings, or recommendations about their care decisions. Most caregivers see the medical record as being under their control. EMR may be perceived as changing the locus of that control from the caregiver to the IT department and its personnel. Caregivers may feel awkward carrying and using a portable notepad and may feel it interferes with the patient-caregiver relationship. Finally, caregivers are strongly socialized into providing services in a certain way; the use of EMR may require them to approach the care encounter in a way for which they have not been trained and it is difficult to change the culture and structure of a trained clinician.

EMR is not the only technology to enhance the quality, efficiency, and productivity of health care. **Computerized Physician Order Entry (CPOE)**, for example, is being seen as a giant step in the direction of enhanced patient safety. It is estimated that 98,000 patients die each year due to medical errors (IOM, 2000, 2001). Medication ordering and administration errors are at the top of the list of causes. The countless medication errors that cause adverse reactions, but not death, are not included in this number. Not included are the errors that have no adverse impacts or errors that go unreported. There are literally thousands of medications, many with similar sounding and similarly spelled names. The changing of one letter in a medication's name can be the difference between life and death. CPOE is a hand-held device that records and reports physicians' orders, thus electronically eliminating the often illegible physician-written prescription orders and any verbal orders. CPOE also incorporates a decision-support system with alerts and queries to ensure that the physician is alerted to possible drug interactions and side effects, dosage issues, and alternative medications and treatment options. CPOE can be a free-standing system, but is most effective when used in concert with EMR, when it can automatically document the physician's orders and activities.

Another tool in the battle against medical errors is **bar coding**. Bar coding has long been used in the retail industry to track and change prices of items, to record the sale of merchandise, and to instantaneously update a store's inventory records. Health organizations must not only track materials (medical and non-medical), but they must also keep close watch over "sharps" such as syringes and scalpels, and controlled substances (opiates and other abused drugs) in their facilities. Bar coding can bring Just In Time (JIT) inventory control to health organizations and help track what is being used and by whom.

Bar coding can be integrated into an organization's medication administration processes and can provide a powerful safety tool. Each patient receives a bar coded wrist band that is encrypted with patient-specific information. The bar code is scanned whenever medication is provided. The provider then scans her or his own bar coded identifier to log the administration of medication to the patient. The bar code device alerts providers to any medication error. Bar coding provides positive identification of the patient, the caregiver, and the medication. In more sophisticated systems, bar coding can also trigger immediate documentation into the EMR, the JIT inventory system, and patient billing.

Up to now our discussion has focused on the use of technology internal to health organizations. Not everyone in our country has fast and easy access to health organizations, regardless of the organization's technology. The problem of ensuring access to high quality medicine to citizens in the vast, rural areas of our country is complex and pressing.

One possible answer to such access in this situation is **Telehealth**, the delivery of health information and actual health care to people in distant locations. Telehealth is a broad umbrella that encompasses topics such as administrative and educational services, remote access to digital health information (such as imaging and health records), on-line, real time, two-way interactive conferencing, consultation, and health exams. Telehealth can even include remote medical care such as telesurgery where the hands-on provider in one location controls a remote robot treating the patient in a different location. Telehealth opens the door to countless possibilities with the opportunity for patients in distant and rural areas to gain access to providers, particularly specialists, and their expert knowledge and skills. Finally, Telehealth can increase efficiency and productivity through its ability to save and store images and information. A group of consultants in different locations can, via teletechnology, conduct a patient visit or consultation either in real-time—with the patient as an active member of the group—or at a later time when all parties are available, using "store and forward" technology. Finally, Telehealth artifacts can become part of the EMR.

Another facet of Telehealth is E-Health. The Internet has become a source of health information for thousands of people. Anyone with Internet access can gather information about diseases, treatments, medications, and prevention at the click of a mouse. E-Health, as health information on the Internet is often called, is a truly wonderful resource to anyone with Internet access. However, as the information on the Internet is not regulated or controlled, users must exercise caution and judgment about the sources, the sites, and the information garnered there.

An often overlooked facet of Telehealth is e-mail for patient-provider communications. It is estimated that 63% of the U.S. adult population use the Internet: 102 million Americans use e-mail and 52 million use instant messaging (Pew, 2003). Seventy percent of physicians say they use the Internet, but only 25% use e-mail to communicate with patients (AMA, 2004). However, many patients would probably welcome e-mail as a way to communicate with their providers.

Providers have legitimate concerns about confidentiality, legal issues, and reimbursement. In addition, they may be concerned about being deluged with hundreds of e-mails and about patients who might learn about abnormal test results electronically. Still, e-mail could be triaged by office personnel and some questions could be answered by providing the appropriate link to medical information. E-mail eliminates the "telephone tag" that commonly occurs when physicians and patients attempt to telephone each other. Also, by avoiding interruptive phone calls or wasting time attempting to contact patients by phone in between patient visits, physicians can better allocate their time (Hassol, Walker, Kidder, Rokita, Young, Pierdon, Deitz, Kuck, & Ortiz, 2004). In addition, e-mail communication automatically documents the conversation, and with a sophisticated EMR, it can be instantaneously entered into the patient's medical record.

EMR is the heart of the clinical care information system. It is a virtual, non-physical location for all appropriate and relevant patient care information. Its rich, interactive information can create an environment where physicians and all other caregivers can provide the most timely, highest quality, and safest care. It is important to remember, however, that not all users of clinical information need, nor should they have access to, complete patient records. There are many people who provide information and enter information into the patient record (admissions, discharge, and business office personnel, for example) that have no need, nor legally should be able to access the total record. Health leaders have a moral, ethical, and legal responsibility to ensure that all users of patient health information have access only to the information needed to complete their jobs—no more and no less. These concerns about access, confidentiality, full information, and information security all come together under the umbrella of the Enterprise system.

An Enterprise system, sometimes called an **Enterprise Resource Planning system (ERP)**, is an overarching system that coordinates and provides interoperability among all the computers and computer information systems in the organization. An Enterprise system can be a large system with multiple facets and add-on systems of its own, or a coordinating system that enables all current information systems in the organization to interoperate.

Health computing systems have, as yet, no universally accepted standards for data definitions, recording, storage, or access protocols. What one proprietary system calls "patient" and identifies with alphabetical characters, another may call "name" and translate into numbers, or multiple fields of first, middle, and last. While one system will record "date" as January 1, 2005, another may record it as 01-01-05, while still another as 1/1/2005. To humans, all three of these dates mean the same thing. To a computer, however, each of these is a completely different thing. In addition, there are a number of ways that software programs can store and access data, making it difficult, and sometimes impossible, for one type of software to interface with another and successfully find, access, and use data.

Enterprise systems have long been the dream, and are sometimes the reality, in many U.S. industries. Health care, with its myriad of freestanding, discipline-specific programs, has been slow to even attempt adopting and implementing Enterprise systems. Health managers dream of a system where each piece of information can be entered once and only once, and then accessed in different ways by different users. Patients would not be asked to fill out dozens of forms asking for the same demographic and basic health history information over and over again with every new provider or visit. Appointments could be scheduled on-line and patients could have access to their own patient records and to state-of-the-art health information. Physicians could access past and current patient records, incorporating all lab, imaging, up-to-the-minute nursing notes, and expert decision support systems from their homes, offices, or the patient's bedside. In cases of traveling or emergency situations, health organizations and providers could share pertinent and appropriate patient information.

THE ROLE OF THE HEALTH MANAGER

If Enterprise systems are the health information systems of the future, EMR appears to be the first step for most health organizations. Purchasing and implementing any new technology can be daunting for either a large or small organization and requires skilled leadership. What kinds of knowledge and skills should health managers have to get the job done? Below is a list of three broad competencies that skilled health IT professionals need to possess:

1. Environmental Knowledge
   - knowledge of the state of the art in our industry and in other industries
   - basic understanding of hardware, software, networks
2. Healthcare Data, Structure, Content
   - understanding of the use of IT to assure quality and safety
3. Administration and Leadership in Information Management
   - systems analysis, selection, design, implementation skills
   - analytic assessment skills

Environmental Knowledge

Few industries change as quickly and as drastically as high technology. From the days when a computer took up an entire large room and data were entered with punch cards, to today when a chip smaller than a postage stamp holds more information and has more computing power than the room-sized computer described above, computers have become an accepted part of all of our lives. It is fair to say that computers are integrated into nearly every aspect of our society. Indeed, computers even control some of our transplanted body parts. It is vital that the skilled health

IT professional keep up with the changes and advances in health technology. At the time of this writing, the "cutting edge" IT systems being implemented in health care are EMR, enterprise systems, and wireless environments. The health IT professional must know the technology environment and be able to make sound and knowledgeable decisions about what her or his organization needs, can implement, and can afford.

Health Data, Content, and Structure

As described earlier in this chapter, health data are multifaceted and can reside in a number of places, both virtual and physical, in a health organization. The healthcare IT professional must understand the data and its location, and ensure that access to that information is easy, fast, and available only to those who have the need and the right to see it. In some circumstances that might mean password and/or firewall protection. In other situations it may be a matter of encoding the data, and in still others it may mean secure and dedicated lines, service carriers, transmission/communication media, and information systems. Finally, all organization staff and employees must not only be well trained in how to access data, but they must be indoctrinated into the ethics and practices of privacy, confidentiality, and data security.

Protection of the privacy, confidentiality, and security of healthcare data in the electronic form has been raised to a new level of consciousness for all health care personnel. Federal Public Law 104-191 (also known as the Kennedy-Kassebaum Bill) Health Insurance Portability and Accountability Act of 1996, also known as **HIPAA**, mandated that, by the year 2000, all healthcare organizations would establish and implement security standards to protect patient confidentiality. The law, which finally went into effect in 2004, states that:

> Each person who maintains or transmits health information shall maintain reasonable and appropriate administrative, technical and physical safeguards to ensure the integrity and confidentiality of the information, to protect against reasonably anticipated threats or hazards to the security or integrity of the information; and unauthorized uses or disclosures of the information.

Penalties for violating this law can be as high as fines of $250,000 and 10 years in jail. Every healthcare manager must be trained in desirable practices to ensure compliance with HIPAA. These practices include: access controls, user identification codes and passwords, authentication/password controls, appropriate authorization for access to patient data, security administration, network controls, audit controls, security policies, and HIPAA training for all healthcare personnel (Massachusetts Health Data Consortium, 2006).

IT has the potential to be our strongest tool in ensuring quality of care. Unlike protocols on paper, a computer can simply not allow further progress in a routine if a step is missed. Fail-safe systems can be built into software. For example, the CPOE will "freeze" until the physician checks for drug interactions; the admissions process will refuse to print admissions papers until proof of insurance has been verified; or the medications cabinet will remain locked until the appropriate caregiver's barcode has been scanned. IT as an organization-wide system is new to most healthcare personnel, particularly as it applies to quality. We have barely scratched the surface of its potential uses and applications in helping create a safer health system.

Administration and Leadership in Information Management

IT professionals are managers, and the skills and principles of management (planning, organizing, directing, controlling) are as germane to IT personnel as they are to any other discipline of management. However, because all employees in the organization will likely need to learn and use the IT system, it behooves the IT manager to have excellent communication and interpersonal skills. The days of the stereotypical IT person who only spoke in programming language are long gone. IT professionals must be able to work with all people in the organization, speak "their language," and be patient. In health care that means training and supporting physicians, nurses, caregivers, other managers, business office personnel, physical plant workers, patients, and many others.

The myriad of IT users in any healthcare organization make the analysis and implementation of IT in health organizations very complex and difficult. Using IT to its greatest effect does not mean simply automating existing tasks and procedures. IT is at its most effective when tasks and procedures first undergo in-depth analysis to see how tasks can best be performed and executed using technology.

An example of simply automating an existing task is to continue to have patients complete information forms on paper, by hand, and then having someone enter that information into the appropriate fields in the computer, produce the appropriate paper document, and have the patient proceed from there. A better IT approach might be to have the patient (with assistance as needed) enter the information directly into a terminal, or better yet, into a hand-held electronic notepad that highlights inconsistent and/or omitted information. When the information is complete, the notepad could be downloaded into the enterprise system, which would automatically search for previous information on that patient and prompt for inconsistent, changed, and/or new information. Once all information has been confirmed, the system would enter the information into the organization's admissions and billing systems, print the patient's bar coded identification bracelet, and enter the appropriate information into the patient's medical record. The patient could then proceed with the notepad to her or his next destination.

The IT professional must assess the scope of the organization's technology, analyze tasks, processes, and procedures, design IT appropriate tasks, implement the software, teach users, and be able to support and troubleshoot.

CHALLENGES

This chapter started with the assertion that "Few topics have more potential to change healthcare delivery, quality, and efficiency than information technology (IT)." Today's healthcare environment is arguably the most complex and fastest changing environment in society. Coupled with the fast and exciting changes in the technology industry, it makes the intersection of health care and technology an exhilarating and challenging place to be.

There is, however, a human side of computing and IT: For every system created to ensure the security of health data and information, there is someone who can find a way around it and break into the system. The regulation of health organizations is second only to the nuclear power industry. New laws and policies regarding insurance and the confidentiality of patient information, such as the Health Insurance Portability and Assurance Act (HIPAA), create new challenges for the use, maintenance, and sharing of privileged health information. For an industry that is steeped in the creation and use of paper documentation and medical records, it is a difficult leap into the virtual world of EMR and Enterprise systems.

Adoption of IT has been slow in health care. There are many barriers. Perhaps the largest hurdle for most organizations is the cost. While the public perceives hospitals and providers as financially secure and sometimes even wealthy, the truth is that many health organizations are struggling with little or no profit margins. The days of easy profits are gone for most health facilities. In today's tight financial environment it is often hard to convince governing boards and owners that they need to spend hundreds of thousands of dollars on a new computer system. To most, it looks like a huge expense which may not pay off now or in the future. Governing boards and owners approach IT purchases with great caution and reluctance.

This widespread perception of IT as a bottomless money abyss needs to be changed to a perception of IT as an investment in quality, efficiency, patient satisfaction, and future profits. IT is a financial investment, much like the building and maintaining of the physical plant, recruitment of medical staff, and the education of employees. It pays off in the long run. In the meantime, however, there are things that might be considered to make the transformation easier and faster.

Other than the faith that an investment in IT will pay off in the long run, there also needs to be the recognition among payers that technologically enhanced care is higher quality, works actively against medical errors, and is more efficient and productive. One idea might be to create incentives for health organizations and providers by reimbursing providers who use EMR, bar codes, and CPOE at higher levels than those who don't. Another idea is for the U.S. Congress to pass legislation similar to the Hill-Burton legislation of the 1940s and 1950s that would offer low interest loans to organizations and providers that invest in IT for the delivery of care.

Two final challenges are **standards** and **interoperability**. These are vital topics, not only within organizations, but across them. Intra-organizational standards of data collection, data definitions, and storage promote quality and efficiency. However, data standards and software interoperability among outside health providers and organizations can allow easy movement of information and transfer of records between hospitals, pharmacies, and ancillary providers in the cases of travel, emergency, or relocation.

Further, there is a vitally important aspect of data standards' interoperability: national security. One of the glaring problems brought to light by the September 11, 2001 terrorist attacks on the United States was that health departments, hospitals, providers, and government organizations could not communicate, transmit information and data, or coordinate their efforts electronically. Some health departments had no electronic systems at all and those that did could not "talk" to each other. In a time rife with national security concerns, the importance of the healthcare industry cannot be underestimated. It is of vital importance to U.S. national security that our industry moves ahead quickly in the areas of information transfer, information security, and interoperability.

CONCLUSION

It has been said that, in health care, the 1980s was the age of the Chief Executive Officer (CEO); the 1990s was the age of the Chief Financial Officer (CFO); and the year 2000 and beyond will be the age of the Chief Information Officer (CIO). Information is power. Other industries have evolved through the creation and implementation of appropriate, industry-specific IT systems, and health care will too. We can focus on the problems and barriers, or we can be excited and exhilarated by the vast possibilities and challenges of IT in our industry. Health care is on the threshold of an information and IT explosion. Those who stand on the sidelines and wring their hands will undoubtedly be left behind. Those who have vision and have the competencies and skills to lead their organizations forward into the realm of IT sophistication will see and help to create a new and better healthcare industry.

DISCUSSION QUESTIONS

1. Describe the initial uses of computers in health care and the evolution of information technology (IT). What was the biggest driver of acceptance of computers and IT in health care?

2. What kind of data do the following patient encounters require for documentation: emergency room visit; sick patient physician visit; well-patient physician visit?

3. In a hospital setting who should have access to patient medical data; patient financial data; employee data?

4. What is the electronic medical record? How can computerized physician order entry decrease medical errors?

5. What is bar coding and how is it helpful for materials management and inventory control?

6. Jane Dough e-mails her physician, Dr. Smith, a medical question. Dr. Smith responds to Jane only. Then Jane forwards the e-mail and the physician's response to all her family and friends. Has the physician violated patient confidentiality? Why or why not?

REFERENCES

American Medical Association (AMA). (2004, September). *Physician internet use jumps*. Retrieved September 2004 from http://www.healthdatamanagement.com/html/PortalStory.cfm?tupe=trend&DID=5704

Hassol, A., Walker, J. M., Kidder, D., Rokita, K., Young, D., Pierdon, S., et al. (2004). Patient experiences and attitudes about access to a patient electronic health care record and linked web messaging. *Journal of the American Medical Informatics Association, 11*(6), 505–513.

Institute of Medicine (IOM). (2000). *To err is human: building a safer health system*. Washington, DC: National Academies Press.

Institute of Medicine (IOM). (2001). *Crossing the quality chasm: a new health system for the 21st century*. Washington, DC: National Academies Press.

Massachusetts Health Data Consortium. (2006). HIPAA overview and summary. Retrieved September 23, 2006 from http://www.mahealthdata.org/hipaa/resources/summary.html

Pew Internet and American Life Project. (2003). Retrieved June 9, 2006 from http://www.pewinternet.org/reports/toc.asp?Report=106

Wager, K. A., Lee, F. W., and Glaser, J. P. (2005). *Managing health care information systems: a practical approach for health care executives*. San Francisco, CA: Jossey-Bass.

CHAPTER 7

Financing Health Care and Health Insurance

Nancy H. Shanks
Suzanne Discenza
Ralph Charlip

LEARNING OBJECTIVES

By the end of this chapter the student will be able to:

- Describe background about healthcare spending, how it has grown and is expected to continue to grow;
- Identify the concepts of healthcare financing and payment for health care;
- Provide an overview of how health insurance works;
- Outline a brief history of how health insurance has evolved;
- Define terms and characteristics of health insurance;
- Compare and contrast the different types of private health insurance;
- Delineate the types of social insurance;
- Obtain data on health insurance coverage and lack thereof;
- Characterize the uninsured; and,
- Explain the implications for management.

INTRODUCTION

As healthcare managers, there are a number of concerns relating to the overall costs of health care, how it is financed, how health insurance works, where the gaps in insurance are, and how to better manage these areas.

NATIONAL HEALTH SPENDING

Healthcare spending in the United States has continued to grow over the last 35 years at what has been characterized as an alarming rate. While the increases have not, as yet, reached the double-digit levels that existed in the 1980s and early 1990s, the Centers for Medicare and Medicaid Services (CMS) are predicting that the expansion in national healthcare spending will continue. Projected expenditures for 2006 were expected to reach $2.2 trillion and to account for 16.5% of Gross Domestic Product (GDP) or $7,110 per capita (Centers for Medicare and Medicaid Services, 2006).

Expenditures for health care were directed to a variety of services, as shown in Table 7-1. Four areas accounted for more than two-thirds of those expenditures. Hospital care accounted for 30.6%, physician and clinical services represented another 21.4%, prescription drug costs made

TABLE 7-1 2006 National Health Spending by Type of Expenditure (in billions)

Hospital Care	$ 662.5
Physician and Clinical Services	463.3
Prescription Drugs	219.2
Other Professional, Dental, and Personal Care Services	216.7
Nursing Home and Home Health Care	181.5
Administrative Costs	151.5
Structures and Equipment	98.4
Public Health Activities	67.0
Other Medical Products	58.7
Research	45.2
TOTAL	$2,164.0

Source: Centers for Medicare and Medicaid Services, 2006.

up 10.1%, and nursing home and home health care comprised 8.4% of total health expenditures.

In addition, CMS has also projected that healthcare spending will double in the next 10 years, reaching $4 trillion and 20.0% of GDP by 2015 (Borger, Smith, Truffer, Keehan, Sisko, Poisal, & Clemens, 2006). This will equate to an estimated $12,320 per capita. In comparison, national health expenditures were $247.3 billion in 1980 and accounted for 8.9% of GDP (Levit, Lazenby, Braden, Cowan, Sensenig, McDonnell, Stiller, Won, Martin, Sivarajan, Donham, Long, & Stewart, 1997).

PAYING FOR HEALTH CARE

Payments to cover these healthcare expenditures are derived from a variety of sources. These include individuals who pay out-of-pocket, private health insurance of a variety of types, other private funds, and public insurance programs. These categories are described further below.

- Out-of-pocket payments include payments by individuals who pay for services themselves or pay for part of those services through co-payments and/or deductibles.
- Private health insurance includes payments made by individuals for their health insurance premiums, which in turn cover the costs of payments made by various health plans, including indemnity plans, preferred provider plans (PPOs), point-of-service plans (POSs), health maintenance organizations (HMOs), and catastrophic plans.
- Other private funds include, among other things, health spending accounts (HSAs).
- Public funds include funding from federal, state, and local government programs, including among others, Medicare, Medicaid, and the State Children's Health Insurance Program (SCHIP).

In 2006 the breakdown of expenditures by these sources of funding (see Figure 7-1) indicated that 34.4% of payments were derived from private health insurance, another 7.3% were from other private funds, and 11.4% came from out-of-pocket payments. The remaining 46.9% of the payments were provided by public (government) funders.

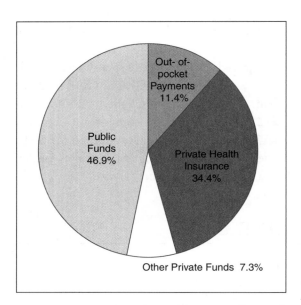

FIGURE 7-1 National Health Expenditures by Source of Funds, 2006

Source: Centers for Medicare and Medicaid Services, 2006.

INTRODUCTION TO HEALTH INSURANCE

As with other types of insurance, the intent of **health insurance** is to provide protection should a covered individual experience an event, adverse or otherwise, that requires healthcare treatment. When individuals purchase coverage, they join together with others and pool their resources in order to protect against losses. In so doing, they pool the potential risk for losses that might be experienced. Two key concepts in insurance are that:

- risk is transferred from the individual to the group; and,
- the group shares the costs of any covered losses incurred by its members.

Fifty years ago health insurance coverage was typically purchased on an individual basis, much like car insurance. Individuals purchased policies to protect themselves and their families against catastrophic types of illness. This was at a time when health care was not as expensive as it is today and individuals paid for routine types of care out-of-pocket, thereby using health insurance to cover catastrophic expenditures and to protect against income loss. The latter, while technically a form of health insurance, is what we now think of as disability income insurance coverage.

During the second half of the 20th century, the demand for and use of health insurance has changed in a number of significant ways. Health insurance products have also changed in response to that demand. Of particular importance were the following facts:

- Most health insurance coverage includes a comprehensive set of healthcare benefits, most frequently including hospital stays and physician care, as well as other types of services and benefits;
- Both the public and private sectors began to have expanded and increasingly important roles in the provision of health insurance coverage;
- Group health insurance policies began to be offered as an employee benefit, with the purchasing of coverage being handled by companies and fewer people taking out individual insurance policies;
- Mechanisms for reimbursing healthcare providers have expanded from solely paying on the basis of costs to reimbursing on a prepaid basis; and,
- The cost of health care began to rise.

BRIEF HISTORY OF HEALTH INSURANCE

During the Great Depression of the 1930s, there were discussions about creating a national health insurance policy that would provide a system of universal health insurance coverage in the United States. While the proposal had some proponents, the American Medical Association (AMA) and others opposed the move. With the Depression and U.S. involvement in World War II, the funding required for such a system was not available. While there continued to be interest in national health insurance after the war, the concept of a universal health insurance mechanism eventually became synonymous with "socialized medicine" during the cold war of the 1950s. The end result was a health insurance system rooted in the private sector (Starr, 1982).

In response to increasing numbers of poor and elderly individuals who had little or no access to health care, the government began to play a role in providing healthcare coverage. In 1965, with the passage of the legislation that created the Medicare and Medicaid programs, government assumed responsibility for providing coverage to millions of poor and aged Americans. Those public programs have had a significant impact in a variety of ways. They have been expanded to bring more eligible individuals into coverage, have added types of benefits, and have changed in a variety of other ways over time. One such major expansion of public sector coverage took place with the creation of the State Children's Health Insurance Program in 1997.

Additionally, the federal government also has an extensive program for providing health care to active duty military personnel, veterans, and their dependents. The military medical system is one of the most sophisticated in the world and has come to serve as a model in many ways.

Private healthcare coverage has evolved significantly in the last 50 to 60 years, as well. A major change came as employers began to provide health insurance as an employee benefit. That is, employers chose to offer the benefit in lieu of providing wage increases to employees. This was primarily the result of collective bargaining agreements, where unions negotiated increased benefits for workers and their families. Over the last 50 years, private insurance has evolved from indemnity policies to pre-paid plans and managed care plans. Today, a variety of different types of coverage are used in the industry.

CHARACTERISTICS OF HEALTH INSURANCE

This section discusses some important aspects of health insurance, including how healthcare services are financed, how costs are controlled, and the types of benefits offered.

Forms of Payment

Two forms of payment provide the basis for all types of health insurance coverage. These are payment on a **fee-for-service** basis versus **prepayment**, which are defined as follows:

- **Fee-for-service**—This approach was developed by Blue Cross-Blue Shield plans and is based on the idea of an insured individual purchasing coverage of a set of benefits, utilizing individual medical services and paying the healthcare provider for the services rendered. The provider is paid either by the insurer or out-of-pocket by the insured who in turn is reimbursed by the insurer. Typically, the insured must meet deductibles and make copayments for their care.

- **Prepayment**—In this approach, an insured individual pays a fixed, pre-specified amount in exchange for services. Routine types of care are typically covered in full, with small copayments for selected services, e.g., prescriptions.

Cost Sharing

Most insurance policies require insured individuals to bear some of the cost of care out-of-pocket. **Cost sharing** may take different forms, but may include some or all of the following:

- **Copayments**—are costs that are borne by the insured individual at the time a service is used. For example, a prescription medication or a physician office visit may require a $15 or $20 copay. Copayments are used in both fee-for-service and pre-paid plans.
- **Deductibles**—are required levels of payments that the insured individual/family must meet before the insurer begins making its payments for care in a fee-for-service plan. Deductibles are regularly met at the beginning of each year and vary by policy type. The amount of the deductible can range from relatively small amounts for traditional types of insurance to quite substantial amounts under catastrophic coverage.
- **Co-insurance**—Under a fee-for-service policy, insured individuals pay a percentage of the cost of care, while the insurer is responsible for the remaining costs. For example, the insured's coinsurance is usually 20%, while the insurer pays 80%.

Policy Limitations

Often the insurance policy has various types of limitations—some that limit payments by the policy holder and some that limit how much total coverage the insurer will provide.

- **Maximum out-of-pocket expenditure**—This is an amount where the insured individual's cost sharing is capped. After reaching this point, the insurer will pick up 100% of the tab.

- **Lifetime limit**—This is a maximum cap that the policy will pay out over the lifetime of the insured individual. This type of limit usually only comes into play when there are catastrophic types of illnesses requiring very costly care. For example, in various types of transplants or spinal cord injuries, the treatment costs can escalate to hundreds of thousands of dollars. The limit is usually $1.0 million or higher.

Moral Hazard

The concept of **moral hazard** refers to the idea that existence of insurance coverage provides an incentive for insured individuals to use the coverage.

Types of Benefits

Different types of benefit packages can be purchased that offer varying types of coverage for individuals and families. These include:

- **Comprehensive policies**—These policies provide benefits that typically include physician and other types of outpatient visits, inpatient hospitals stays, outpatient surgery, medical testing and ancillary services, medical equipment, therapies, and other types of services. Prescription drugs are sometimes covered, as are rehabilitation services, hospice, and mental health care. Despite the name "comprehensive," most policies do not cover everything and thus have exclusions; in particular most types of experimental treatments are excluded.
- **Basic, major medical, or hospital-surgical policies**—Referred to by several different names, the benefits provided by these policies are limited to types of illness that require hospitalization. Benefits include inpatient hospital stays, surgery, associated tests and treatments, related physician services, and other expenses incurred during an illness. There usually are limits on hospital stays and caps on expenditures.
- **Catastrophic coverage policies**—Benefits under these policies are intended to cover extraordinary types of illness; policies typically carry very sizeable deductibles ($15,000 or higher) and lifetime limits on coverage.
- **Disease-specific policies**—In these policies the benefits cover only the specific disease(s) covered (e.g., a cancer care policy).
- **MediGap policies**—These policies provide supplemental coverage of certain benefits that are excluded from other types of policies (e.g., prescription drugs).

Other Issues of Concern Regarding Health Insurance

There are a number of issues that are important when managers and/or individuals are making decisions about healthcare coverage. These include the following:

- **Provider Choice**—The concern here is whether the insured individuals have choices when they select providers or whether there are limitations on which providers can be chosen.
- **Access to vs. Restrictions on Care**—The concern here is whether access to care is limited or controlled for the insured individual. Under some insurance policies there is unlimited access, while under others, it is restricted by a gatekeeper.

The remaining sections of the chapter explore the different types of insurance coverage in greater depth. The chapter includes a discussion of the numbers and demographics of specific segments of the population who do and do not have health insurance coverage. Finally, the chapter concludes with a discussion of the implications of health insurance for healthcare managers.

PRIVATE HEALTH INSURANCE COVERAGE

Each type of private health insurance is described briefly below. Additionally, consideration is given to the pluses and minuses of the type of insurance with respect to access to care, choice of providers, and cost.

Indemnity Insurance

Most **indemnity insurance** products are based on the **fee-for-service model**. When the insured individuals utilize healthcare services, they pay for those services and seek reimbursement from the insurer. Care is rendered by independent healthcare providers, without gatekeeping or other restrictions. Management of care only comes into play in elective admissions, which require pre-authorization. Table 7-3, provided later in this section, delineates the pluses and minuses of indemnity and other types of health plan coverages.

Managed Care Plans

Unlike indemnity plans, these health plans seek to manage the cost, quality, and access to health services through control mechanisms on both patients and providers. These delivery systems attempt to integrate both the financing and provision of health care into one organization. The primary types include **HMOs, PPOs,** and **POS plans** and are described further below.

Health Maintenance Organizations (HMOs)—Individuals become members of the organization by paying a fixed prepayment amount. Once they become members they are enrolled in the HMO. Enrollees are eligible to get care from the providers and facilities that are aligned with the HMO. Services are used at no charge, although minor copays are often required for prescription medications. Administration is centralized with providers typically being reimbursed under a **capitated rate**. This means that the providers are paid a set amount no matter how much care they need to provide. Various types of contracting arrangements exist with providers, which may take the form of:

- **Closed-panel HMO**—physicians practice only with the HMO, frequently in a HMO-owned health center;
- **Open-panel HMO**—physicians practice within and outside of the HMO;
- **Group Model HMO**—the HMO contracts with a multi-specialty group practice to care for their enrollees;
- **Staff Model HMO**—groups of physicians are either salaried employees of the HMO or salaried employees of a professional group practice contracting exclusively with the HMO;
- **Independent Practice Association or IPA model**—the HMO contracts with an association of physicians practicing independently in their own offices; and,
- **Network Model HMO**—the HMO contracts with several groups of physicians or with individual physicians or multi-specialty medical clinics (physicians and hospitals) to provide a full range of medical services.

Preferred Provider Organizations (PPOs)—These plans reflect a combination of **indemnity insurance** and **managed care** options. In PPOs insured individuals purchase coverage on a fee-for-service basis, with deductibles, copays, and coinsurances to be met. Care is managed in the sense that insured individuals pay less if care is obtained from a network of preferred provider organizations with which the insurer contracts for discounted rates. These preferred provider organizations include physicians, hospitals, diagnostic facilities, and other types of service providers. If care is not provided by a preferred provider, the insured individual pays at a higher and undiscounted rate, and must meet higher deductibles and co-insurances for these services.

Exclusive Provider Organizations (EPOs)—These plans are very similar to PPOs, with the primary differences being limitations in terms of access. The provider network is limited to a specific group of in-network providers. Like HMOs, described previously, EPOs use primary care physicians to serve as gatekeepers for referrals to specialty care. EPOs do not provide coverage if the insured individual is treated outside of the plan.

Point-of-Service (POS) Plans—These plans provide some flexibility to the HMO model described above and are sometimes referred to as open-ended plans. Under the POS plan, an enrollee can use services that are out of plan, in exchange for deductibles and coinsurance payments. The plan tries to address some of the shortcomings of the pure HMO approach.

In the mid-1990s, many people thought managed care was the solution to the rising healthcare cost problem. While initially there was tremendous growth in managed care, particularly in HMOs, in recent years that trend has slowed. Additionally, consumer perceptions indicate negative views of managed care plans, concerns about the restrictions imposed in the plans, and the quality of care provided (Kaiser Commission on Medicaid and the Uninsured/Kaiser Family Foundation, 2006).

Recent evidence also suggests that PPOs have become the dominant form of coverage (Hurley, Strunk, & White, 2004). This represents a radical change in choice of plan since 1988, as shown in Table 7-2. At that time 73% of covered workers were enrolled in conventional health insurance plans, 16% were in HMOS, 11% were in PPOs, and POS plans weren't even an option. By 2005, 61% of workers enrolled in health plans opted for a PPO, while only 21% and 15% were in HMOs and POSs, respectively. Only a very small percentage, 3%, remained in conventional health plans (Kaiser Family Foundation and the Health Research and Educational Trust, 2005).

Other types of plans have also been pursued in recent years, although data on them are scant.

TABLE 7-2 Health Plan Enrollment by Type of Plan, 1988–2005

Type of Plan	1988	1993	1998	2003	2005
Conventional	73%	46%	14%	5%	3%
HMOs	16%	21%	27%	24%	21%
PPOs	11%	26%	35%	54%	61%
POSs	0%	7%	24%	17%	15%

Source: Kaiser Family Foundation and the Health Research and Educational Trust, 2005.

Physician–Hospital Organizations (PHOs)—These plans are essentially joint ventures developed between hospitals and physicians in order to provide more bargaining power in healthcare markets. They set up their own organizational and reimbursement structures, eliminating the added costs of intermediaries.

Direct Contracting Plans—Considered the "wave of the future," these plans are on the rise in several states. Large employers contract directly with **integrated delivery systems**, which are networks of healthcare providers accepting financial risk and delivering a full range of healthcare services. These also eliminate the costs of intermediaries.

The primary types of private health insurance coverage, excluding the last two types of plans listed above, are compared across a number of important dimensions in Table 7-3. These include issues of access to care in general and to specialists, choice of providers, cost-sharing, restrictions on utilization, administrative costs, paperwork, and several other dimensions. It is clear from reviewing this information that there are tradeoffs between plans. For example, those that provide unlimited access tend to have difficulties controlling costs, but afford higher quality. Those that are able to manage and control costs do so by limiting access and utilization.

CONSUMER-DRIVEN HEALTH PLANS

In addition to these trends, another relatively new direction for healthcare benefits coverage has begun to focus on **consumer-driven health plans**. Wilensky (2006, p. 175) has defined the term as "a high-deductible insurance plan that is paired with some type of tax-advantaged account."

TABLE 7-3 Comparison of Insurance Plan Characteristics

	Indemnity Plans	Health Maintenance Organizations (HMOs)	Preferred Provider Organizations (PPOs)	Point-of-Service Plans (POSs)
Access to Care	Unlimited	Limited and controlled; may require waiting for care	Unlimited	Unlimited
Geographic Limitations	None	Limited to geographic regions served by HMO, except in emergencies	Unlimited	Unlimited
Choice of Provider	Unlimited choice of providers	Limited to in-network providers	Unlimited, but pay less when preferred (in-network) providers used	Can go out-of-network, but pay more
Access to Specialist	Unlimited; can self-refer	Limited; need referral from gatekeeper	Unlimited; can self-refer	Unlimited; may self-refer out-of-plan at a higher cost
Utilization Restrictions	None	Limitations may be imposed on certain services	Mostly unlimited; plan may place annual dollar or visits limits	Mostly unlimited; plan may place annual dollar or visits limits
Deductibles/ Copayments	Both typically must be met	No deductibles/small copays	Deductibles and copays required	Deductibles and copays required
Coinsurance	Required	None	Required	Required for services received out-of-plan
Quality Issues	Likely to be high	May be lower, if patients have to wait for care	Likely to be high	Likely to be high, if patient gets second opinions
Paperwork	Insured must complete to be reimbursed	Minimal; billing only needed on a small number of procedures	Excessive	Moderate for out-of-plan services
Administrative Costs	Moderately high	Low; controlled by not having to bill for most services	High; uncontrolled	Moderate to high
Management of Costs	Costs difficult to manage; plans are cost inducing	Costs are known and can be managed	Costs are difficult to manage, costs are based on utilization	Costs are partially known for in-plan care; out-of-plan care is less known

Various options have been created to assist employees in paying for their health care. These strategies are discussed further below.

Flexible Spending Accounts—provide employees with the option of setting aside pretax income for use in paying for out-of-pocket healthcare expenditures. Employees submit claims for these expenditures and are reimbursed from their spending accounts for approved items. A drawback to these accounts is that all dollars must be spent in the year that they were set aside—any unspent dollars are forfeited at the end of the year.

Medical Savings Accounts (MSAs)—are another vehicle mandated as part of the Health Insurance Portability and Accountability Act of 1996. MSAs allow workers, who are employed in firms with 50 or fewer employees and who have high deductible health insurance plans, to set aside pretax funds to be used to pay for health insurance premiums and "unreimbursed healthcare expenses" (Saleem, 2003).

Health Reimbursement Arrangements (HRAs)—also referred to as "personal care accounts," are accounts where "the employer funds the account, the account is 'owned' by the employer, and the money remains with the employer if the employee leaves the company" (Wilensky, 2006). This approach has been criticized for the absence of portability.

Health Savings Accounts (HSAs)—Among the many provisions of the Medicare Prescription Drug, Improvement, and Modernization Act (MMA) of 2003 are provisions that are intended to address the shortcomings underlying HRAs. HSAs were mandated to "pair high-deductible plans that meet certain requirements with fully portable, employee-owned, tax-advantaged accounts" (Wilensky, 2006). The underlying ideas behind HSAs are that consumers will:

- become more educated users of health care;
- be more likely to utilize preventive and chronic care services;
- become more cognizant of the costs of care;
- be less likely to make poor decisions about using care that is not necessary or not appropriate; and,
- be more prudent when using an account that is seen as containing "their own funds."

As Wilensky (2006) pointed out, these plans are relatively new and it is not entirely clear how quickly they will be adopted and what their impacts will be. While it is anticipated that this trend will increase, only 1 to 2 million people were using HRAs and HSAs in 2004 and 2005. The impact of consumer-driven health plans is also unknown at this time. Wilensky does suggest that they may have a large impact on hospital pricing and the potential to propel the movement toward increased transparency in hospital pricing.

THE EVOLUTION OF SOCIAL INSURANCE

As with private insurance, many changes have taken place in how individuals can access care via social insurance or federal entitlement programs. The changes in both areas are discussed below.

THE CONVERGENCE OF POLITICAL OPPORTUNITY AND LEADERSHIP

Although the expansionist social policies of President Lyndon B. Johnson's Great Society in the 1960s are credited with development of the largest social health insurance programs this country has ever known, now known as Medicare and Medicaid, the seeds of these programs were actually sown by Congress during the Eisenhower administration in the 1950s. At a time when private health insurance coverage was increasingly being provided for workers by their employers, the elderly had virtually no such coverage and yet were the group in society with the largest health costs and often the most limited financial resources. The ultimate passage of the Kerr-Mills Act by Congress in 1960 provided for federal matching grants to the states for a new category of "medically indigent" individuals, but still did not cover elders other than those who had become poor. However, this piece of legislation played a pivotal role as the precursor to Medicaid.

It was actually President John F. Kennedy, backed by senior interest groups and supported by labor unions and nurses, who proposed the first Medicare bill to Congress in 1962 in keeping with his strong belief in the need for federal health care for the elderly. Although this measure was defeated by legislative opponents in the Senate, it did serve to raise public awareness of the issues and thus to build future public support. This set the stage for President Johnson to utilize his considerable political popularity, legislative liaisons, and persuasiveness in small groups (such as the AMA) to lead the charge for passage of the Medicare and Medicaid legislation in 1965.

Unlike the above programs, development and implementation of the Veterans Administration medical system, initially established to ensure access to medical care for veterans with service-related medical problems, were accomplished much more directly and smoothly. This program, and other programs directed toward insuring military personnel and their families, will be discussed later in this section.

MAJOR LEGISLATION

The social health insurance programs of Medicare and Medicaid, as they exist today, have continued to evolve over the past 40 years since their inception. The following discussion will address some of the major pieces of legislation shaping this evolution.

Social Security Acts of 1965

The 1965 Amendments to the Social Security Act of 1935 established the two largest government-sponsored health insurance programs in the history of the United States. **Medicare, Title XVIII** of the Act, entitled persons 65 and over to coverage of hospital care under Part A and physicians' and other outpatient health services under Part B. Further eligibility for Medicare benefits has since been extended to younger people with permanent disabilities, individuals with end stage renal disease (ESRD), and persons under hospice care. **Medicaid, Title XIX**, set up a joint federal-state program entitling financially-qualified indigent and low-income persons to basic medical care. This program, too, has undergone numerous iterations at both the state and federal levels as these governments have attempted to strike a balance between equity in coverage for certain services (mandated at the federal level) and states' rights in controlling use of public funds. Medicare and Medicaid eligibility, benefits, financing, and expenditures will be described in greater depth in future sections of this chapter.

TEFRA 1982 and OBRA 1989

In response to rapidly rising healthcare costs, Congress passed the **Tax Equity and Fiscal Responsibility Act (TEFRA)** in 1982, with particular emphasis on Medicare cost controls. Among its key provisions were the following:

- a mandate for a **prospective payment system (PPS)** for hospital reimbursement, with payment rates established up front for conditions known as **Diagnosis-Related Groups (DRGs)**;
- the option of providing managed care plans to Medicare beneficiaries; and,
- the requirement that Medicare become the secondary payer when a beneficiary had other insurance.

Similar payment arrangements have been mandated for other types of providers, such as compensation for physician office services to Medicare beneficiaries using the **Resource-Based Relative Value System (RBRVS)**, mandated as part of the Omnibus Reconciliation Act (OBRA) of 1989 and implemented in 1992. Under RBRVS, payments are determined by the cost of resources needed to provide each service, including physician work, practice expenses, and professional liability insurance.

Balanced Budget Act of 1997

Despite reductions in reimbursements for hospital admissions and physician visits, Medicare expenditures continued to soar throughout the 1990s. Congress passed the Balanced Budget Act (BBA) of 1997 in an attempt to control costs for other healthcare services, mandating some 200 changes (primarily restrictive) to the Medicare program alone, as well as changes to the Medicaid program. Medicare prospective payment systems were phased in and implemented in other healthcare settings beginning in 1998 as follows:

- **Skilled nursing facilities (SNFs)**, in 1998, with **RUGs (Resource Utilization Groups)**;
- **Home health agencies (HHAs)**, in 2000, with **HHRGs (Home Health Resource Groups)**;
- **Hospital outpatient department services**, in 2002, with **OPPS (Hospital Outpatient Prospective Payment System)**; and,
- Payment reductions and prospective payment arrangements for hospice care, rehabilitation hospitals, ambulance services, and durable medical equipment.

Other key provisions of the BBA, providing for cost controls in some areas and expansion of coverage in others, were:

- the creation of **Medicare Part C**, known as **Medicare+Choice** and referred to as **"Medicare managed care,"** which was designed to move Medicare recipients into alternative forms of coverage, including HMOs and PPOs;
- anti-fraud and abuse provisions;
- improvements in protecting program integrity;
- restrictions on public benefits for illegal immigrants;
- addition of Medicare prevention initiatives (such as mammography, prostate cancer, and colorectal screenings);
- addition of rural initiatives; and,
- establishment of the **State Children's Health Insurance Program (SCHIP)** for low-income children under Medicaid.

Medicare Prescription Drug Improvement and Modernization Act of 2003

This Act (also known as the Prescription Drug Benefit, **Medicare Part D**, and MMA) produced the largest additions and changes to Medicare in its almost 40-year history and was projected to cost $395 billion in its first decade alone. Barely passed by Congress but signed into law by President George Bush in 2003, this controversial entitlement to prescription drugs for eligible Medicare beneficiaries became effective January 1, 2006. This law instigated a flurry of activities by individual states to mitigate uncertainties in its implementation and to temporarily provide prescription coverage for millions of seniors still in the process of meeting eligibility requirements. Tax breaks, subsidies, and other incentives to pharmaceutical companies and private, managed care insurers, along with significant pressure on seniors to enroll in so-called **Medicare Advantage Plans** (administered by managed care health plans) or risk significant out-of-pocket costs, are among the most controversial provisions of the drug benefit portion of this legislation.

With so much attention focused on the drug benefit, it has become easy for other provisions of this legislation to become lost in the discussion. Some of the more important ones include:

- increased prevention benefits;
- an extra $25 billion boost to the often severely under-funded rural hospitals;

- a requirement for higher fees to be collected from wealthier seniors; and,
- the addition of a pretax health savings account for working people.

Finally, in a proactive attempt toward privatizing Medicare as one solution to its current financial woes, the Act mandates a six-city trial of a partly-privatized Medicare system by 2010.

MAJOR "PLAYERS" IN THE SOCIAL INSURANCE ARENA

Three key areas of social programs provide access to health care for different population groups. These include the social insurance programs, Medicare and Medicaid, as well as the federal entitlement programs for veterans, active and retired military personnel and their families. Each program is described in this section.

Medicare

As discussed previously, **Medicare** is a federal program that provides healthcare coverage for the elderly over 65 years of age, for permanently disabled younger adults, and for those suffering from end-stage renal disease (ESRD). Further end-of-life "palliative" care (or comfort care) is also provided for terminally ill patients in their last 6 months of life. The primary benefits of this program, intermittently examined above, can best be summarized through description of its four "parts":

- **Part A**—Hospital Insurance (HI), allowing 90 days inpatient hospital coverage per benefit period (with a 60-day life-time inpatient hospital reserve), up to 100 days per episode in a skilled nursing facility (SNF) (with a 90-day life-time SNF reserve), currently prequalified home healthcare services, and (since 1982) hospice care for the terminally ill.
- **Part B**—Supplemental Medical Insurance (SMI), with coverage for physician visits, outpatient treatments, and preventive services, including flu and Hepatitis B vaccines, mammography, and pap smears.
- **Part C**—Medicare+Choice, allowing beneficiaries to enroll in a variety of private health insurance plans that are generally required to provide the same types of services covered under traditional Medicare

plans, with the option of additional benefits such as prescription drugs.

- **Part D**—The Prescription Drug Benefit, with drug coverage available only through Medicare Advantage Plans administered through private managed care insurance companies.

Administered federally by the Centers for Medicare and Medicaid Services (CMS), formerly known as the Health Care Financing Administration (HCFA), Medicare has been financed through three primary means. The first has been through assessments to employers and employees, contributing 2.9% of payroll (1.45% each), and is dedicated entirely to paying Part A benefits. While this fund currently is showing a surplus ($269 billion in 2002), it is expected that the fund will break even (with program receipts being equal to benefit payments) around 2012 and will become insolvent in 2020 (American Academy of Actuaries, 2005, p. 2). The second means of financing Medicare has involved increased cost sharing by beneficiaries, including premiums (financing about 25% of all Part B benefits), deductibles, co-insurance, and balance billing, amounting to approximately 16.5% of all expenditures in 2002. The third and largest financing source has increasingly been derived from allocations from general revenues (federal taxes), which, combined with interest on the assets of the Medicare Trust Fund, now finances close to 75% of Part B expenditures (Kaiser Family Foundation, 2005a, p. 60). Figure 7-2 summarizes the relative percentages from major Medicare revenue sources.

Public policy circles have become increasingly concerned about the growth in the number of enrollees in the Medicare program and the concomitant rise in expenditures. According to figures provided by the 2005 Annual Reports of the Boards of Trustees of the HI and SMI Trust Funds, 19.1 million individuals were enrolled in Medicare at its inception in 1966; this number grew to 40.6 million in 2002 and is projected to grow to 78 million by 2030. This growth translates from a mere $1.6 billion (in current dollars) of spending in 1966 to $265.7 billion in 2002, with a projected figure of $439.5 billion in 2006. As a percentage of the gross domestic product (GDP), Medicare's share of the U.S. economy is expected to increase from 2.7% in 2005 to 6.8% in 2030 (Medicare Boards of Trustees, 2005). More than one-third of this increase is expected to result from addition of the prescription drug benefit in 2006 (Kaiser Family Foundation, 2005a, p. 65). Another issue of concern surrounding

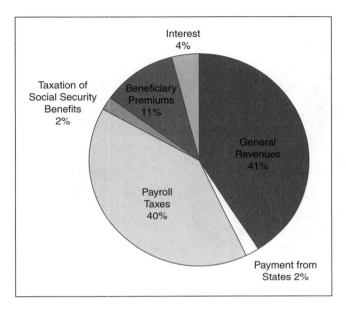

FIGURE 7-2 Distribution of Medicare Revenues, 2005

Source: Centers for Medicare and Medicaid Services, 2004.

Medicare expenditures is the distribution by percentages of dollars allocated to various sectors of the healthcare arena. Figure 7-3 summarizes this distribution, using data from the 2004 Mid-Season Review, Office of the Actuary, Centers for Medicare and Medicaid Services.

These numbers are partially indicative of the aging of the population, with increased life expectancy. Healthcare services are being used by those 65 and older at a much higher rate than other age groups, and the huge Baby Boomer generation (born between the years of 1946 and 1964) is beginning to turn 65 in 2011. Yet these factors do not tell the entire story. Why else have Medicare expenditures grown so dramatically? The following are among the most frequent and significant factors:

- a shift from treatment of acute illnesses to more chronic care as society ages and lives longer, with more substantial outlays of money to treat the latter;
- tremendous growth in hospital expenditures;
- initial lack of cost-conscious Medicare reimbursement, using retrospective fee-for-service (payments based on charges) methods;

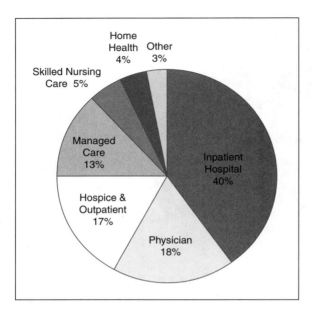

FIGURE 7-3 Distribution of Medicare Expenditures, 2004
Source: Medicare Boards of Trustees, 2005.

- huge growth in pharmaceutical costs and in technological innovations in the medical field;
- increased payments to Medicare Advantage plans and rural health providers; and,
- rising medical malpractice premiums related to increasing litigation.

During the early 1990s, federal policy makers were already alarmed by the dramatic rise in healthcare expenditures, particularly concerning Medicare. In fact, during the first Clinton administration in the early 1990s, there was a push toward legislation providing for a national healthcare system. While this solution to rising expenses was defeated in Congress, largely through the lobbying efforts of the American Medical Association and the American Association of Retired Persons (AARP), it continues to be touted as a possible solution for the future. Meanwhile, legislation to slow the rate of growth, such as with controls enacted through the Balanced Budget Act of 1997, initially served to reduce Medicare and overall healthcare expenditures in general. With this means of reducing costs largely exhausted, new solutions have come to the forefront in order to maintain Medicare's solvency. Feldstein (2005, p. 475–76) enumerates the pros and cons of a number of these, including: phasing in an increase in the eligibility age to age 67, increasing the Medicare payroll tax, further reducing payments to the suppliers of Medicare services, making Medicare an income-related program, and changing Medicare from an entitlement program to a defined contribution, where government pays a fixed dollar amount toward a health plan. Another suggestion has included privatizing the Medicare system.

Medicaid

Medicaid, the second largest provider of socialized health insurance in the United States, provides healthcare coverage to the medically indigent (those below certain poverty-level determinations) and is jointly funded by the federal government and individual states. Mandatory services required by the federal government include a relatively small number of basic health services, including inpatient hospitalization, outpatient hospital, lab and x-ray, nursing facilities, and home health services. Beyond this, each state has significant authority in administering Medicaid programs, including amount and scope of services and differences in eligibility requirements. More recently, through enactment of the Balanced Budget Act of 1997, the State Children's Health Insurance Program (SCHIP) began providing matching funds to states that finance health insurance for other low-income children.

There is a huge variation in the types of benefits provided by various states. For example, some states provide a wide array of dental benefits to its beneficiaries. Others provide mental health benefits and/or drug and alcohol treatment. Similarly, there are significant variations in states' coverage of the poor. Thus, some "bare bones" Medicaid programs cover only individuals mandated by the federal government, while other states cover individuals with higher incomes. These differences, as well as differences by ages of individuals covered, result in wide gaps in Medicaid coverage from state to state, creating a phenomenon known as "welfare magnets," in which low-income individuals from less generous states travel across the borders to more generous ones.

Despite the considerable discretion given to the states in terms of eligibility requirements in relation to income, the following categories of medically indigent and low-income individuals must be included in state Medicaid programs:

- The medically indigent, historically linked to two federal assistance programs, TANF (Temporary Aid to Needy Families, which replaced AFDC, Aid to Families with Dependent Children, in 1996) and SSI (Supplemental Security Income);
- Low-income pregnant women, children, and infants, as mandated through the Omnibus Reconciliation Act (OBRA) of 1986; and,
- Children whose parents have income too high for Medicaid but too low for private insurance, through the SCHIP (formerly Kids Care) program of the Balanced Budget Act of 1997.

The primary problems caused by allowing such liberal state discretion have been the huge inequities in the numbers and percentages of residents being served and the types of benefits being received. Part of these discrepancies may be related to the differences in how Medicaid is financed. The federal government finances 50–77% of Medicaid costs in any given state, depending on the **poverty status**, i.e., the number of individuals living below the federal poverty level, of the given state. This leaves state contributions ranging from 23% to 50%, with the poorer states contributing the lowest percentage. Many "richer" states, often feeling the pinch of reduced state coffers related to factors other than income, feel it is unfair that they must shoulder 50% of the health insurance burden of their poorest members and thus often contribute a smaller proportion of their General Fund to the provision of Medicaid services. Finally, it should be noted that there are two categories of costs that must be considered when financing Medicaid services. These include:

- costs for **provider services**, using a formula in which the state or local governments are responsible for at least 40%; and,
- costs for **administrative services**, divided equally between the federal and state governments.

Over time, the population covered by Medicaid has remained relatively stable, with poor individuals, families and children being eligible for benefits. What has changed radically, however, is the dollars consumed by different groups. For example, the aged, blind, and disabled account for less than 27.2% of Medicaid beneficiaries, but accounted for 69.6% of available Medicaid spending in 2000 (Centers for Medicare and Medicaid Services, 2003).

As with Medicare expenses, Medicaid expenditures have grown dramatically over the past couple of decades. Medicaid has experienced annual increases averaging 19.3% (versus private insurance with 6%, and Medicare, with 10.5% for Part A and 7.2% for Part B). Although this growth had slowed to 10.6% in 2001, increases in Medicaid spending began to climb again in 2002, with 11.7% growth in Medicaid spending (Prologue, 2004, p. 142). In 1966, at the inception of the Medicaid program, there were only 10 million recipients of Medicaid, with total spending at only $1.7 billion (in 1966 dollars). By 2004, total spending had risen to over $288 billion, with over 50 million recipients of Medicaid services, four times the level of 35 years prior (Kaiser Family Foundation, 2005b). Other ways of looking at expenditures are in terms of types of services provided and populations served. Figure 7-4 summarizes the distribution of Medicaid expenditures by service, and Figure 7-5 summarizes the distribution of Medicaid expenditures by population, as percentages of total spending (Kaiser Family Foundation, 2005b, and Centers for Medicare and Medicaid Services, 2004).

As previously asked for Medicare expenditures, why have Medicaid expenditures grown so dramatically? The following are illustrative of the

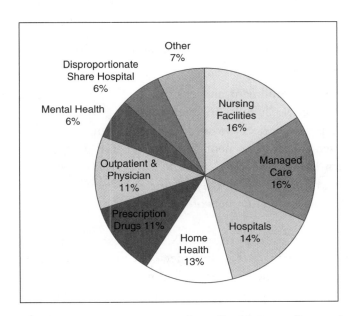

FIGURE 7-4 Distribution of Medicaid Expenditures by Service

Source: Extrapolated from data from the Kaiser Family Foundation (2005b) and Centers for Medicare and Medicaid Services (2004).

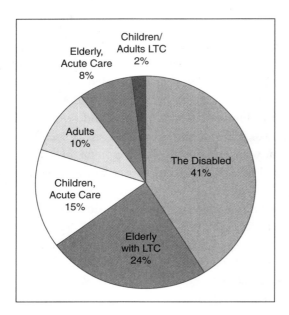

FIGURE 7-5 Distribution of Medicaid Expenditures by Population

Source: Kaiser Commission on Medicaid and the Uninsured, 2005. Kaiser Family Foundation, 2005b.

most significant reasons given for growth in spending and numbers of Medicaid recipients:

- Increased Medicaid enrollment and changes in Medicaid policies, including expansion of eligibility requirements.
- Expansion of types of services provided, including dental care, rehabilitation, preventive services, mental health care, and drug and alcohol treatment, in more generous states.
- Downturns in the economy and rising unemployment rates that have resulted in increasing numbers of the poor and uninsured since 2001.
- The unexpected significant increases in Medicaid expenditures as a result of higher payment rates to providers and more spending on those who "deserve" public support, including the aged blind, disabled, and children, according to some Republican governors.

As the federal government has been attempting to control escalating Medicare costs, the Centers for Medicare and Medicaid Services and individual states alike have been active in implementing cost controls and reductions in Medicaid eligibility and benefits. At the federal level, one of the most significant measures enacted has been the provision in the Balanced Budget Act of 1997 allowing states to enroll Medicaid recipients in managed care health plans. Additionally, the Deficit Reduction Act of 2005 has attempted to reduce expenditures even more dramatically by calling for net Medicaid reductions of $4.8 billion over the next 5 years and $26.1 billion over the next 10 years (Kaiser Family Foundation, 2006, p. 1). These changes, if implemented as proposed, would primarily shift costs to beneficiaries, limiting access to services and healthcare coverage for low-income recipients. As this chapter is being written, these concerns have been the subject of intense debate in Congress.

Insuring Veterans, Active and Retired Military Personnel, and Their Families

This section covers federal health benefits for veterans, military personnel, and their family members under the Department of Defense's (DOD) medical facilities and **TRICARE plan**, the medical facilities of the **Department of Veterans Affairs (VA)** and **VA's Civilian Health and Medical Program (CHAMPVA)**, and other specialized programs. While everyone who served in the military is a veteran, only those who served for an extended period (normally 20 years) are retired. Health benefits described in this section are federal benefits or entitlements—technically, not insurance.

TRICARE and DOD

TRICARE is not an abbreviation; it is the title of the military health program. It covers active duty personnel, retired military personnel, and family members of both. DOD's medical facilities are considered part of TRICARE—there are 536 hospitals and clinics worldwide (Office of the Secretary of Defense, n.d.). DOD has contracted with various companies to provide health care in the private sector both in the United States and overseas. Figure 7-6 shows the demographics of the population covered by TRICARE.

TRICARE offers three separate programs: an HMO, a PPO, and a fee-for-service option. All active duty members are automatically enrolled at no cost in the HMO option called PRIME. Other categories must enroll. Retirees and their families pay an annual enrollment fee; active duty families do not. All enrollees (except active duty) have copays for office visits, prescription medication, diagnostic tests and hospitalization. Most preventive

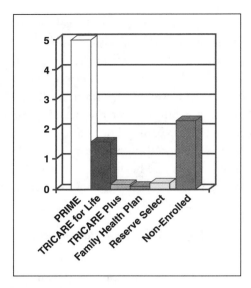

FIGURE 7-6 DOD Demographics (in millions)
Source: TRICARE, 2006b.

services are free. Individuals who do not elect to enroll in PRIME pay an annual deductible and have copays. Those that use the PPO (called **TRI-CARE Extra**) have a 20% copay, while those that use the fee-for-service option (called **TRICARE Standard**) are subject to a 25% copay. DOD offers all participants a mail-order pharmacy program. Dental services for active duty members are free; for others, there is an insurance plan where enrollees pay a monthly premium for covered services. There is no long-term care coverage under TRICARE.

The US Army, Navy, and Air Force operate military medical facilities around the world and afloat. DOD (versus the three military services organizations) manages the contracted arrangements, except in the limited case where contracts are issued by a medical facility—these are managed by the medical facility. Medical personnel from each of the three services provide staff to the DOD organizations that oversee the contracted arrangements.

Problems with TRICARE primarily focus on:

- the limited network of providers in rural areas;
- providing care to National Guard and Reserve personnel who alternate from active duty to inactive duty; and,

- ensuring there are sufficient providers to meet the needs of the 9.2 million beneficiaries (Office of the Secretary of Defense, n.d.).

These problems are normally addressed within DOD and the services, but veterans' organizations and the Congress take an active role in helping to ensure that beneficiaries receive access to quality services at a reasonable cost.

Veterans Affairs

The VA, through the Veterans Health Administration (VHA), operates the nation's largest healthcare system with over 160 medical centers and 1000 community clinics. Every VA medical center is affiliated with a national medical school. Unlike DOD, the VA does not differentiate between veterans who retired from the military and those that did not. Virtually all veterans are eligible for care in the VA, although those receiving less than honorable discharges or who left the service before serving 180 days, may have limited or no benefits. VHA operates its medical facilities in 22 regions called **Veteran Integrated Service Networks (VISN)**. VISN directors are responsible for providing or arranging care for enrolled veterans, as well as some who are not enrolled. Individuals who enroll are placed in one of eight categories based on disability or service, as shown in Table 7-4. VHA also purchases care from private providers when the VA does not have the needed service.

TABLE 7-4 VA Enrollment Categories (abbreviated explanation)

Category 1: Service connected (SC) veterans—50% or more disabled.

Category 2: SC veterans—30–40% disabled.

Category 3: SC veterans—10–20%; former Prisoners of War; Purple Heart Recipients.

Category 4: Vets receiving aid and attendance allowance or catastrophically disabled.

Category 5: Low income SC veterans with 0% disability and non-SC vets, vets receiving VA pension, vets eligible for Medicaid.

Category 6: WWI vets; Mexican Border War vets; compensable SC vets with 0% disability; vets seeking care for herbicide exposure (Vietnam), exposure to ionizing radiation, Gulf War illness, or who participated in Project SHAD (Shipboard Hazards and Defense).

Category 7: Vets with income above a certain limit and below the HUD (U.S. Department of Housing and Urban Development) geographic index who agree to pay copays for services.

Category 8: Same as Category 7 except above the HUD geographic index.

Source: US Department of Veterans Affairs, 2006.

Veterans who are in category 4 and above are provided virtually all their medical needs by the VA. Those in categories 5 through 8 are provided care primarily for conditions that the veteran incurred while in the military—called **service connected** conditions.

The VA leads the nation in providing quality care to veterans, as described in Table 7-5, and in its use of electronic medical records. When New Orleans was devastated by hurricanes in late 2005, not one veteran's medical record was lost.

Family members of selected veterans are provided care through the VA's special health benefits programs. If the veteran is not retired from the military and is rated permanently and totally disabled or died from a service connected condition, family members are eligible for the **CHAMPVA program**. CHAMPVA is a fee-for-service program patterned after the TRICARE fee-for-service option with an annual deductible and a 25% copay. Unlike TRICARE, CHAMPVA is operated completely by the VA

TABLE 7-5 VHA Performance Compared to Non VA

Clinical Performance Indicator	VA FY 05	HEDIS[2] Commercial 2004	HEDIS[2] Medicare 2004	HEDIS[2] Medicaid 2004
Breast cancer screening	86%	73%	74%	54%
Cervical cancer screening	92%	81%	Not Reported	65%
Colorectal cancer screening	76%	49%	53%	Not Reported
LDL Cholesterol < 100 after AMI, PTCA, CABG	Not Reported[3]	51%	54%	29%
LDL Cholesterol < 130 after AMI, PTCA, CABG	Not Reported[3]	68%	70%	41%
Beta blocker on discharge after AMI	98%	96%	94%	85%
Diabetes: HgbA1c done past year	96%	87%	89%	76%
Diabetes: Poor control HbA1c > 9.0% (lower is better)	17%	31%	23%	49%
Diabetes: Cholesterol (LDL-C) Screening	95%	91%	94%	80%

(*continued*)

TABLE 7-5 (*Continued*)

Clinical Performance Indicator	VA FY 05	HEDIS[2] Commercial 2004	HEDIS[2] Medicare 2004	HEDIS[2] Medicaid 2004
Diabetes: Cholesterol (LDL-C) controlled (<100)	60%	40%	48%	31%
Diabetes: Cholesterol (LDL-C) controlled (<130)	82%	65%	71%	51%
Diabetes: Eye Exam	79%	51%	67%	45%
Diabetes: Renal Exam	66%	52%	59%	47%
Hypertension: BP <= 140/90 most recent visit	77%	67%	65%	61%
Follow-up after Hospitalization for Mental Illness (30 days)	70%[4]	76%	61%	55%

Clinical Performance Indicator	VA FY 2005	HEDIS[2] Commercial 2004	HEDIS[2] Medicare 2004	BRFSS[2] 2004
Immunizations: influenza, (note patients age groups)[6][7]	75% (65 and older or high risk)	39% (50-64)	75% (65 and older)	68%
Immunizations: pneumococcal, (note patients age groups)[6]	89% (all ages at risk)	Not Reported	Not Reported (65 and older)	65%

Source: Office of Quality and Performance Updated 11-01-05.

1) Beginning with Qtr 4 of FY 2004 VA comparison data was obtained by abstracting medical record data using methodologies that matched HEDIS methodologies. The scores presented here are from those HEDIS mirrored extractions performed in the 4th Qtr of FY 04.

2) HEDIS Data was obtained from the 2005 "State of Health Care Quality Report" available on the NCQA website: www.ncqa.org

3) HEDIS mirrors for these measures were changed to include vascular diseases in addition to AMI. VHA initiated capture of expanded definition in FY 06. Scores will be posted when sufficent size threshold has been obtained.

4) HEDIS calculates score for MH follow-up on a calendar year (Jan-Dec), VHA calculates on FY (Oct-Sept).

5) BRFSS reports are available on the CDC website: www.cdc.gov

6) BRFSS (survey) scores are median scores. VA scores are averages obtained by medical record abstraction in 2003 - 2004 Influenza seasons (Sept 03 to Jan 04 and Sept 04 to Jan 05).

7) The influenza vaccine shortage in the fall of 2004 resulted in disparities in distribution and a change in targeted populations that impacted scores.

Source: U.S. Department of Veterans Affairs, 2005.

and not through contractors. If a veteran is a Vietnam veteran or served in Korea between 1967–1971 near the Demilitarized Zone (DMZ) and his or her child has **spina bifida**, a disorder involving incomplete development of the brain, spinal cord, and/or their protective coverings, (except for spina bifida occulta), the VA provides 100% coverage for conditions associated with spina bifida under the Spina Bifida Healthcare Program. For women Vietnam veterans who have children with certain birth defects, the VA provides 100% coverage for the related condition under the Children of Women Vietnam Veterans Healthcare Program. Both the Spina Bifida Healthcare Program and the Children of Women Vietnam Veterans Healthcare Program were established because of veteran's exposure to **Agent Orange**, a defoliant used extensively in Vietnam and near the DMZ in Korea. Figure 7-7 displays the VA population demographics.

Problems with VA health programs are addressed through typical patient advocate activities. As with DOD, veteran organizations and the Congress play very active roles in the oversight of the VA's health system. The VA has problems providing services in rural areas, much like the DOD. Also, the large number of Guard and Reserve members serving in Operation Iraq Freedom and Operation Enduring Freedom, who contin-

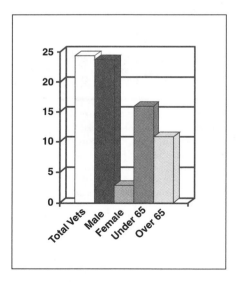

FIGURE 7-7 VA 2005 Demographics (in millions)
Source: U.S. Department of Veteran's Affairs, 2005.

ually change status from active to inactive, sometimes have problems with continuity of care issues.

Financing for DOD and VA Health Programs

To obtain funds for their programs, the DOD and VA submit budgets to the Office of Management and Budget (OMB). OMB validates the requests and includes them in the President's request to the Congress, which appropriates funds for the operation of the health systems. Figure 7-8 shows the FY06 appropriations for DOD and VA health programs.

STATISTICS ON HEALTH INSURANCE COVERAGE AND COSTS

As a part of the U.S. Census Bureau's Current Population Survey, health insurance coverage data are collected on an annual basis. The data from 2004 indicated that 84.3% of the population had some type of coverage. The data presented in Figure 7-9 show the breakdown of health insurance by type of coverage.

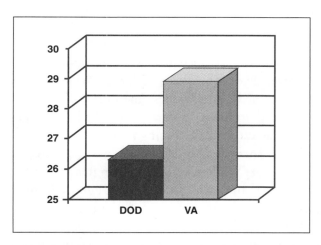

FIGURE 7-8 Appropriations, Fiscal Year 2006 (in billions)

Source: Department of Defense and VA, 2006. Note: these data do not include $10.B for the Medicare eligible retiree accrual fund. The VA appropriate includes only the appropriation for Veterans Health Administration and excludes information technology expenses.

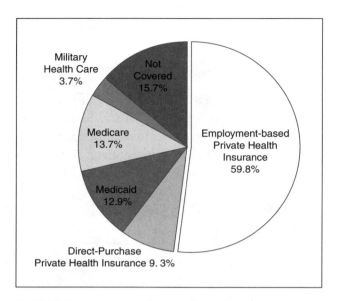

FIGURE 7-9 U.S. Health Insurance Coverage, 2004
Source: U.S. Census Bureau, 2005.

These data reflect only modest changes from the previous year. The individuals covered by some form of insurance increased by 2.0 million between 2003 and 2004. Coverage of individuals with employment-based private health insurance remained virtually the same during that time - period, while government health insurance programs absorbed the majority of this increase, with the largest increase coming in Medicaid.

At the outset of this chapter there was a brief discussion of the increases in the expenditures for health care. While government programs are funded primarily from taxes, payments to the Social Security Trust Fund, and cost-sharing by recipients, private health insurance must be financed by employers and employees. The costs of premiums for different types of health insurance, presented in Table 7-6, show the variation in the contributions toward premiums paid by employees and employers. Data are provided for individual policy holders, as well as for individuals opting for family coverage. These data also only reflect premiums and do not include deductibles, coinsurance, and/or copayments.

TABLE 7-6 Premiums Paid by Employees and Employers, 2005

Type of Plan	Employee Contribution	Employer Contribution	Total Premium
Individual coverage			
All plans	$ 610	$3,413	$ 4,024
Conventional	$ 498	$2,284	$ 3,782
HMO	$ 563	$3,203	$ 3,767
PPO	$ 603	$3,548	$ 4,150
POS	$ 731	$3,183	$ 3,914
Family coverage			
All plans	$2,713	$8,167	$10,880
Conventional	$2,321	$7,658	$ 9,979
HMO	$2,604	$7,852	$10,456
PPO	$2,641	$8,449	$11,090
POS	$3,250	$7,551	$10,801

Source: Kaiser Family Foundation and the Health Research and Educational Trust, 2005.

THOSE NOT COVERED—THE UNINSURED

As indicated earlier in Figure 7-9, 15.7% of the U.S. population was not covered by health insurance in 2004. This represented a slight increase in the uninsured population over 2003.

A breakdown of the data, as shown in Figure 7-10, indicates differences in those who are uninsured by racial group. For example, while Blacks made up 12.5% of the population in 2004, they accounted for 16.4% of the uninsured, and while Hispanics comprised only 14.3% of the population 30.2% of the uninsured were from this ethnic group. These disparities are a function of many things, among them differences in employment, eligibility for public programs, and income.

Additionally, when these numbers are broken down by age, the distribution shows that those without insurance coverage spanned all age groups in 2004. Figure 7-11 indicates that, while only a small number of those 65 and over were uninsured (as would be expected due to Medicare coverage), all other age groups include several million uninsured individuals, with more than 81% being adults. The largest groups were individuals under 35 years of age and the 8.7 million young adults aged 18 to 24 years. Another 8.3 million of the uninsured were children.

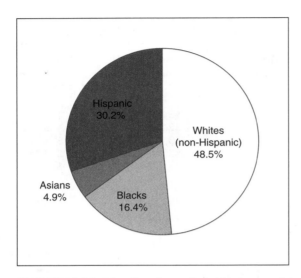

FIGURE 7-10 Distribution of the Uninsured by Race, 2004
Source: U.S. Census Bureau, 2005.

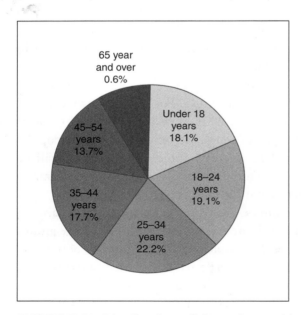

FIGURE 7-11 Distribution of the Uninsured by Age, 2004
Source: U.S. Census Bureau, 2005.

Research (Abel, 1998; Rowland, Lyons, Salganicoff, & Long, 1994) about other characteristics of the uninsured also helps us to understand who this population includes. The following are some of the key characteristics of these individuals.

- Approximately 25% were in families with incomes below the poverty level.
- Most were individuals from families with incomes above the poverty level, but many had incomes below 300% of the poverty level.
- More than four-fifths were workers or dependents of workers who were employed in industries that do not typically provide health insurance coverage.
- The percentages of individuals without health insurance coverage vary across the states. More people in states in the South and the West tend be uninsured than those living in the Midwest and East.
- Those who are uninsured have been shown to use the healthcare delivery system in different ways. Without coverage and/or ability to pay, studies have shown that the uninsured:
  - do not typically have a primary care physician;
  - delay seeking care until they are sicker; and,
  - utilize hospital emergency departments, the most expensive entry point to the healthcare system, to receive health care.

Additionally, the Kaiser Commission on Medicaid and the Uninsured has identified 10 myths associated with those who are uninsured as shown in Table 7-7.

Providing health care to the uninsured falls primarily to hospitals where much of it becomes uncompensated care. There are some funds available to assist hospitals through the federal government's disproportionate-share program that provides some funding for providing large amounts of uncompensated care. There are also state and local programs that help to support these hospitals. The cost of care provided to the uninsured is borne by the taxpayers, as well as by insured patients, with the costs of that care being passed along in the form of higher taxation and higher health insurance costs.

Addressing the problem of the uninsured has periodically been on the forefront of national health policy. Many policy analysts believe that developing a universal health insurance system is the only way to bring these individuals into coverage, while others think that we should let the market

TABLE 7-7 Ten Myths about the Uninsured

Myth	Fact
The uninsured go without coverage because they believe they do not need or do not want it.	The majority of uninsured, regardless of how young they are, say they forgo coverage because they cannot afford it, not because they do not need it.
Most of the uninsured do not have health insurance because they are not working, so they do not have access to health benefits through an employer.	Most of the uninsured are either working full-time or have someone in their immediate family who does—the problem is that the majority of the uninsured are not offered benefits through their employers.
Most of the growth in the uninsured has been among those with higher incomes.	The majority of the growth in the uninsured since 2000 has been among people earning less than $38,000 a year for a family of four (commonly considered low-income).
Most of the uninsured are new immigrants who are U.S. citizens.	The large majority of the uninsured (79%) are American citizens.
The uninsured often receive health services for free or at reduced charges.	Free or even discounted health services are not common and when the uninsured are unable to pay the full costs, the unpaid medical bills add to their providers' costs.
The uninsured can get the care they need when they really need it and are able to avoid serious health problems.	The uninsured are more likely to postpone and forgo care with serious consequences that increase their chances of preventable health problems, disability, and premature death.
Buying health insurance coverage on your own is always an option.	Individually purchased policies—vs. job-based group policies with similar benefits—are more expensive and coverage can be limited or even denied to persons in less than good health.
We do not really know how large the uninsured problem is and many are only uninsured for brief periods.	Depending on whether we count the number of people who are uninsured during a specific month, for an entire year, or just for short periods, the numbers will differ; and all measures are useful.
The health care the uninsured receive, but do not pay for, results in higher insurance premiums.	The large majority of uncompensated care is subsidized through a mix of federal and state government dollars not cost-shifts to private payers.
Expanding health insurance coverage to all, or even a large share of the uninsured, will cost far more than the country currently spends on health care.	Because both the uninsured and government subsidies pay for a good share of their healthcare costs already, the amount of additional health spending to cover all of the uninsured is relatively small.

Source: Kaiser Commission on Medicaid and the Uninsured/Kaiser Family Foundation, n.d.

address the problem. As the problem of the uninsured becomes increasingly worse and access to healthcare coverage begins to impact middle class Americans, it is likely that politicians will address this issue.

CONCLUSION

There are two primary ways that health insurance issues impact healthcare managers. The first relates to managing the health insurance benefit for employees and their dependents. In this regard, managers need to understand the options available to them in selecting plans that meet the needs of their employees, as well as meet the needs of the company. In the case of the latter, the affordability of providing health benefits to employees is becoming an increasingly difficult proposition. As part of this issue, managers are increasingly being called on to try to reduce the costs of coverage, to select cost-effective health plans, to encourage employees to manage their care better, and to take steps to have employees bear more of the cost of coverage.

The second way that health insurance is important for managers is related to patients—their insurance coverage and how they receive reimbursement from their insurers. Managing the patient health insurance function well is clearly critical to the financial success and viability of the organization. Issues relating to coding, billing, and other aspects of this are discussed further in Chapter 8.

DISCUSSION QUESTIONS

1. What factors make it difficult to provide healthcare coverage for everyone in the United States? How could more people be brought into coverage?

2. Compare and contrast fee-for-service and prepaid health plans.

3. What types of cost sharing in health insurance are most effective?

4. What are the pros and cons of the different types of health insurance benefit packages that someone might purchase?

5. What is the best type of health insurance? Justify your answer.

6. Compare and contrast Medicare and Medicaid in terms of eligibility, benefit packages, access to care, and other key dimensions.

7. How does the SCHIP add to coverage provided under the Medicaid Program?

8. What issues and concerns have arisen relating to Medicare Part D? How can they be resolved?

9. Discuss the different types of healthcare coverage/health insurance that are provided to military personnel and their dependents.

REFERENCES

Abel, P. (1998, April). *1997 Colorado health source book: insurance, access & expenditures*. Denver, CO: Colorado Coalition for Health Care Access and Coalition for the Medically Underserved.

American Academy of Actuaries. (2005, March). *Medicare's financial condition: Beyond actuarial balance*. Issue Brief. Washington, DC: American Academy of Actuaries.

Borger, C., Smith, S., Truffer, C., Keehan, S., Sisko, A., Poisal, J., et al. (2006, January/February). Health spending projections through 2015: Changes on the horizon. *Health Affairs, 25*(2), 61–73.

Centers for Medicare and Medicaid Services. (2003). *Data compendium, 2003 edition*. Retrieved May 21, 2006, from http://www.cms.hhs.gov/DataCompendium/02_2003_Data Compendium.asp

Centers for Medicare and Medicaid Services. (2004). *2004 Mid-season review*. Baltimore, MD: Centers for Medicare and Medicaid Services, Office of the Actuary, 2004.

Centers for Medicare and Medicaid Services. (2006, February). *National health care expenditures projections: 2005–2015*. Baltimore, MD: Centers for Medicare and Medicaid Services, Office of the Actuary. Retrieved March 29, 2006, from http://www.cms.hhs.gov/NationalHealthExpendData/03_NationalHealthAccountsProjected.asp

DeNavas-Walt, C., Proctor, B. D., & Lee, C. H. (2005). *Income, poverty, and health insurance coverage in the United States: 2004*. Current Population Reports. U.S. Census Bureau. Washington, DC: U.S. Government Printing Office, 60–229.

Feldstein, P. J. (2005). *Health care economics (6th ed.)*. Clifton Park, NY: Thomson Delmar Learning.

Hurley, R. E., Strunk, B. C. & White, J. S. (2004, March/April). The puzzling popularity of the PPO. *Health Affairs, 23*(2), 56–68.

Kaiser Commission on Medicaid and the Uninsured/Kaiser Family Foundation. (2006, January). *The public, managed care, and consumer protections*. Menlo Park, CA: Kaiser Family Foundation.

Kaiser Commission on Medicaid and the Uninsured/Kaiser Family Foundation. (n.d.) *Myths about the Uninsured.* Menlo Park, CA: Kaiser Family Foundation.

Kaiser Family Foundation. (2005a). *Medicare chart book* (3rd *ed.*). Menlo Park, CA: Kaiser Family Foundation.

Kaiser Family Foundation. (2005b). *Total Medicaid spending, FY 2004.* Kaiser Commission on Medicaid and the Uninsured. Retrieved March 29, 2006, from http://www.statehealthfacts.org

Kaiser Family Foundation. (2006, February). *Deficit Reduction Act of 2005: Implications for Medicaid.* Menlo Park, CA: Kaiser Commission on Medicaid and the Uninsured.

Kaiser Family Foundation and the Health Research and Educational Trust. (2005, September). *Employer health benefits 2005 annual survey.* Menlo Park, CA: Kaiser Family Foundation and Health Research and Educational Trust.

Levit, K. R., Lazenby, H. C., Braden, B. R., Cowan, C. A., Sensenig, A. L., McDonnell, P. A., et al. (1997, Fall). National health expenditures, 1996. *Health Care Financing Review, 19,* 161–200.

Office of the Secretary of Defense. (n.d.). *Health affairs senior leaders briefing.*

Medicare Board of Trustees. (2005, March). *2005 Annual Report of the Boards of Trustees of the Federal Hospital Insurance and Federal Supplementary Medical Insurance Trust Funds.* Baltimore, MD: Centers for Medicare and Medicaid Services.

Prologue: Medicaid in the health insurance market. (Prologue). (2004, March/April). *Health Affairs, 23*(2).

Rowland, D., Lyons, B., Salganicoff, A., & Long, P. (1994, Spring). A profile of the uninsured in America. *Health Affairs,* 13, 283–289.

Saleem, H. T. (2003, December). *Health Spending Accounts.* U.S. Bureau of Labor Statistics.

Starr, P. (1982). *The social transformation of American medicine.* New York: Basic Books.

TRICARE. (2006a). *Stakeholders report—Military medicine transforming the future.* Falls Church, VA: TRICARE Management Activity. Retrieved June 9, 2006, from http://www.tricare.osd.mil/stakeholders/downloads/stakeholders_2006.pdf

TRICARE. (2006b). *Understanding TRICARE for life.* Retrieved September 28, 2006, from http://www.military.com/Resources/ResourcesContent/0,13964,30818—0,00.html

U.S. Department of Veterans Affairs. (2005, April). *VetPop 2004 Version 1.0.* Retrieved June 9, 2006, from http://www.va.gov/vetdata/

U.S. Department of Veterans Affairs. (2006, March). Health Care Enrollment Priority Groups, Fact Sheet 163-2. Retrieved June 9, 2006, from http://www.va.gov/healtheligibility/Library/EPG/Enrollment Priority Group.pdf

U.S. Department of Veterans Affairs, Veterans Health Administration Office of Quality and Performance. (2005). VA's Performance Compared to Non-VA. Retrieved June 9, 2006, from the VA Intranet website.

Wilensky, G. R. (2006, January/February). Consumer-driven health plans: Early evidence and potential impact on hospitals, *Health Affairs, 25*(1), 174–185.

CHAPTER 8

Managing Costs and Revenues

Suzanne Discenza

LEARNING OBJECTIVES

By the end of this chapter the student will be able to describe:

- The importance, purpose, and major objectives of financial management in healthcare organizations;
- Tax status implications of for-profit versus not-for-profit healthcare entities and the organizational structure of the financial components of these organizations;
- The primary methods of reimbursement to providers from private health plans and from government-sponsored programs such as Medicare and Medicaid;
- Methods for classifying and controlling costs, including the processes of cost allocation, determining product costs, and break-even analysis;
- Determinants and initial processes considered by healthcare managers in setting charges/prices for the products and services provided by their organizations;
- The purposes, primary sources, and major problems associated with managing working capital;
- Some of the important issues and major processes involved in managing accounts receivable in healthcare organizations;

- The importance, basic tenets, and commonly accepted methods for managing materials and inventory in hospitals and other healthcare entities; and,
- The major characteristics and types of budgets utilized by healthcare managers, and the major processes involved in cash versus capital budgeting.

INTRODUCTION

Students in healthcare management and administration frequently become apprehensive about that portion of their academic preparation and career progression dealing with the financial management aspects of the field. It is the goal of this chapter to dissect, clarify, and provide a general overview of the various components of financial management within healthcare organizations, providing examples and application that are user-friendly to students with a non-financial orientation.

WHAT IS FINANCIAL MANAGEMENT AND WHY IS IT IMPORTANT?

Healthcare financial management may be defined as the process of providing oversight of the healthcare organization's day-to-day financial operations as well as planning the organization's long-range financial direction. Put even more simply, it is involved in increasing the revenues and decreasing the costs of the organization.

To accomplish these goals, the finance departments of most healthcare organizations have been charged with two primary functions, accounting and finance:

- *Accounting* consists of two types:
  1. **Managerial accounting,** in which financial data are provided concurrently or prospectively to internal users (managers, executives, and the organization's governing board).
  2. **Financial accounting,** in which data are provided retrospectively to external users (stockholders, lenders, insurers, government, suppliers).

- *Finance* generally includes:
  1. Borrowing and investing funds.
  2. Analyzing accounting information to evaluate past decisions and make sound future decisions.

While Nowicki (2004, p. 4) emphasizes financial management's primary purpose as being "to provide both accounting and finance information that assists healthcare managers in accomplishing the organization's purposes" Berger (2002, p. 7) takes this description of purpose one step further by noting that "a primary role of financial management [is] helping to analyze the financial implications of the data across the healthcare organization's setting." The latter implies the importance of involving managers at all levels of the organization in financial analysis and decision making. For example, the manager in the radiology unit of a hospital should be directly involved in looking at both the revenues generated by procedures performed in the department (X-rays, ultrasound procedures, CT scans, etc.) and the expenses incurred in running the department, in order to be involved in hiring personnel, managing appropriate staffing ratios, making decisions involving the replacement or purchase of equipment, and so on.

TEN MAJOR OBJECTIVES OF FINANCIAL MANAGEMENT

Numerous experts on healthcare financial management have attempted to enumerate the major objectives of healthcare financial management (Gapenski, 2003; McLean, 2003; Nowicki, 2004; Zelman, McCue, Millikan, & Glick, 2003; and Berger, 2002). The following "Top Ten" list includes some of the most-commonly mentioned:

- *Generating a reasonable net income*, through billing and collecting revenues generated by the operation, and by effectively managing current assets.
- *Setting prices* (gross charges) for services provided by the healthcare organization.
- *Facilitating relationships and managing contracts with third-party payers* (i.e., Medicare, Medicaid, managed care organizations, and other insurers) and *influencing method and amount of payment,*

including discounts and capitated prices in exchange for large volumes of patients.

- *Recording and analyzing cost information* across the organization and at the department level, including comparing actual to budgeted costs.
- *Investing in long-term capital assets,* including new plant and equipment acquisition, to not only support operations but also to keep the healthcare organization competitive in today's rapidly-changing healthcare environment.
- *Preparing, auditing, and disseminating the financial reports* for the healthcare organization to allow stakeholders to determine the organization's financial performance and to help guide the organization's future goals.
- *Ensuring that the payroll is covered and that the suppliers are paid.*
- *Protecting the healthcare organization's tax status:*
  1. If not-for-profit, protecting its tax-exempt status.
  2. If for-profit, seeking ways to reduce its tax liability.
- *Responding to government regulators, accrediting agencies, external auditors, and quality consultants* in a timely and cost-effective manner.
- *Controlling financial risk to the organization,* through monitoring medical staff and their potential financial liability to the organization (in terms of ordering patterns and possible negligence), and through following accepted accounting practices, implementing compliance and risk management programs, etc.

Based on this list alone, it is no wonder that financial management is often considered "the most important predictor of whether healthcare organizations will survive in the current competitive climate and beyond" (Nowicki, 2004, p. 15).

TAX STATUS OF HEALTHCARE ORGANIZATIONS

In order to fully comprehend the financial needs and constraints of any given healthcare organization, it is important to first determine the tax status of that organization. Although primarily categorized as either for-profit or not-for-profit, Berger (2002, p. 29–30) discusses three major types of healthcare organizations, one for-profit and two not-for-profit. For clearer understanding by the student, they have been arranged somewhat differently below, and additional comments have been included:

- *For-profit, Investor-owned Healthcare Organizations:*
  These organizations are owned by investors or others with a private equity interest, provide goods and services with the objective of maximizing profits for the owner's benefit, and pay taxes. Traditionally this has included most physician practices and skilled nursing facilities.
- *Not-for-profit Healthcare Organizations:*
  Historically, these organizations have taken care of the poor, needy, and indigent residents of communities and thus have been granted tax-exempt status. They include the following two groups:
  1. *Business-oriented (private) organizations:*
     Private enterprises with no ownership interests; self-sustaining from fees charged for goods and services; exempt from income taxes and may receive tax-deductible contributions from those who support their mission; must provide a certain amount of charity care or community service. Based on its roots with many religious-affiliated organizations, it is not surprising that this group has included an overwhelming majority of hospitals.
  2. *Government-owned organizations and public corporations:*
     Influenced by political interests, but exempt from taxation; includes organizations that have the ability to issue directly (rather than through state or municipal authority) debt that pays interest exempt from federal taxation. Included in this group are government-owned hospitals (especially research and training institutions, or those serving the medically indigent) and public health clinics.

Table 8-1 delineates the primary differences between for-profit and not-for-profit healthcare organizations:

In addition, there are significant differences in financial management goals based on tax status, which can be summarized as follows:

- *Financial Goals in For-profit Organizations:* According to Berman, Weeks, and Kukla (1986, p. 4), "management must administer the assets of the enterprise in order to obtain the greatest wealth for the owner," that is, the goal is to maximize earnings and profits while minimizing risk to the organization.

TABLE 8-1 Comparison of For-Profit and Not-for-Profit Organizations

For-Profit	Not-for-Profit
Serve private interests.	Serve public or community interests.
Pay federal and state income taxes on profits, state and local sales taxes, and property taxes.	Are tax-exempt; healthcare organizations receive 501(c)(3) designation if meet federal IRS criteria.
Must file an annual for-profit tax return.	Must file the IRS 990 annual corporate tax return, including a community service benefits report.
Are motivated by profit, with income benefiting individuals.	Revenues cannot benefit individuals beyond reasonable salaries.
Must pay business fees	Are exempt from paying most business fees and licenses.
Must adhere to taxable bond yields.	Can access tax-exempt bond markets to raise capital.
May participate in political campaigns and influence legislation.	May not participate in political campaigns nor influence legislation.
Able to issue stock to raise capital and offer stock options to recruit and retain staff.	May not issue stock or offer stock options to staff.
Have limited obligation to provide indigent care.	Must provide designated amounts of community benefit, including indigent care.

- *Financial Goals in Not-for-profit Organizations:* According to Berger (2002, p. 6), while management must still "produce the best possible bottom line . . . they simply need to do so in the context of providing optimal patient care in the most efficient manner." However, Berger and Nowicki (2004) both emphasize that nonprofit healthcare providers still place somewhat greater emphasis on community services and other social goals.

FINANCIAL GOVERNANCE AND RESPONSIBILITY STRUCTURE

Finally, the organizational structure of these healthcare organizations may also be affected by their tax status, although the largest differences are probably seen in the structure of their governing bodies, or Boards of Directors. While similar types of professionals (or "volunteers," in the case of not-for-profit Boards) are specifically charged with financial accountability and stewardship, in smaller organizations one individual may perform several of the separate functions. Knowing the organizational structure of the financial components of the organization will allow all managers to access the appropriate individual(s) in order to make judicious financial decisions for their departments or divisions. In order of responsibility:

- *The Governing Body, or Board of Directors:* As described by the American Hospital Association (AHA, 1990) and reiterated by Nowicki (2004, p. 30), in its "fiduciary" role (persons in a position of trust) the Board is ultimately "responsible for the proper development, utilization, and maintenance of all resources in the healthcare organization." In for-profit organizations, Board members may be paid, but Board members serve strictly as "volunteers" in not-for-profit organizations.
- *The Chief Executive Officer (CEO)* is hired and delegated authority by the Board and serves as chief administrator of the operations of the entire organization. The CEO's fiscal performance is monitored through the Board's Finance Committee.
- *The Chief Operating Officer (COO),* often the Senior Vice President, is responsible for the day-to-day operations of the organization.
- *The Chief Financial Officer (CFO),* who may also serve as a vice president, is responsible for the entire financial management function of the organization. The CFO is in charge of two primary financial branches, involving: 1) the accounting function, and 2) management of financial assets. The CFO directly supervises two officers (and occasionally one other) directly in charge of these functions:
  - *The Controller* (also called the Comptroller) is the chief accounting officer responsible for the accounting and reporting functions, including financial record keeping. He/she oversees such departments and activities as patient accounts, accounts payable, accounts receivable, cost analysis, budgets, tax status, the generation of financial reports, and sometimes internal auditing.
  - *The Treasurer* is charged with the stewardship of the organization's financial assets, including cash management, commercial bank relations, investment portfolios, management of pensions or endowment funds, capital expenditures, management of working capital, and long-term debt obligations.
  - *The Internal Auditor* is often a separate staff position from the CFO in large healthcare organizations and is responsible for ensuring that the accounting, bookkeeping, and reporting processes are performed in accordance with **Generally Accepted Accounting**

Principles (GAAP), the nationally accepted rules that determine how financial information is recorded and reported. GAAP includes, among other things, the overarching ideas of conservatism, consistency, and matching of revenues and costs. The internal auditor protects the organization's assets from fraud, error, and loss.

- *The Chief Information Officer (CIO),* present in many large healthcare organizations, is the corporate officer responsible for all information and data processing systems, including medical records, data processing, medical information systems, and admitting. The CIO reports either to the CFO or directly to the CEO.
- *The Independent Auditor,* generally a large accounting firm, is retained by the healthcare organization to ensure that all financial reports sent to external entities are accurate as to format, content, and scope in presenting the organization's true financial position.
- *All Managers* in a healthcare organization are financial managers to the extent that they consider asset selection, charges, financing, reimbursement, and/or department budgets. This shared responsibility at all levels of the organization serves to maximize efficiency and accountability.

MANAGING REIMBURSEMENTS FROM THIRD-PARTY PAYERS

As discussed above, as one of the ten major objectives of financial management, facilitating and managing third-party reimbursements is vital to generating revenues for the daily operations, growth, and competitiveness of the healthcare organization. This section will discuss both the methods of payment to providers by managed care organizations (MCOs) and other private insurers and reimbursements to providers from public entities such as Medicare and Medicaid.

WHAT ARE THE PRIMARY METHODS OF PAYMENT USED BY PRIVATE HEALTH PLANS FOR REIMBURSING PROVIDERS?

Private healthcare plans use a variety of methods for reimbursing the providers servicing the plan's enrollees. Some are utilized more frequently than others for payments to different provider groups. They are classified according to the amount of financial risk assumed by healthcare organizations, and whether reimbursements are determined after or before health-care services are delivered.

Retrospective Reimbursement

With retrospective reimbursement, the amount of reimbursement is determined *after* the delivery of services, providing little financial risk to providers in most cases. It can involve the following methods:

- *Charges*, most commonly called **fee-for-service**: Healthcare providers are paid close to or at 100% of their submitted prices or rates for care provided. Because there is virtually no financial risk to providers, these are no longer common. Unfortunately, where full charges persist is with uninsured individuals who have not had insurance companies that negotiated discounted rates on their behalf.
- *Charges Minus a Discount* or *Percentage of Charges:* Healthcare organizations offer discounted charges to third parties in return for large numbers of patients. This is the second most common form of reimbursement to hospitals.
- *Cost Plus a Percentage for Growth:* Healthcare institutions receive the cost for care provided plus a small percentage to develop new services and products.
- *Cost:* The organization is reimbursed for the projected cost, expressed as a percentage of charges. While this method provides the smallest amount of reimbursement to providers, there is little risk unless full costs (direct plus indirect) are not recognized.
- *Reimbursement Modified on the Basis of Performance:* The provider is reimbursed based on quality measures, patient satisfaction measures, etc. Obviously, this method poses more risk for providers.

Prospective Reimbursement

This method of reimbursement to providers is established *before* the services are provided to patients. These are the primary methods utilized by managed care organizations (MCOs):

- *Per Diem*, in which a defined dollar amount per day for care is provided. This is the most common method of reimbursement to hospitals. It presents risks and incentives. It tends to be bad for acute only patients for which greater costs are incurred earlier in care, without the opportunity to make up differences later when less intense services may be needed.

- *Per Diagnosis*, in which a defined dollar amount is paid per diagnosis. It provides risks and incentives. Most common are those similar to the rates utilized by CMS (Centers for Medicare and Medicaid) for Medicare reimbursements, including DRGs for hospitals, RUGs for nursing homes, and HHRGs for home health care. Additional rates have more recently been determined for outpatient and inpatient rehabilitation hospital services. In virtually all cases, fewer patient treatments or visits, and/or shorter hospital stays, are now being provided for any given diagnosis.
- *Bundles for Hospital and Physician Services*, in which a fixed amount is paid by the MCO for treatment of a patient and is to be shared by all providers.
- *Fee Schedule by CPT Code*, or procedure code, which is the most common method for reimbursement of specialty physicians. The more complex and time-consuming the procedure, generally the higher will be the rate of reimbursement.
- *Capitation*, which is an agreement under which a healthcare provider is paid a fixed amount per enrollee per month by a health plan in exchange for a contractually specified set of medical services in the future. Negotiated capitated payments are based on perceptions of expenses for a population. Thus, capitation shifts the risk of coverage from the insurer to the provider of care, providing the most financial risk but also the most opportunity. It is the most common reimbursement method for primary care physicians in MCOs, providing penalties and withholdings for too much care and bonuses as an incentive for ordering lower levels of care.

The third-party reimbursement system in the healthcare arena has become so complex that many healthcare providers (including hospitals and large physician practices) have been forced to hire employees specializing in different contract types within their insurance/finance departments to negotiate the labyrinth of rules and regulations. While the following quote could easily apply to government-sponsored payers (e.g., Medicare or Medicaid), Berger (2002, p. 109) addresses the reimbursement methods of MCOs:

Not only do managed care companies have all of these ways to reimburse providers, but also the providers could contract with dozens of managed care companies during any given year. This means that the provider, whether a hospital, a physician, a home health agency, or a SNF, needs a mechanism or tool to keep track of the deal being signed. Otherwise, it cannot prepare monthly financial statements that include managed care contractual adjustments. Providers have had to make significant adjustments in operating structure to accommodate the decreased reimbursements from MCOs.

WHAT ARE THE PRIMARY METHODS OF PAYMENT USED FOR REIMBURSING PROVIDERS BY MEDICARE AND MEDICAID?

The largest government-sponsored healthcare programs in the United States, known as Medicare and Medicaid, were signed into law in 1965 in an effort to provide health insurance for the growing numbers of uninsured elderly and for the otherwise medically indigent. As described in Chapter 7, "Financing Health Care and Health Insurance," the number of Medicare and Medicaid enrollees increased much more rapidly than had been anticipated and was accompanied by an exponential rise in healthcare expenditures. By the early 1980s the federal government became aware of the need to pass additional legislation to start reining in the skyrocketing costs in these programs. The current regulations regarding reimbursement to providers in these programs are reflective of various cost containment efforts.

Reimbursement to Hospitals and Contractual Allowances

Due to rapidly rising healthcare expenditures based on an initial retrospective, charge-based reimbursement system to providers, Congress passed the Tax Equity and Fiscal Responsibility Act (TEFRA) in 1982, with particular emphasis on Medicare cost controls. Among its provisions included a mandate to hospitals for a prospective payment system (PPS) with reimbursement rates established up-front for certain conditions, the option of providing managed care plans to Medicare beneficiaries, and the requirement that Medicare become the secondary payer when a beneficiary had other insurance.

Like most third-party payers for hospital services, the Centers for Medicare and Medicaid Services (CMS, formerly known as HCFA) substantially reduces reimbursement to hospitals (from original hospital charges to beneficiaries) based on a system of contractual allowances. As defined by McLean (2003, p. 53), a **contractual allowance** is the "difference between the charge for a bed-day in the adult medicine unit and the amount that the hospital has agreed to accept from the patient's insurance carrier."

In the case of Medicare-eligible patients, CMS reimburses a fixed amount *per admission* and *per diagnosis*, based on the patient's **diagnosis-related group**, or **DRG** (a prospective payment system for hospitals established through the Social Security Amendments of 1983). In this scenario, for example, a patient being admitted for heart bypass surgery would receive a higher reimbursement rate than a patient admitted for observation after a fall in which he/she suffered a fractured humerus (arm bone). Berger (2002, p. 127) asserts that the International Classification of Diseases, ninth edition (ICD-9 codes), is "the most important element" in creating the DRG for reimbursement of an inpatient stay. Further, the Omnibus Budget Reconciliation Act of 1990 later folded capital costs into DRG rates as well, with hospitals risking significant reimbursement losses if their buildings and equipment are not properly utilized (Nowicki, 2004).

On the other hand, the Medicaid reimbursement rate to hospitals for any given service varies from state to state, but in all cases includes a substantial contractual allowance. Individual states implement cost controls for Medicaid payments, using either DRGs (like Medicare) or **case mix** to set reimbursement rates. Case mix, also referred to as **patient mix**, is usually related to the mix of patients served by an organization based on the severity of illnesses. An example of differences in this type of reimbursement would be a nursing unit primarily serving patients on ventilators that would be reimbursed at a substantially higher rate than a nursing unit serving patients with orthopedic problems due to the greater expenses incurred by the former. In all cases, providers must accept reimbursement as payment in full and follow designated efficiency and quality standards.

Reimbursement to Physicians

Concerning reimbursement for physician office services to Medicare beneficiaries, the Resource-Based Relative Value System (RBRVS) was implemented in 1992. This system pays a prospective flat fee for physician visits, and is based on HCPCS (Healthcare Common Procedure Coding System) codes used by outpatient healthcare providers and medical suppliers to code their professional services and supplies. *The Physician's Current Procedural Terminology*, fourth edition (CPT-4), is the generally accepted coding methodology utilized. An example of this system is the higher reimbursement rate afforded to a physician for an extended initial patient visit to fully assess a patient's medical condition, versus the lower reimbursement provided for a brief follow-up visit to assess how well a prescribed medication was working.

Similarly, state Medicaid programs have implemented cost controls for reimbursement to physicians, initially through fee schedules, but with many states more recently following the state option (as provided by the Balanced Budget Act of 1997) to require beneficiaries to enroll in capitated managed care plans. As defined by Gapenski (2003, p. 576), **capitation** is "a flat periodic payment per enrollee to a healthcare provider; it is the sole reimbursement for providing defined services to a defined population . . . Generally, capitation payments are expressed as some dollar amount per member per month (PMPM)."

Medicare Reimbursements to Other Providers

Despite reductions in reimbursements for hospital admissions and physician visits, Medicare expenditures continued to soar throughout the 1990s. Congress passed the Balanced Budget Act of 1997 in an attempt to control costs for other healthcare services. Prospective payment systems were implemented in other settings beginning in 1998, as follows:

- Skilled nursing facilities (SNFs), in 1998, with RUGs (Resource Utilization Groups);
- Home health agencies (HHAs), in 2000, with HHRGs (Home Health Resource Groups); and,
- Outpatient hospitals and clinics, in 2002, with OPPS (Outpatient Prospective Payment System).

HOW ARE PROVIDERS REIMBURSED BY INDIVIDUALS WITH NO HEALTH INSURANCE?

As discussed above, those individuals who are not covered by any type of health plan, whether private or public, are often billed for full charges (generally well above costs) by the healthcare organization delivering the care. This is largely due to the inability of the uninsured individual to negotiate a discounted rate for his/her care that is usually afforded patients covered by group health plans. This phenomenon has had the unfortunate consequence of substantially increasing the number of personal bankruptcies related to medical bills. As revealed in a frequently-cited article in the journal *Health Affairs*, approximately half of the 1.458 million personal bankruptcies filed in 2001 were related to medical bills caused by injury and illness (Himmelstein, Warren, Thorne, & Woolhandler, 2005, w5.63). As a direct result, there have been increases in the amount of uncompensated, or unreimbursed, care.

Not Covered, or **Uncompensated Care**, is a measure of total hospital care provided without payment from the patient or an insurer. This accounted for 5.6% of hospital total expenses in 2004, down from 6.2% in 1999 (AHA 2005). The two major types include:

- *Bad Debt*, in which the healthcare organization bills for services but receives no payment. These operating expenses are based on charges, not costs, and are written off by the organization. This term is usually used with for-profit organizations.
- *Charity Care*, in which the not-for-profit organization provides care to a patient who it knows will be unable to pay. Level of charity care (based on either costs or charges) must be documented in footnotes to the financial statements, otherwise the organization's tax status can be questioned.

Although uncompensated care may be written off as bad debt or charity care by the healthcare organization, and is even required to a certain extent with a not-for-profit organization to maintain its 501(c)(3) status, it is important for managers to recognize that providing too much of this type of care could serve to financially cripple the organization, both in terms of difficulty in maintaining current operations and inability to maximize investment opportunities. Some for-profit organizations question the tax status of not-for-profit organizations and their ability to write off debt as "charity care." They also decry the use of the term "bad debt," because it implies that the manager who extended the credit used poor judgment. This is a controversial topic and one that bears watching.

CONTROLLING COSTS AND COST ACCOUNTING

Historically, healthcare organizations, especially hospitals, have been provided strong financial incentives to maximize reimbursements rather than to control costs. However, as can be seen in the preceding discussion, there has been a major movement during much of the past two decades to decrease the levels of reimbursement to providers in almost all sectors of the industry. It has thus become increasingly important for these organizations to understand how to estimate and manage their costs. This changing environment has also resulted in separation of "cost accounting systems from financial accounting systems" and movement "from traditional allocation-based cost systems to activity-based cost systems" (Zelman et al. 2003, p. 15).

While Nowicki (2004, p. 145) describes its purpose as providing managers with cost information for such reasons as "setting charges and profitability analysis," it is important to note that cost accounting ultimately leads to decision making. This might include enhancing departments that are making money, eliminating services that are losing money, and carefully managing **loss leaders** (i.e., procedures provided cheaply or below cost to attract customers to the organization). Cost accounting also provides methods for classifying and allocating costs, as well as more precisely determining product costs, all of which will be described briefly in this section.

CLASSIFYING COSTS

Although there are a number of ways in which costs may be classified, the purpose of the following table (Table 8-2) is to illustrate a sampling of the most frequently-utilized methods. The importance of such systems is merely to provide a point of departure for controlling costs.

While many authors provide a concise summary of the major methods of classifying costs such as those shown above (Zelman et al., 2003; Nowicki, 2004), they do not show how these classifications are often combined by managerial accountants to demonstrate the complexity of cost analysis within healthcare organizations. For example, concerning salaries and wages in hospitals, the salaries of radiology department managers are both

TABLE 8-2 Frequently-utilized Methods of Classifying Costs

Method	Classification	Example
By Behavior	Fixed Costs—stay the same in relation to changes in volume of services	Electricity for lighting
	Variable Costs—change directly in relation to changes in volume	Number of sutures used to close incisions
By Traceability	Direct Costs—can be traced to a particular patient, product, or service	Gauze pads used in dressing a wound
	Indirect Costs—cannot be traced to a particular patient or service	Amount of water used during a typical hospital stay
	Full Costs—both direct costs and indirect costs	Treatments provided plus utilities used
By Decision-Making Capability	Controllable Costs—under the manager's influence	Wages of CNAs per shift
	Uncontrollable costs—cannot be controlled by the manager	Upper administrative hours allocated to department
	Sunk costs—already incurred and cannot be influenced further	Costs of insurance paid in advance
	Opportunity costs—proceeds lost by rejecting alternatives	No purchase of x-ray machine if money spent on new ultrasound machine

direct and fixed, the wages of on-call nurses are direct but variable, and the salaries of the CEO and CFO are fixed but indirect.

ALLOCATING COSTS

Cost allocation involves the determination of the total cost of producing a specified healthcare service through assigning costs into revenue-producing departments and then further allocating the costs down to the unit-of-service or procedure level based either on departmental revenue or volume. The purpose of this methodology is:

- To ensure that patients are paying [theoretically] "for only the costs of the services and products they received" (Nowicki, 2004, p. 147).

- To separate costs at the unit-of-service level to allow managers to:
  - Measure the effects of change in intensity and case mix;
  - Identify those costs that can be converted from fixed to variable; and,
  - Identify inefficient functions and demonstrate the nature of the problem, such as price, volume, or practice (Berger, 2002, p. 216).

Although a number of methods have been identified for cost allocation purposes, in each case the process ends when all of the organization's costs (including those generated in non-revenue producing departments such as housekeeping and medical records) are allocated to the cost centers of revenue-producing departments (radiology, pediatrics, and so forth). These methods have been widely used for pricing and reimbursement purposes in the past, but are beginning to be replaced by more accurate methods of determining product costs.

DETERMINING PRODUCT COSTS

A number of methods for determining product costs (e.g., home health visits or patient days) have been posed, each of which crosses department lines of responsibility. However, one method, **activity-based costing** (the ABC method), has enjoyed increasing popularity in healthcare organizations because of its greater accuracy. This change in methodology is also due to the fact that cost allocations are no longer made on the basis of cost center characteristics (e.g., number of office visits or percentage of square feet) but rather on the basis of **cost drivers**, or "the activities that go on in preparation for and during a unit of service" (McLean, 1997, p. 142). As explained by Zelman et al. (2003, p. 426), "ABC is based on the paradigm that activities consume resources and products consume activities. Therefore, if activities or processes are controlled, then costs will be controlled."

BREAK-EVEN ANALYSIS

The ultimate goal of managing costs is minimally to break even and not run a deficit. **Break-even analysis** is the method of determining at what level of volume the production of a good or service will break even. It is used by healthcare managers for the purpose of determining profit or loss. The **break-even point** is the volume of production in units and sale of goods or services where total costs equal total revenue. As noted by Nowicki (2003, p. 159), "After the break-even point has been reached and fixed costs have been covered, each subsequent unit produced contributes to profit." McLean (2003, p. 142), however, emphasizes that the break-even quantity (e.g., total number of visits) does not necessarily need to be reached for a healthcare organization to decide to keep a specified service. He states, "If [a] unit covers its direct costs (fixed and variable) and makes *any* contribution to overhead, it is worth keeping, even in the long run" since the organization would incur overhead expenses even without the unit. However, in the long run, "if the unit cannot meet its own (direct) total costs, it should be eliminated unless some outside entity or another revenue center is to subsidize it" (McLean, 2003).

SETTING CHARGES

Only after costs have been determined can healthcare organizations go about the business of setting rates or charges for their services and products. While the earlier section on "Managing Reimbursements from Third-Party Payers" describes a number of methods used by third-party payers and healthcare organizations to negotiate payments for services, a more complete picture of what is involved when setting charges should be taken into consideration by any provider.

A first step in this discussion might be to differentiate the meanings of *charges* versus actual *prices* set by the organization. *Pam Pohly's Net Guide*, in its "Glossary of Terms in Managed Health Care," defines **charges** in terms of "published prices." The entire, more revealing definition reads:

> These are the published prices of services provided by a facility. HCFA [now CMS] requires hospitals to apply the same schedule of charges to all patients, regardless of the expected sources or amount of payment. Controversy exists today because of the often wide disparity between published prices and contract prices. The majority of payers, including Medicare and Medicaid, are becoming managed by health plans which negotiate rates lower than published prices. Often these negotiated rates average 40% to 60% of the published rates and may be all inclusive bundled rates (Pohly, 2005).

Prices in health care, on the other hand, involve that which is given up by consumers or third-party payers to acquire medical goods or services on behalf of patients, including:

- Money actually spent;
- The perceived value of these goods or services;
- Lost time and/or lost "dignity" in acquiring these services; and,
- Other opportunities foregone (purchases, activities).

In other words, charges posted by the organization do not necessarily translate into actual prices paid for services.

OTHER DETERMINANTS OF SETTING CHARGES AND PRICES

Although not claiming to be all-inclusive, the following factors are provided to make sure that the healthcare manager gives due consideration to each when involved in setting prices for services or products.

- *Consider legal and regulatory issues*
  - State and federal regulations,
  - JCAHO and other accrediting body regulations, and
  - Anti-trust and other fair pricing laws.
- *Establish pricing goals and objectives*
  - Efficient and effective use of resources,
  - Profit-oriented pricing, including profit maximization, satisfactory profits, or break-even strategies,
  - Sales-oriented pricing, including market share or sales maximization,
  - Equity and fairness issues,
  - Positive consumer attitudes, and
  - Maximum participation in third-party payer opportunities.
- *Estimate the economic market conditions* involving supply and demand factors
  - Awareness of the basic principles of supply and demand.
  - Awareness of **elasticity of demand**, in which ineffective pricing can cause surpluses or shortages. The more **inelastic** the products, the better for the organization in terms of price (less need to drop prices). For more **elastic** products, dropping price will generally increase demand.

- Awareness that the availability and prices of substitutes, or product durability and quality, may affect elasticity of demand as well.
- *Estimate costs*, including fixed costs, variable costs, and the break-even point below which healthcare services or goods should not be priced, recognizing that during slow periods, it is important to charge anything above variable costs to absorb some of the overhead.
- *Consider penetration and policies of third-party payers*, including managed care, Medicare, Medicaid, and other insurers, including the effects of discounts, **allowable** or **approved charges** (limits of charges approved for payment by Medicare or private health plans), or rebates.
- *Consider other competitors in the market*, including their prices, product lines, market share, proximity, etc.
- *Consider the effects of over- or under-pricing*, in that:
  - Over-pricing leads to lost sales and
  - Under-pricing leads to lower returns on sales.
- *Take into consideration allowable costs*, including:
  - *Case mix*, which addresses patient eligibility,
  - *Service mix*, focusing on necessity or appropriateness of care, and
  - *Staff mix*, addressing appropriateness of who provides the care.
- *Utilize pricing tactics*, where appropriate, including:
  - *Geographic pricing*, taking into consideration variances in costs associated with shipping, place of service (urban vs. rural, home vs. facility), etc.,
  - *Professional charges*, in which fees are based on performance of a particular service rather than the time or equipment involved, and
  - *Flexible or variable pricing*, in which different prices may be set for the same items or same services (e.g., discounts offered during slow census periods).

Setting charges or rates remains a highly complex activity within any healthcare organization due to the need to consider a huge number of variables, both internal and external to the organization. While individual healthcare managers may be involved in providing substantial input into this process, larger organizations employ experts dedicated to this task in order to sustain revenue maximization and competitiveness in the healthcare market.

MANAGING WORKING CAPITAL

Working capital has been defined in a couple of different ways by financial experts in the field. Some define working capital simply as **total current assets**, which are the "cash and other short-term assets that the organization expects to convert to cash within one year" (Nowicki, 2004, p. 177). Current assets also include accounts receivable (patient accounts), inventory, and prepaid expenses (such as insurance premiums). Others assert that "working capital refers both to current assets and to **current liabilities**, with the latter being "those liabilities that will be paid within the current accounting period" (McLean, 2003, p. 288). Virtually all experts, however, define **net working capital** as "current assets *minus* current liabilities," a concept which seems to remind us that healthcare organizations are never without accumulation of debt.

The primary sources of working capital include:

- *Permanent working capital:* The initial amounts of working capital to cover start-up costs, and ultimately the minimum amount always kept on hand.
- *Net income:* Working capital provided at that point in which collected revenues surpass expenses. In for-profit organizations, working capital is said to be taken from the organization's profits.
- *Temporary working capital:* Additional monies needed to respond to unanticipated or seasonal increases in business, financed through:
  - Equity or net assets;
  - Short-term debt or loans; and,
  - Trade credit from delayed payments to vendors.

What Are the Purposes of Working Capital Management?

The end result of the first set of purposes is to increase revenues and reduce expenses:

- To serve as the "catalyst" to make capital assets (buildings and equipment) productive by wisely managing such current assets as labor and inventory.
- To control the volume of resources committed to current assets. McLean (2003, p. 288) states that "financing working capital by the least costly means available can allow one's organization to deliver the

same amount of care at lower cost, or can allow an organization with a limited budget to deliver a greater amount of care."

- To conserve cash by cutting the organization's financing costs in order to take advantage of short-term investments.
- To manage **cash flow**, i.e., the amount of inflows and outflows, and the **cash conversion cycle**, i.e., the process (measured in days) through which initial cash is converted into the inventory, labor, and supplies needed in healthcare operations that in turn generate accounts receivable and that finally are collected in the form of cash revenues.
- To manage the **liquidity** of an organization, i.e., "a measure of how quickly assets can be converted into cash" (Zelman et al., 2003, p. 488).

The second set of purposes involves enhancing "good will" toward the organization:

- To pay vendors and employees on time.
- To demonstrate to lenders that the organization is "credit-worthy," by showing it has sufficient resources to repay loans or at least pay interest on short-term funds.

Why Is Working Capital Management in Healthcare Environments Problematic?

Managing working capital tends to be more problematic with healthcare organizations because they generate very little immediate cash. This is largely due to the huge preponderance of third-party payers for healthcare services, leading to substantial delays in payment. Also, even if paid by private parties, the large costs incurred for most medical services result in payment after the billing cycle, by credit card, or in negotiated installments.

Another area of concern for many healthcare financial managers is how best to make decisions in managing working capital when faced with such a wide array of options. Even new and inexperienced managers might take heart by heeding the advice of Sachdeva and Gitman (1981, p. 45), who offer a simple decision rule when faced with alternative choices between possible means of managing current assets and liabilities: "Undertake changes in working capital management practices that add value to the organization."

MANAGING ACCOUNTS RECEIVABLE

Accounts receivable (AR) have been defined as a "current asset, created in the course of doing business, consisting of revenues recognized, but not yet collected as cash" (McLean, 2003, p. 352). Zelman et al. (2003, p. 175) estimate that AR comprise "approximately 75 percent of a healthcare provider's current assets." Also called "patient accounts" in many healthcare organizations, accounts receivable provide no interest for the provider unless they have been converted into interest-bearing loans to allow patients to pay out their debts for services over time. Therefore, management of AR becomes exceedingly important in order to collect revenues generated to insure cash flow for management of the operations of the organization. It is essential to note that the ultimate collection of AR becomes less likely as the amount of time since services are rendered increases.

A number of other important insights concerning accounts receivable have been offered by Nowicki (2004), Zelman et al. (2003), McLean (2003) and others and are listed below.

- Willingness to *extend credit* to patients and/or to wait for third-party payers to pay the bill is a way of attracting business and gaining contracts with insurers.
- The importance of *MCO contracts* cannot be overstated since they represent 20% to 50% of most healthcare organizations' net revenues.
- A healthcare organization's *collection period* is determined largely by the payment practices of its patients' managed care companies and other third-party insurers. This typically ranges from 30 to 90 days, with collection periods becoming longer over the past several years.
- Having large dollar amounts in AR means lost opportunities for other investments.
- There are *costs* associated with AR, including carrying costs, delinquency costs, routine credit and collection costs, and opportunity costs to use the cash for other purposes.
- Healthcare organizations often need to receive *cash advances* on outstanding accounts receivable in order to continue operations. Two methods utilized to finance AR include: **factoring receivables** (selling AR at a discount) and **pledging receivables as collateral** to negotiate a line of credit to cover temporary cash shortfalls.

- The *primary goal* of managing AR is to reduce the **collection period** (also known as "days in AR"), which is calculated by dividing net accounts receivable by patient revenues per day. The shorter the collection period, the smaller the opportunity cost of assets tied up in accounts receivable. This is a good situation for the organization!

MAJOR STEPS IN ACCOUNTS RECEIVABLE MANAGEMENT

Managing accounts receivable involves collaboration and cooperation among almost all departments of a healthcare organization although some departments are more directly involved than others. The following table (Table 8-3) provides examples of involvement in a typical hospital setting.

Some additional thoughts and clarification are warranted concerning the "overriding importance" of all departments in managing accounts receivable:

- Documentation capture emphasizes the importance of the quality of the written record of patient care by all healthcare professionals.

TABLE 8-3 Hospital Departmental Involvement in Managing Accounts Receivable

Department	AR Involvement
Contracts	Relationships and contract negotiation with third-party payers
Admissions/Registration	Precertification, preadmission, insurance verification
Patient Care Unit (Nursing, Lab, Radiology, Rehab, etc.)	Documentation capture, charge capture for services rendered
Medical Records	Coding, utilization review, QA (quality assurance) audits
Billing	Bill preparation, billing audits
Compliance	Fraud and abuse internal audits
Collections	Collection policies and procedures, financial counseling, third-party and self-pay follow-up
Legal	Contracts, litigation policy, federal regulations, patient rights

- Ultimately, interdependence among departments impacts the reduction in the AR collection period. For example, accurate documentation supports the coding, and the timeliness of the coding greatly impacts the ability of the billing department to send out a timely bill. Cooperation among managers is essential.
- AR outcomes are often measured by first determining a baseline of the progress to be measured and then monitoring the outcomes periodically by looking at the organization's balance sheet and income statements. This process is often referred to as **benchmarking**, in which the current year's results can be measured against prior results to see whether things are getting better or worse.

MANAGING MATERIALS AND INVENTORY

Formerly referred to as "inventory management" and more recently designated as "supply chain management," **materials management** refers to the process of managing the clinical and non-clinical goods and inventory purchased and used by the personnel of a healthcare organization in order to perform their duties.

Why Is Materials Management Important?

There are at least three important reasons why materials management is so important to the healthcare organization. The first involves delivery of *appropriate patient care*, in which the organization must have the right kind and right amount of supplies, delivered in the right time frame. Stock-outs (not having enough of a product) are considered totally unacceptable in healthcare organizations, as they may result in unnecessary deaths or poor outcomes. A second involves *cost control*. Inventory, a non-productive asset, loses value over time, increasing the costs to the healthcare facility. If items spend too much time in inventory, they may become contaminated, lost, stolen, or expired. Further, cash tied up in excessive inventory cannot be used for assets that produce income. The third reason involves *improvement of the organization's profitability*. Skillful materials management can improve the organization's bottom line through such techniques as reducing utilization of overused supplies, obtaining best pricing for supplies and equipment through negotiation, and standardizing the organization's supplies to provide purchasing discounts (Berger, 2002).

What Are the Basic Tenets of Materials Management?

In addition to the above, the following guidelines can be utilized to improve the bottom line through reduction in materials and inventory costs:

- *Develop close relations with distributors*, who consolidate the supplies of many manufacturers, and control the availability, pricing, and receiving schedule for the goods.
- *Adopt the consignment method of equipment acquisition* (whenever possible), in which the provider acquires the goods from the supplier, but payment is made only if the item is used. This is most often used for relatively expensive and specialized equipment.
- *Understand the costs of inventory* in order to minimize the inefficiencies and unnecessary costs associated with having the wrong amount of inventory. These include: purchasing costs, ordering costs, carrying costs (opportunity costs and holding costs), stock-out costs (not having enough), overstock costs (having too much), and total costs.
- *Calculate the economic order quantity (EOQ) and reorder point (RP)* in order to know the right quantity of items that should be ordered at the most appropriate point in time to minimize total inventory costs.
- *Evaluate inventory performance* through such methods as the inventory turnover ratio in order to minimize overstocking or understocking, especially under conditions of uncertainty.
- *Create in-service training programs* for the organization's entire management group covering both internal and external issues, such as the processes and procedures for requesting purchase orders, negotiating with vendors, etc.
- *Implement E-commerce*, in which the provider accesses suppliers and distributors on the Internet, to help streamline materials management. This is frequently utilized for ordering goods, pricing and processing orders, tracking and receiving orders, invoicing, and payments.
- *Facilitate annual review by the Finance Committee*, involving thorough materials management analysis.

It is also important to adopt the most appropriate method for stocking inventory. This includes keeping a **safety stock level** of inventory, below which the healthcare facility will not allow units on hand to fall. It further involves understanding and adopting one of the commonly accepted methods for **valuing inventory**:

- *FIFO*, or "first-in, first-out," in which the first item put in inventory is the first taken out; it produces an inventory of newer items and thus values the cost of inventory at the price paid for the newest items;
- *LIFO*, or "last-in, first-out," in which the last item put in inventory is the first taken out; it produces an inventory of older items and thus values the cost of inventory at the price paid for the oldest items;
- *Weighted average*, in which the average cost of inventory items is multiplied by the number of units in inventory; and,
- *Specific identification*, in which the actual cost of each item is included. This tends to be used with high-cost (and relatively few) items.

Finally, adopting the most appropriate method for stocking inventory includes application of either the JIT or ABC inventory methods in terms of when to order or deliver products to the healthcare facility:

- *Just-in-time (JIT):* With this technique, products are literally delivered to the organization "just in time" for use. This method is preferred by Berger (2002, p. 306) in order to decrease the "chance for obsolescence and shrinkage (theft)" and to reduce **holding costs** associated with warehousing items in the healthcare facility.
- *ABC Inventory Method:* With activity-based costing (ABC), each supply item is categorized as belonging to one of three groups. Group A includes very expensive items that must be monitored closely, such as certain expensive drugs. Group B consists of intermediate-cost items, where order and inventory quantities change "as interest rates and unit prices vary." Group C, the largest group, consists of items representing little cost but which are important to the day-to-day operations of the healthcare organization (e.g., bandages, tissues, pain relievers). Zelman et al. (2003, p. 424–37) and Nowicki (2004, p. 154–57) describe the ABC method in detail, providing examples of how it is applied.

While it may be the ultimate responsibility of the materials manager to insure that all goods needed by both the clinical and non-clinical users in a healthcare facility are available when required and in the most cost-efficient manner, every manager in the organization must be held accountable for timely ordering and judicious use of materials. Physicians, and other users of high-cost equipment and supplies, should also be trained on the procedures involved in the ordering and stocking process.

MANAGING BUDGETS

One of the most critical functions for managers in healthcare organizations is management of the departmental or division budget. While the facility's Finance Department is generally involved in working with the manager in developing both operational and capital budgets for her/his department, it is the responsibility of each manager to insure that expenditures (in terms of such items as labor, equipment, and supplies) and revenues (if the department supplies services or products for patients/consumers) are monitored carefully on an ongoing basis.

Sorting Out the Definitions and Distinguishing Characteristics of Budgeting

Budgeting means different things to different people, even in healthcare organizations, and it further does not help that not all authors or organizations utilize the same terms in discussing their budgeting process. The purpose of the current section is to try to sort out some of the commonly used budgeting terms that are used in the financial management departments of healthcare entities.

Budgeting is, quite simply, the process of converting the goals and objectives of the organization's operating plan into financial terms: expenses, revenues, and cash flow projections. The **budget**, then, is a financial plan for turning these objectives into a program for earning revenues and for expenditure of funds. Listed below are characteristics of budgeting important to healthcare managers.

- The budget should be a dynamic working document, to be utilized on an ongoing basis by every manager in the organization.
- Managers must have access to a budget manual and last year's data regarding volumes, revenues, expenses, and cash flows on a monthly basis to provide guidance for their departments' budgeting process.
- Budgets provide a tool for ex post facto evaluation of managers concerning their performance in efficiently running their departments and for assessing how well the organization as a whole has met its financial performance goals.
- The **budget period** is the period of time for which a budget is prepared, often one fiscal year (McLean 2003, p. 353).

- The **budget calendar** is a planning tool used to design and maintain all of the organization's projects falling under the budget, with separate calendars being prepared for the operating and capital budgets (Berger, 2002, p. 148). Included in this calendar are the budget activities, time-frame expectations, the parties responsible, and follow-up meeting times.

What Are the Specific Types of Budgets?

The **operating budget** generally refers to the annual budget that follows the strategic financial and operating plan. Berger (2002, p. 145–148) describes 24 steps in preparing the operating budget, including 5 distinct "segments": strategic planning, administrative segments, communications, operational planning, and budgeting segments. He further asserts that these steps "involve managers in every facet of operations. In addition, a critical set of stakeholders who must be accessed, solicited, and appeased are the physicians linked to the organization, either in an employment capacity or in an affiliate relationship."

Cash budgets, a term sometimes used interchangeably with operating budgets, are specifically distinguished from the latter by some authors and organizations. Prepared by the finance department staff, this budget is described by Berger (2002, p. 235) as "the necessary step that allows the organization to determine how to optimize the value of the cash being generated by its operations." McLean (1997, p. 355) more specifically defines a cash budget as "a forecast of cash inflows, cash outflows, and net lending or borrowing needs for the months ahead." This 52-week budget attempts to forecast the receipts (most often from third-party payers) and disbursements (expenses) of the organization. These budgets are comprised of:

- An *expense budget*, which is a prediction of the total expenses that the organization will incur. It typically includes such items as labor, supplies, and acuity levels (case mix) and is included on the left-hand side (the debit side) of accounting entries.
- A *revenue budget*, shown on the right-hand (credit) side of accounting entries, which includes data on forecasted utilization of specific services within the organization and third-party payer mix.

Three other terms generally associated with cash budgets are:

- *Cash outflows,* which include such expenses as mortgage payments or rents, salaries and wages, benefits, utilities, supplies, and interest paid out.
- *Cash inflows,* which include cash payments up front, 30-day and 60-day collections, government appropriations, donations, and any interest earned each month.
- *Ending cash,* which comprises both the cash balance at the end of the month and the following month's beginning cash level. The following formula is used to determine this amount: *Ending cash = Beginning cash + Cash inflows – Cash outflows.*

There are two other types of budgets with which healthcare managers should become familiar. The term **statistics budget** is given to the initial statistics delineated in the operating plan that forecasts service utilization (by service type, acuity level or case mix, and payer mix), resource use, and policy data (employment data, occupancy rates, staffing ratios, etc.). The **capital budget** refers to the plan for expenditures for new facilities and equipment (often referred to as **fixed assets**) whose expected useful life is longer than one year. The following discussion will focus on the latter.

The Importance of Capital Budgeting

Capital budgeting may be defined as the process of selecting long-term assets, whose useful life is greater than one year, according to financial decision rules. The capital budget determines funding amounts, what capital equipment will be acquired, what buildings will be built or renovated, depreciation expenses, and the estimated useful life to be assigned to each asset. Berger (2002, p. 157) states that its main purpose "is to identify the specific capital items to be acquired. The problem in almost all healthcare organizations is which capital projects should be funded" in light of scarce resources. McLean (2003, p. 189) further asserts that "[t]he *basic question* that any capital budgeting system must ask is, 'Does this asset or project, in a time value sense, at least pay for itself? If not (if it requires a subsidy), is there a subsidy forthcoming?' If the answer is yes, then the project is worth doing."

The following are types of items typically included in such budgets:

- *Land acquisition,* including land to be used for expansion of service offerings.
- *Physical plant or facility construction, expansion, acquisition, renovation, or leasing.* This may include medical office space for physician

practices.

- *Routine capital equipment*, including items used in clinical areas (radiology, lab, surgery, rehab, and nursing departments).
- *Information technology infrastructure or upgrades* for financial systems, medical records, and clinical use.
- *Recruitment and acquisition of staff physicians* (more recently included), either through purchasing existing physician practices or establishing new practices by employing physicians.

While the capital budgeting process often involves substantial outlays of time by managers at different levels of the organization, it is important to consider some essential steps that are frequently followed. Determination of the capital budget often begins with a wish list of various items requested by staff, physicians, or any other individuals who must obtain or use equipment within the department. It is important to note that engaging physician leaders in this process cannot be overemphasized because they ultimately make the majority of diagnostic and clinical decisions regarding patient care in healthcare organizations. The basic wish list includes:

- Any new equipment that offers a new line of revenue to the organization or could improve patient outcomes.
- Any updated items to replace current equipment that has become worn out, obsolete, harmful to patient care, or is no longer "state-of-the-art."

Department managers, the "proposal writers," must then complete and submit designated capital budget requests to the Finance Department. Land acquisition and facility construction, on the other hand, are most often approved by the Governing Body, with such requests also being submitted to the Finance Department. Once all proposals have been submitted, the *finance staff* must review all capital proposals for consistency and completeness of all required information. *Proposal reviewers*, assigned to review the technical aspects of all capital requests, must make sure each proposal contains all of the data required. This group often includes accounting staff, information systems management, materials management, and facilities management. Next, designated *proposal evaluators* must evaluate the merits of each proposal, how each compares to all other project requests on a criteria basis, and whether each adheres to strategic plan criteria. *Administrative* approval and approval by the *governing body* completes the process.

While there are a number of methods utilized to make capital budgeting decisions, most healthcare organizations establish criteria-based **decision rules**. These range from a simple **accept/reject decision**, which merely addresses "whether or not to acquire an asset or initiate a project," to **capital rationing**, in which a fixed dollar amount is placed on annual capital spending by governing bodies and those with the highest **profitability index** are selected (McLean 2003, p. 193–195). However, as a "safety valve" in the decision process, it is necessary to include a mechanism that allows some needed capital acquisitions "to be purchased no matter what," i.e., despite not being able to meet formal evaluation criteria. Berger (2002, p. 205) calls this **non-criteria-based capital budgeting.**

CONCLUSION

Managing costs and revenues in the healthcare arena is a complex and often technical process that involves understanding of the interrelatedness of the processes involved, the interplay of many departments and managers within the organization, and the importance of influences external to the organization. This chapter has addressed the importance and objectives of financial management, the impacts of tax status and organizational structure, and a cursory look at how effective management of a variety of organizational support functions contribute to maximizing revenues and controlling costs. More specifically, the healthcare administration student with a nonfinancial career path should have at least a basic understanding of managing costs, reimbursements from third-party payers and other sources, budgeting, capital acquisition, working capital, accounts receivable, setting charges and prices, and managing materials and inventory. Managers at all levels of the organization are often involved in addressing these functions.

What this chapter did not address more specifically were investment decisions, short-term versus long-term financing, managing endowments, financial ratios, or financial statement preparation and analysis. This is largely due to the fact that these functions are most often handled by professionals within the Finance Department of the healthcare organization, who in turn provide managers with pertinent related information on an as-needed basis. However, for healthcare managers more directly involved in financial management as a major part of their jobs, it is imperative that they avail themselves of this and other detailed financial management information to help ensure the financial viability of the organizations within which they work.

DISCUSSION QUESTIONS

1. What are the major objectives of financial management in healthcare organizations?

2. How do financial objectives differ between for-profit versus not-for-profit healthcare entities?

3. What are the primary methods of reimbursement to providers from private health plans and government-sponsored programs such as Medicare and Medicaid?

4. What are the major categories of costs? How are product costs determined?

5. A 350-bed, suburban hospital is considering purchasing a robotic surgical system. What should the CFO include in her break-even analysis to determine if it will be a good investment?

6. What are some of the major problems associated with managing working capital?

7. The operating room in the same hospital noted above is having a problem with controlling the costs of surgical scrubs. What should the OR manager do?

REFERENCES

American Hospital Association (AHA). (1990). *Role and functions of the hospital governing board.* Chicago, IL: AHA.
American Hospital Association (AHA). (2005, November). *Uncompensated hospital care cost fact sheet.* Retrieved June 9, 2006, from http://www.aha.org/ahapolicy forum/resources/content/0511UncompensatedCareFactSheet.pdf
Berger, S. (2002). *Fundamentals of health care financial management: A practical guide to fiscal issues and activities, 2nd ed.* San Francisco, CA: Jossey-Bass.
Berman, H. J., Weeks, L. E., & Kukla, S. F. (1986). *The financial management of hospitals, 6th ed.* Chicago, IL: Health Administration Press.

Gapenski, L. C. (1996). *Financial analysis and decision making for healthcare organizations*. Chicago, IL: Irwin Professional Pub (McGraw-Hill).

Gapenski, L. C. (2003). *Understanding healthcare financial management, 4th ed.* Chicago, IL: Health Administration Press.

Himmelstein, D. U., Warren, E., Thorne, D. & Woolhandler, S. (2005, February). Market watch: Illness and injury as contributors to bankruptcy, *Health Affairs, 10*(W5), 63–73, Web Exclusive.

McLean, R. A. (1997). *Financial management in health care organizations*. Clifton Park, NY: Thomson Delmar Learning.

McLean, R. A. (2003). *Financial management in health care organizations, 2nd ed.* Clifton Park, NY: Thomson Delmar Learning.

Nowicki, M. (2004). *The financial management of hospitals and healthcare organizations, 3rd ed.* Chicago, IL: Health Administration Press.

Pohly, P. (2005). Glossary of terms in managed health care. *Pam Pohly's Net Guide*, 1997–2005. Retrieved June 9, 2006, from http://www.pohly.com/terms.html

Sachdeva, K. S., & Gitman, L. J. (1981). Accounts receivable decisions in a capital budgeting framework, *Financial Management, 10*(4), 45–49.

Zelman, W. N., McCue, M. J., Millikan, A. R., & Glick, N. D. (2003). *Financial management of health care organizations: an introduction to fundamental tools, concepts and applications, 2nd ed.* Malden, MA: Blackwell Publishing.

CHAPTER 9

Managing Healthcare Professionals

Sharon B. Buchbinder
Dale Buchbinder

LEARNING OBJECTIVES

By the end of this chapter the student will be able to describe:

- The education, training, and credentialing of physicians, nurses, nurses' aides, midlevel practitioners, and allied health professionals;
- The supply of and demand for healthcare professionals;
- Reasons for healthcare professional turnover and costs of turnover;
- Strategies for increasing retention and preventing turnover; and,
- Issues associated with the management of the worklife of physicians, nurses, nurses' aides, midlevel practitioners, and allied health professionals.

INTRODUCTION

Healthcare organizations employ a wide array of clinical, administrative, and support professionals to deliver services to their patients. The Bureau of Labor Statistics (BLS), which lists over thirty different categories of healthcare professionals at its website, notes that "as the largest industry in 2004, healthcare provided 13.1 million jobs for wage and salary workers" and that "most workers have jobs that require less than four years of college education, but health diagnosing and treating practitioners are among the most educated workers" (BLS, 2006a).

The largest category of healthcare workers is registered nurses, with 2.4 million jobs, 60% of which are in hospitals (BLS, 2006b). In 2006, there were 884,974 physicians, with the majority working in metropolitan areas (Smart, 2006). In 2004, physician assistants held 62,000 jobs, about a quarter of which were in hospitals, and the rest in outpatient care centers (BLS, 2006c). Allied health professionals constitute a broad array of twenty health science occupations, including anesthesiologist assistants, medical assistants, respiratory therapists, and surgical technologists (CAAHEP, 2006).

These statistics mean that, as a healthcare manager, in many instances you will be working with a mix of people with either more or less education than you have. It also means that you will not have the clinical competencies that these healthcare providers have, an intimidating scenario, to say the least. Instead of clinical expertise, you will bring a background that enables you to enhance the environment in which these highly specialized personnel deliver healthcare services. You will be the person responsible for making sure that nurses, doctors, and other healthcare professionals have the resources to provide safe and effective patient care. Your role will be to provide and monitor the infrastructure and processes to make the healthcare organization responsive to the needs of the patients and the employees. The more you understand clinical healthcare professionals, the better prepared you will be to do your job as a healthcare manager. The purpose of this chapter is to provide you with an overview of who your future colleagues are, how they were trained, and ways to manage the quality of their work environment.

PHYSICIANS

Physicians begin their preparation for medical school as undergraduates in premedical programs. Premedical students can obtain a degree in any subject; however, the American Association of Medical Colleges (AAMC) indicates that the expectation is that they will graduate with a strong foundation in mathematics, biology, chemistry and physics (AAMC, 2006). Entry into medical school is competitive; applicants must have high grade point averages and high scores on the Medical College Admission Test (MCAT).

There are some shorter, combined Bachelor of Science/Medical Doctor (BS/MD) programs, however, the majority of medical school graduates will have had 8 years of post-high school education before they go through the National Residency Matching Program (NRMP, 2006), a matching process whereby medical students interview and rank their choices for Graduate Medical Education (GME), also known as residencies, and the residency training programs do the same. Once matched with a residency training program, physicians are prepared in specialty areas of medicine. Depending on the specialty, the length of the residency training program can be as short as 3 years (for family practice) or as long as 10 years (for cardiothoracic surgery or neurosurgery). According to the Accreditation Council for Graduate Medical Education (ACGME), "When physicians graduate from a residency program, they are eligible to take their board certification examinations and begin practicing independently. Residency training programs are sponsored by teaching hospitals, academic medical centers, healthcare systems and other institutions" (ACGME, 2006a). Depending on the type of healthcare organization where you are employed, you may be working with residents-in-training and medical students, as well as physicians who have been in independent practice for decades.

In addition to having a long length of time before they can practice independently, residents work extensive hours as part of their training programs. At one time, it was not uncommon for residents to be on-call continuously for forty-eight hours, because ceilings on hours of work for residents varied by residency training program. However, that all changed due to the death of Libby Zion, an 18-year-old college student, who was seen at the Cornell Medical Center in 1984 and allegedly died due to resident overwork (AMA-MSS, 2006). Although the hospital and resident were exonerated in court, the battle over resident work hours had begun. New York was the first state to institute limits on resident work hours in 1987. Over the past two decades, various specialty societies, medical associations, and legislators fought over the definition of "reasonable" work hours for physicians in training. Effective July 1, 2003, all specialty and subspecialty residency training programs were required to limit resident work hours to no more than 80 hours per week, inclusive of in-house call activities (ACGME, 2006b). And, for all ACGME-approved residency training programs, in-house continuous on-site duty must not exceed 24 consecutive hours (ACGME, 2006c). These new work-hour rules underscore the fact that residents are in the hospital for education, not to provide service to the hospital, a major departure from the way graduate medical education was conducted a few decades ago.

The implications of limits on resident work hours are multifold. While Residency Training Program Directors are responsible for monitoring resident work hours, they must be in compliance with the healthcare institutions policies as well. You may be responsible for ensuring that compliance, by collecting work-hour data for your managers. Healthcare managers are obligated to ensure adequate coverage of the hospital with physicians. Resident work hour restrictions may mean that you need to hire physicians or **midlevel practitioners**, physician assistants and nurse practitioners, as employees. And, your organization may need to hire **ancillary staff** and **allied health professionals**, such as intravenous therapists and surgical assistants, to do tasks previously covered by resident physicians.

Most physicians are eligible to obtain a license to practice medicine after one year of post-graduate training. **Licensure** is granted by the state, required for physicians, nurses and others to practice, and demonstrates competency to perform a scope of practice (NCSBN, 2006). State Boards of Physician Quality Assurance (BPQA) establish the requirements for medical licenses. These requirements are lengthy and strenuous. For example, the State of Maryland requires the following (Annotated Code of Maryland, 2006):

- Good moral character;
- Minimum age of 18 years;
- A fee;
- Documentation of education and training; and,
- Passing scores on one of the following examinations:
  - All parts of the National Board of Medical Examiners' examinations, and/or a score of 75 or better on a FLEX exam, or a passing score on the National Board of Osteopathic Examiners, or a combination of scores and exams; or,
  - State Board examination;
  - All steps of the U.S. Medical Licensing Examination (USMLE).

Candidates must demonstrate oral and written English language competency and supply the following:

- A chronological list of activities beginning with the date of completion of medical school, accounting for all periods of time;

- Any disciplinary actions taken by licensing boards, denying application or renewal;
- Any investigations, charges, arrests, pleas of guilty or *nolo contendere*, convictions, or receipts of probation before judgment;
- Information pertaining to any physical, mental, or emotional condition that impairs the physician's ability to practice medicine;
- Copies of any malpractice suits or settlements, or records of any arrests, disciplinary actions, judgments, final orders, or cases of driving while intoxicated or under the influence of a chemical substance or medication; and,
- Results of all medical licensure, certification, and recertification examinations and the dates when taken.

Some states now require criminal background checks (CBCs) for physician applicants for licensure (NCSBN, 2006a). The reasons are multifold, and include, but are not limited to: increasing societal concerns about alcohol and drug abusers, sexual predators, and child and elder abusers. If a CBC contains information about convictions, the licensure board will examine the application on a case-by-case basis. The reviewers will be looking for level and frequency of the criminal behavior, basing their decision on that, along with other materials submitted by the applicant, such as proof of alcohol and drug rehabilitation.

In addition to obtaining a license, physicians may voluntarily submit documentation of their education, training, and practice to an American Board of Medical Specialists (ABMS) Member Board for review (ABMS, 2006). Upon approval of the medical specialty board (i.e., successful completion of an approved residency training program), the physician is then allowed to sit for examination(s). Successful completion of the examination allows the physician to be granted certification, and she is designated as **board certified** in that specialty (e.g., a board certified pediatrician or a board certified general internist). Certificates are time-limited; physicians must demonstrate continued competency and retake the exam every 6 to 10 years, depending on the specialty. The purpose of the recertification examinations is to ensure that physicians remain up-to-date in their specialties. Board certification is a form of **credentialing** a physician's competency in a specific area. For staff privileges and hiring purposes, most hospitals, HMOs, and other healthcare organizations require a physician to be board certified or **board eligible** (i.e., preparing to sit for the exams) because board certification is used as a proxy for determining the quality of health professional's services. This assumption of quality is based on research that more education and training leads to a higher quality of service (Donabedian, 2005; Tamblyn, Abrahamowicz, Brailovsky, Grand'Maison, Lescop, Norcini, Girard, & Haggerty, 1998).

Most states require that physicians complete a certain number of **continuing medical education (CME)** credits to maintain state licensure and to demonstrate continued competency. Additionally, hospitals may require CME credits for their physicians to remain credentialed to see patients (NIH, 2005). Seven organizations, the American Board of Medical Specialists (ABMS), the American Hospital Association (AHA), the American Medical Association (AMA), the Association of American Medical Colleges (AAMC), the Association for Hospital Medical Education (AHME), the Council of Medical Specialty Societies (CMSS), and the Federation of State Medical Boards, Inc. (FSMB) are members of the **Accreditation Council for Continuing Medical Education (ACCME)** (AMA, 2005). The ACCME establishes criteria for determining which educational providers are quality CME providers and gives its seal of approval only to those organizations meeting their standards (ACCME, 2006). The ACCME also "recognizes state or territorial medical societies that accredit intrastate providers of CME" (AMA, 2005).

Physician credentialing is the process of verifying information that a physician supplies on an application for staff privileges at a hospital, HMO, or other healthcare organization. Most healthcare organizations have protocols that they have established, and, as a healthcare manager, you will be required to follow that protocol. Physicians are tracked by the AMA from the day they graduate from medical school until the day they die. Information about every physician in the United States is in the AMA Physician Masterfile, which has been in existence for 100 years. Originally created on paper index cards to establish biographic records on physicians, it is now a computer database, "used by the medical community for credentials verification, research, manpower planning, and other public good efforts" (Eiler, 2006).

Physician credentialing is a time consuming, labor intensive, costly process that must be repeated every 2 years. When physicians apply for privileges at a hospital, they must specify what they want, not only by specialty, but in the surgical specialties, by procedure. For example, a general surgeon who wants to do laparoscopic cholecystectomies (i.e., removal of the gall bladder through a very small incision, using an instrument like a tiny telescope) would apply for both general surgery privileges and for that specific procedure. Using extensive documentation, the surgeon must demonstrate competency for those privileges. The hospital must conduct diligent research on that surgeon before granting privileges, or it can be held liable in a court of law for allowing an incompetent physician on its staff, should there be a bad outcome.

It is preferable to obtain primary verification and documentation by contacting each place of education, training and employment individually by phone and obtain original documents, such as transcripts with raised seals. Verification can include, but is not limited to, the following elements (AMA, 2006):

- Name, address(es) and telephone numbers;
- Birth date, place of birth;
- Medical school;
- Residency training program and other graduate education, including fellowships;
- State licensure details, including date of issue and expiration;
- Specialty and subspecialty, including board certification and eligibility;
- Continuing medical education;
- Educational and employment references;
- Drug Enforcement Agency (DEA) registration status; and,
- Licensure, Medicare/Medicaid, and other state or federal sanctions.

As a healthcare manager, you may find yourself working in the physician relations and credentialing department of a hospital, HMO, or other healthcare delivery organization, and you may be responsible for determining whether the credentials offered by a physician are legitimate. Physician credentialing requires excellent interpersonal skills, organizational skills, persistence, an eye for details, and the ability to identify inconsistencies in data.

Since physicians are tracked from the moment they graduate from medical school, the first thing you want to verify is that there are no gaps in their resumes. Physicians rarely take time off "to find themselves." If there is a significant gap between educational or employment placements (e.g., nothing on the resume for 4 years between a residency training program and an evening shift job working at a clinic with a poor reputation), you need to question what has transpired in this individual's life. Physicians are human and could have had events in their life such as mental illness, addiction, or imprisonment. Since you will be responsible for safe, effective patient care, you must be mindful about who is providing that care. The first clue will be in the credentials, especially in the chronology of life events.

Occasionally, you will come across an individual who claims to be a physician, but who is not. In this Internet and computer age, physician imposters can obtain fraudulent credentials from medical schools in other countries, or even in the United States. Physician imposters are rare, but potentially dangerous individuals. There is no substitute for personal interaction with the institution where someone claims to have been educated or to have been employed. This is where an eye for details and inconsistencies and interpersonal skills come into play. You will be required to handle telephone inquiries with the utmost of tact to ensure that you obtain verification. If no one at an institution knows the individual, or if the medical school has "burned down, leaving no records," alarm bells should be ringing in your head and you should notify your manager immediately that there may be a problem with the application.

A comprehensive review of a physician's credentials involves making electronic queries to the **National Practitioner Data Bank (NPDB)**. At one time, physicians who were disciplined or lost their license in one state, could simply move to another state, and get a license there. Other than person-to-person contacts, there were few ways to track "bad docs" who moved across state borders. The NPDB was created to have a system, whereby state licensing boards, hospitals, professional societies, and other healthcare entities could identify, discipline, and report those who engage in unprofessional behavior. "The intent of the NPDB is to restrict the ability of incompetent physicians, dentists, and other healthcare practitioners to move from state to state without disclosure or discovery of previous medical malpractice payment and adverse action history. Adverse actions can involve licensure, clinical privileges, professional society membership, and exclusions from Medicare and Medicaid" (NPDB, 2006). One of the main criticisms of the NPDB is that a physician can be reported for having been sued, but the outcome of the lawsuit, even when dismissed, is not reported and the lawsuit remains on the physician's record. In an era of increasingly litigious consumers of health care, this is not a minor complaint. Physicians may dispute the report, but it can take much time and effort, much like trying to get a correction on a credit report. Per the NPDB, "The information contained in the NPDB should be considered together with other relevant data in evaluating a practitioner's credentials; it is intended to augment, not replace, traditional forms of credentials review" (NPDB, 2006).

When credentialing physicians, it is critical to have other physicians review the application to ensure that experts who understand the nuances of the data contained in an application render the final judgment whether to approve or disapprove privileges. Using the example of a surgeon applying for general surgical privileges at a hospital, after the physician credentialing department receives a physician's application for privileges, and does due diligence in verifying each and every claim on the application, the materials are submitted to a surgical credentialing committee. Unless the hospital is very small, each department will have its own credentialing committee. In this case, if the Department of Surgery's credentialing committee approves the application, the documents are forwarded to a Medical Executive Committee, which is a subcommittee of the hospital board of directors (BOD). The subcommittee then makes a recommendation to the BOD, which then approves or disapproves the application. Under certain circumstances, temporary credentials can be granted. Usually, however, the time from submission of the application to final approval can take 3 to 6 months. If there are problems with the application or missing documents, the process can take even longer.

Physician credentialing is one of the most important jobs in any healthcare delivery setting. By approving a physician's privileges, the healthcare organization indicates that it believes that this MD will provide safe, effective patient care. It is not a responsibility to be taken lightly. The lives of patients and the financial survival of the healthcare organization depend on how well this process has been done.

International Medical Graduates

International Medical Graduates (IMGs), formerly referred to as Foreign Medical Graduates (FMGs), can be U.S. citizens who attend school abroad, or foreign-born nationals who come to the United States seeking educational and professional opportunities and filling voids in healthcare services delivery for the U.S. population. IMGs represent 25% of the U.S. physician workforce, or approximately 180,000 physicians (Smart, 2006). The top three countries for sending foreign-born physicians to the United

States are India, the Philippines, and Cuba, trailed by Pakistan, Iran, Korea, Egypt, China, Germany, and Syria (McMahon, 2004).

Researchers have repeatedly demonstrated that IMGs are more likely to go where U.S. medical graduates (USMGs) prefer *not* to go (i.e., inner-city and rural areas) and to serve populations increasingly at risk of medical abandonment (Hagopian, Thompson, Kaltenbach, & Hart, 2003; Hallock, Seeling, & Norcini, 2003; Mick & Lee, 1999a, 1999b; Mick, Lee & Wodchis, 2000; Polsky, Kletke, Wozniak, & Escarce, 2002). At one time, the quality of care provided by non-USMGs was a major concern. Over the past decade, however, a formidable system of checks and balances has been implemented, and foreign-trained and foreign-born medical graduates (FBMGs) are now required to pass rigorous English language and written and clinical skills assessments examinations prior to being allowed to apply for GME, i.e., residency training positions (Whelan, Gary, Kostis, Boutlet, & Hallock, 2000). This arrangement has improved the quality of the IMG applicant pool that continues to fill graduate medical education positions still left unfilled by USMGs (McMahon, 2004; Cooper & Aiken, 2001).

Recent research indicates that the U.S. primary care physician (PCP) workforce of the future will include more IMGs, most of whom will be citizens or permanent residents of the United States, and graduates of Caribbean medical schools (Brotherton, Rockey, & Etzel, 2005). In addition, contrary to previous predictions of a glut in the medical labor pool, many experts now predict a shortage of physicians resulting, in part, from the aging of the baby boomer population, physician retirements, changing ethnic and racial demographics, increased utilization of services, a hostile malpractice environment, and an increasing number of medical school graduates (both female and male) who desire reasonable work hours (Cooper, 2002, 2003; BHPR, 2003). Newspapers have begun to report on difficulties some PCPs are encountering in seeing patients and shortages in internal medicine (Bell, 2005). In response to these pressures, some authors and organizations—including the Association of American Medical Colleges (AAMC)—are calling for increases in the number of US medical schools and the expansion of U.S. medical school classes to increase the number of graduates (Blumenthal, 2003; AAMC, 2005).

Some authors question the ethics of a country that continues to rely heavily on IMGs (AAMC, 2005, 2006; Biviano & Makarehchi, 2002). Mullen (2002) has pointed out that, in a global economy, the United

States and other developed countries have a disproportionate share of physicians compared to lower-income nations. Others have reported on the expense involved in an IMG coming to America, only to be exploited and placed in poor or unfair working conditions—a situation not unlike indentured servitude (Hagopian et al., 2003). Clearly, these abuses and ethical concerns must be addressed. And, at a time when our nation is escalating the production of physicians, it might seem to some that we don't need to import more. In fact, the AAMC (2006) has asked "whether it is appropriate to have more than 5,000 IMGs enter American medicine every year."

Regardless of politics, as the United States comes to terms with the knowledge that its physician supply is not keeping up with demand, healthcare managers will struggle with recruitment, retention, and optimal utilization of physicians, whether USMG or IMG. Some of the issues you will be most likely to encounter with IMGs will surround the physician credentialing process and the J-Visa, which provides legal entry to the United States for training purposes. Physicians who graduate from foreign medical schools will have to provide, in some instances, additional documentation and verification that the information they have provided is true and correct. The Educational Commission for Foreign Medical Graduates (ECFMG) now offers on-line credential verification services (ECFMG, 2006), which will ease some of the burden, but not all of the responsibility or liability in the granting of privileges.

In summary, physicians are critical to the provision of safe, effective patient care. Ensuring the quality of the physicians practicing in an organization is one of the roles of the healthcare manager. To fulfill this responsibility, you will need to know all the steps in the education, training, and credentialing of physicians. It will take attention to detail, organizational skills, and excellent interpersonal skills to do it well.

Employed Primary Care Physicians and Turnover

At one time the majority of physicians in the United States were self-employed, solo practitioners, or in partnership with one or two other physicians. In 1983, 23% of all patient care Primary Care Physicians (PCPs), excluding residents in training, reported being employed (AMA, 1996). In 1998, the AMA reported that 45% of all physicians in Family Practice (FP), 38.6% of those in Internal Medicine (IM), and 50% of Pediatricians (Peds) reported that they were employees (Zhang, & Thran, 1999).

Much of this change in physician employment is due to consolidation of physicians' practices and enrollment growth in managed care organizations. Buchbinder, Wilson, Melick, and Powe (2001), using data from a nationally representative sample, studied a cohort of 533 post-resident, nonfederal, employed PCPs who were younger than 45 years of age, had been in practice between 2 and 9 years, and had participated in national surveys in 1987 and 1991. They combined data from this sample with a national study of physician compensation and productivity and physician recruiters to estimate recruitment and replacement costs associated with **turnover** (i.e., the proportion of job exits or quits from a facility in a year).

The authors found that by the 1991 survey, slightly more than half (N = 279 or 55%) of all PCPs in this cohort had left the practice in which they had been employed in 1987; 20% (N = 100) had left two employers in that same 5-year period. In an earlier article, these authors estimated that recruitment and replacement costs for individual PCPs for the three specialties were $236,383 for Family Practice (FP); $245,128 for Internal Medicine (IM), and $264,645 for Pediatrics (Peds). Turnover costs for all PCPs in the cohort by specialty were $24.5 million for FP; $22.3 million for IM; and $22.2 million for Peds (Buchbinder, Wilson, Melick, & Powe, 1999). They concluded that turnover was an important phenomenon among the PCPs in this cohort and that PCP turnover has major fiscal implications for PCP employers. Loss of PCPs causes healthcare organization systems to lose resources that could otherwise be devoted to patient care.

A recent physician retention study conducted by Cejka Search and the American Medical Group Association (AMGA, 2005, p. 6) reported that "physician turnover is a top concern and important priority for practice leaders." In addition, the report indicates that nearly half of all physicians who leave do so within 3 years; the effects of turnover burden remaining physicians; the majority of leavers are voluntary, due to practice issues; and compensation is a larger issue in small groups. These are clearly management issues related to physician turnover.

Employee turnover has been clearly linked to job dissatisfaction and job burnout. **Job satisfaction** is the "pleasurable or positive emotional state resulting from the appraisal of one's job or job experiences" (Locke, 1983). **Job burnout** is "a prolonged response to chronic emotional and interpersonal stressors on the job" (Maslach, 2003). In the past, most solutions to job burnout involved removing the affected individual from the job. However, it is the *organization* that is the primary cause of job burnout (due to heavy workload, poor relations with co-workers, etc.) and job dissatisfaction. Therefore, it is the healthcare manager's role to address these issues. Healthcare managers employed in these kinds of settings must be alert to signs of physician job dissatisfaction and burnout, the harbingers of turnover. As a healthcare manager in a medical group practice, you will be expected to work with the physicians to help create a positive practice environment and to provide recommendations for interventions to improve retention.

REGISTERED NURSES

At one time, all nurses were trained in hospital-based programs and received diplomas upon graduation. Before 1917, nursing was essentially an apprenticeship, without a set curriculum (Hilliard, 2004). That changed, however, when "Miss Adelaide Nutting became the first nurse appointed to a university professorship at Teacher's College of Columbia University, and developed the first standard curriculum for schools of nursing" (Hilliard, 2004, p. 5). The hospital-based diploma nursing school is part of a passing era; in 2004, there were only 69 left in the United States (BLS, 2006b). Currently, the majority of nursing education is provided in degree-based settings. Nurses are educated in community colleges, earning an associate degree in 2 to 3 years, or university and college baccalaureate programs for professional nursing practice, earning a Bachelor of Science in Nursing (BSN) in 4 years. Many graduates of associate degree programs go back to school while they work full-time to earn a BSN to improve their opportunities for career advancement (Health Resources & Services Administration, 2004).

Nurses with BSNs can continue their education and enter a wide array of graduate educational programs including, but not limited to: post-baccalaureate certificates, Master's of Science in Nursing (MSN) degrees for community health nursing and nurse education, advanced practice degrees (nurse practitioner, clinical nurse specialist, nurse midwife, nurse anesthetist); and doctoral degrees, such as the Nursing Doctorate (ND), Doctorate in Nursing Science (DNS), or a Doctor of Philosophy (PhD).

The undergraduate nursing school curriculum (BSN) is rigorous and demands a good understanding of the biological sciences. Using Towson University as an example, students are eligible to apply for admission to the major only after completing a minimum of 42 undergraduate credits, including at least four laboratory sciences and an English composition course. Admission is based on the cumulative grade point average and only one grade below a C is allowed in prerequisite or general education courses, and no more than two non-nursing courses may be repeated (Towson University, 2006).

The current shortage of nursing faculty means fewer slots for nursing students—there are fewer faculty to teach (AACN, 2003). Many nursing programs are so competitive that there are three applicants for every acceptance. Due to a crisis-level national nursing shortage and demands for workers, state legislators are pressuring universities and colleges to increase the number of graduates from nursing programs. However, unlike other undergraduate degrees, nursing students must learn clinical skills and be carefully supervised in healthcare organizations by master's or doctorally-prepared nursing faculty. The nursing faculty clinical supervisor is only allowed to have a specific number of student nurses. Exceeding that number could endanger the lives of patients and the faculty member's nursing license.

As nursing students progress through their program of study, meeting state requirements for licensure, and passing the National Council Licensure Examination (NCLEX) is uppermost in everyone's minds. A student must pass the NCLEX to become a licensed registered nurse (RN) in the United States, and nursing programs' pass rates on the NCLEX are used as a proxy for the quality of their educational curriculum. With the current nursing shortage, most graduating nurses have a job offer in hand before they graduate—contingent upon obtaining state licensure and passing the NCLEX (NCSBN, 2006b, c).

As noted before in the section on physicians, some states now require criminal background checks (CBCs) for nurse applicants for licensure (NCSBN, 2006a). Again, the reasons are multifold, and include, but are not limited to: increasing societal concerns about: alcohol and drug abusers, sexual predators, and child and elder abusers. If a criminal background check contains information about convictions, the licensure board will examine the application on a case-by-case basis. As noted previously, the reviewers will be looking for level and frequency of the criminal behavior, basing their decision on that along with other materials submitted by the applicant, such as proof of alcohol and drug rehabilitation.

After graduation, RNs, unlike physicians, do not have post-graduate programs that last from 3 to 10 years. In the past, new RNs have been hired by hospitals or other healthcare organizations, given a brief orientation, then placed on a nursing unit and left to sink or swim. This Darwinian approach to nurse staffing, has led, in part, to massive turnover. Although the vast majority of nurses are female (only 5% are male), women now have career choices other than nursing, teaching, or home-making, and older nurses are retiring faster than new ones are coming into the field (Steiger, Auerbach, & Buerhaus, 2000; HRSA, 2004). Nursing turnover costs have been estimated to be from $46,000 to $65,000 per lost nurse (Kemski, 2002; Kosel & Olivo, 2002). Multiply that by the number of nurses who quit their jobs and the costs can be in the millions of dollars for healthcare organizations. Healthcare managers cannot afford to ignore the loss of nurses from the workforce.

Any strategy that improves the retention of nursing staff saves the organization the costs of using agency or traveler nurses, replacing lost nurses and training new ones, as well as the loss of productivity from burdening the remaining staff. A survey conducted among 67 new nurses from 13 hospital departments indicated that new graduates were concerned about communicating with physicians and were afraid of "causing accidental harm to patients." Additionally, this group identified a desire for "comprehensive orientation, continuing education and mentoring" (Boswell, Lowry, & Wilhoit, 2004, p. 76). Nurse residency programs (NRPs) have been identified by the Joint Commission on Accreditation of Healthcare Organizations (JCAHO, 2002) and the Robert Wood Johnson Foundation (Kimball & O'Neil, 2002) as a strategy for improving RN retention. One study of an NRP for intensive care unit (ICU) nurses demonstrated increased job satisfaction, improved retention, and decreased turnover (Williams, Sims, Burkhead, & Ward, 2002). Another study describing the planning, implementation, and evaluation of a model NRP for ICU and medical-surgical nurses found that new RNs who participated in the NRPs "demonstrated improved retention, critical thinking, socialization, ability to manage stress, and problem-solving skills" (Herdrich & Lindsay, 2006, p. 55).

A difficult transition into practice isn't the only reason that nurses leave healthcare organizations. Nurses quit jobs where they feel overworked, underpaid, and disrespected by their co-workers and managers. Using national focus groups, on behalf of the Robert Wood Johnson Foundation, Kimball and O'Neil (2002) found that RNs are concerned about being unable to physically continue to do the work, increases in their daily workloads, and the lack of ancillary staff to support them. These groups also indicated that they were confused about healthcare financial issues, felt powerless to change things in their work environments, and thought their nurse managers were over-extended and unable to help them. The respondents gave a list of suggestions to improve the retention of nurses, including (Kimball & O'Neil, 2002, p. 46):

- Decreasing workloads;
- Providing support staff;
- Empowering nurse managers;
- Increasing salaries;
- Encouraging physicians to treat nurses as colleagues;
- Improving the orientation process; and,
- Providing paid continuing education.

Overwork of nurses and high patient-to-nurse ratios lead to patient mortality, nurse burnout, and job dissatisfaction (Aiken, Clarke, Sloane, Sochalski, & Silber, 2002). Aiken et al. (2002) benchmark article demonstrated that each additional patient per nurse was associated with a 7% increase in the likelihood of dying within 30 days of hospital admission. The JCAHO (2002, p. 6) report called a high patient-to-nurse ratio "a prescription for danger," and indicated that "staffing levels have been a factor in 24% of 1608 sentinel events (unanticipated events that result in death, injury, or permanent loss or function)." In addition, in 2003, Aiken et al. reported that more nurse education and training leads to a higher quality of service and lower patient mortality. In light of these data, it makes financial sense to employ more RNs per patient, and to hire RNs with a baccalaureate level or higher. Given the nursing shortage, the healthcare manager's next best choice would be to hire RNs with an associate degree, provide tuition assistance, and create incentives for them to return to school for their BSN.

Encouraging physicians to treat nurses as colleagues has always been a challenge. Recommendations for collaborative practice between physicians and nurses have been in place for decades, going back to nursing shortages in the 1980s and the National Commission on Nursing's (1983) *Summary Report and Recommendations*, calling for nurse-physician joint practice. One of the problems in this dyad has been the gap between physician and nursing education. In previous years, when diploma schools dominated nursing education, physicians had at least 20 more years of formal education than the RNs they worked with. In that era, when a physician walked into a room, nurses stood up, as a sign of respect—and to give him her chair. Nurses now have formal educational programs in degree-granting settings, and the educational gap between the two healthcare professional groups is diminishing. Women have also "come of age" since the women's rights movement in the 1970s, and nurses are no longer the doctor's handmaiden. They, too, are healthcare professionals.

Physician resistance to acknowledging nurses as professionals and colleagues leads to poor teamwork, interpersonal conflict, and can lead to poor patient outcomes. One study found that physicians and nurses differed widely in their opinions about teamwork in an ICU setting. Almost three quarters of the physicians reported high levels of teamwork with nurses, but less than half of the nurses felt the same way (Sexton, Thomas, & Helmreich, 2000). As noted in a subsequent chapter on teamwork, despite demonstrated need and effectiveness of interdisciplinarity, formal teamwork, educational training for physicians and nurses is rare (Baker, Salas, King, Battles, & Barach, 2005; Buchbinder et al., 2005). A poll conducted in 2004 by the American College of Physician Executives (ACPE) revealed that about one quarter of the physician executive respondents were seeing problem physician behaviors almost weekly (Weber, 2004). Thirty-six percent of the respondents reported conflicts between physicians and staff members (including nurses) and 25% reported physicians refused to embrace teamwork.

Organizational climate is critical to promoting job satisfaction and retention of nursing staff. Laschinger and Finegan (2005) found that nurses who perceived that they had access to opportunity, experienced honest relationships and open communication with peers and managers, and trusted their managers, were more likely to be retained and to have higher job satisfaction. The American Association of Colleges of Nursing (AACN, 2002) published a white paper titled, *Hallmarks of the Professional Nursing Practice Environment*. The attributes of hospitals with work environments that support professional nursing practice were reviewed and the questions a new graduate should ask were listed. They are: Does your potential employer:

- manifest a philosophy of clinical care, emphasizing quality, safety, interdisciplinary collaboration, continuity of care and professional accountability?
- recognize the contributions of nurses' knowledge and expertise to clinical care quality and patient outcomes?

- promote executive level nursing leadership?
- empower nurses' participation in clinical decision-making and organization of clinical care systems?
- maintain clinical advancement programs based on education, certification, and advanced preparation?
- demonstrate professional development support for nurses?
- create collaborative relationships among members of the healthcare provider team?
- utilize technological advances in clinical care and information systems?

The AACN also recommends that applicants inquire about RN staff education, vacancy, tenure and turnover rates, patient and employees satisfaction scores, and percentage of registry/traveler nurses used. The questions posed by the AACN challenge healthcare organizations to rise to higher standards, and to reach for American Nurses' Credentialing Center Magnet Recognition Program® status (ANCC, 2006a). Unless these questions are answered in the affirmative, nursing turnover will continue to be one of the largest human and financial costs that the healthcare manager will be forced to control.

Like physicians who sit for board certification examinations, RNs can take ANCC or other nursing specialty organizations (e.g., the Wound, Ostomy, and Continence Nurses' Society; the American Association of Critical Care Nurses, etc.) examinations to demonstrate additional competence in a specialty, after they have practiced for a specific number of hours (usually 1,000 hours or about a year) in a specialty area. Nursing Professional Development requires 2,000 hours of practice. Thus nurses can be certified in a large number and variety of specialty areas, including, but not limited to:

- Ambulatory Care;
- Cardiac Rehabilitation;
- Cardiac Vascular;
- Case Management;
- Critical Care;
- Gerontological;
- High-Risk Perinatal;
- Maternal Child;
- Medical-Surgical;
- Nursing Administration;
- Nursing Professional Development;

- Pain Management;
- Pediatric;
- Perinatal;
- Psychiatric and Mental Health;
- School;
- Vascular; and,
- Wound Care.

Nurses who are credentialed in specialty areas must demonstrate continuing competency by fulfilling requirements for certification renewal via one or several of the following mechanisms: continuing education hours, academic courses, presentations and lectures, publications and research, or preceptorships.

In many states, nurses are required to obtain nursing continuing education units (CEUs) to renew and maintain their nursing license. The ANCC Commission on Accreditation, the credentialing unit of the American Nurses Association (ANA), reviews and approves providers of nursing CEUs (ANCC, 2006b). There are, literally, hundreds of providers of nursing CEUs and multiple way to obtain nursing CEUs, including, but not limited to: on-line courses; magazine or journal articles; workshops and conferences; audiotapes, CDs, DVDs; and the above noted academic courses, presentations and lectures, publications and research, or preceptorships. Nurses can even attend other healthcare providers' workshops that have been approved for awarding nursing CEUs. There is no dearth of opportunities for nurses to obtain continuing education. It is the responsibility of the RN to maintain her license. Your role as healthcare manager will be to ensure that resources (i.e., money and time) are available for nurses to participate in these educational opportunities.

Foreign Educated Nurses

The nursing shortage, caused by a confluence of the aging of the U.S. nursing workforce, declining enrollments in nursing schools, higher average age of new graduates from nursing school, and organizational retention and turnover difficulties would have been difficult enough for healthcare managers on its own. However, we have what some people call "the perfect storm" in health care because the nursing shortage is now combined with demographic forces and market forces, such as aging baby boomers, increasing racial and ethnic diversity, increased demand for healthcare services, increasing longevity of U.S. citizens, new treatments for chronic diseases that used to kill people (like asthma, diabetes, hypertension), and educated and demanding healthcare consumers (HRSA, 2003).

Since U.S. healthcare organizations are experiencing a crisis in the nursing workforce, and cannot survive without nurses to deliver care, it is not surprising that foreign-educated nurses are coming to the United States to fill gaps in nursing services. In 2004, about 3.5% (100,791) of the RNs practicing in the United States received their basic nursing education outside the country (HRSA, 2004). A little over 50% of these nurses come from the Philippines, 20% from Canada, 8% from the United Kingdom, and the remaining from a variety of countries. About half of the foreign-educated nurses have a baccalaureate degree or higher.

Most U.S. state nursing boards require foreign-educated nurses to successfully complete the Commission on Graduates of Foreign Nursing Schools (CGFNS) certification program (CGFNS, 2006). This program consists of three parts: a credentials review, a Qualifying Exam of nursing knowledge, and an English language proficiency examination. The CGFNS program is designed to predict an applicant's likelihood of passing the NCLEX-RN® examination and becoming licensed as a registered nurse in the United States. The CGFNS Certification Program removes a major burden from an employer. However, as a healthcare manager your job may require you to ensure that foreign-educated nurses have fulfilled all the requirements of the State Board of Nursing and that they are legally allowed to work in the United States.

Some of the issues you encounter may include interpersonal conflicts between U.S. educated and foreign-educated nurses, and between physicians and foreign-educated nurses. Different cultures bring varying expectations to the work setting. These expectations may well be at odds with those of their co-workers. Excellent interpersonal skills, conflict management, cultural competency, and sensitivity to diversity issues are critical for you to be able to be an effective healthcare manager for these employees.

LICENSED PRACTICAL NURSES/LICENSED VOCATIONAL NURSES

In 2004, there were about 726,000 **Licensed Practical Nurses (LPNs) or Licensed Vocational Nurses (LVNs)** working under the supervision of physicians and nurses in the United States. According to the Bureau of Labor Statistics (2006d), about one quarter were employed in hospitals, about one-quarter in nursing care facilities, and another 12% worked in physician's offices. Others worked for home health services, employment services, community care facilities for the elderly, public and private educational services, outpatient centers, and federal, state, and local government services. After graduation from high school, LPNs are trained in 1-year, state-approved programs. Most are trained in technical or vocational schools, although some high schools offer it as part of their curriculum. In order to be employed as an LPN, students must graduate from a state-approved program, then pass the LPN licensing exam, the NCLEX-PN (BLS, 2006d). LPNs are trained to do basic nursing functions, such as vital signs, observing patients, assisting patients with **activities of daily living (ADLs)**, such as bathing, dressing, and feeding. With additional training, where state laws allow, they can also administer medications. LPNs are the backbone of the long-term care (LTC) sector of the healthcare industry, providing around the clock care and supervision of **certified nurse's aides (CNAs)** in nursing homes and convalescent centers. Many LPNs go on to earn their RN, and in some states, LPNs can take challenge examinations to earn their RN licensure. LPNs are an important part of the healthcare team, and should be included in the healthcare manager's tuition assistance plan to encourage key personnel to return to school for additional education.

NURSING, PSYCHIATRIC, AND HOME HEALTH AIDES

In 2004, there were about 2.1 million nursing, psychiatric, and home health aides employed in nursing and residential care facilities, hospitals, psychiatric and substance abuse facilities, and home health agencies (BLS, 2006e). Nursing aides, nursing assistants, CNAs, orderlies, and other unlicensed patient attendants work under the supervision of physicians and nurses. They answer call bells, assist patients with toileting, change beds, serve meals, and assist patients with ADLs. Regardless of employment setting, aides are front line personnel. Since nursing aides held the most jobs, at 1.5 million, and were employed most often by nursing care facilities, that will be the focus of the remainder of this section.

Nurse's aides have made the news in negative ways in recent years. In the past, CNAs were not required to have criminal background checks (CBCs), and elder abusers, sexual predators, and thieves saw the elderly population as easy prey (New York State Office of the Attorney General, 2000). Now the majority of states and employers require CBCs. However, a clean CBC doesn't guarantee that the person hasn't or won't abuse a patient. Therefore, it is incumbent upon the healthcare organization to have policies about neglect and abuse prevention in place, and the healthcare manager must enforce them. Some nursing homes have installed "granny-cams," video surveillance systems, to keep an eye on caregiver behavior and to document misbehavior. When working with vulnerable populations, it is incumbent upon the healthcare manager to be in a state of constant vigilance for neglect and abuse.

CNAs are often trained on the job in 75 hours of mandatory training and are required to pass a competency examination. CNAs provide direct care to patients over long periods of time and are often the most overlooked group of workers in terms of pay, benefits, and opportunities for advancement. Seavey (2004) conducted a literature review and found estimates of turnover from LTC facilities ranged from 40% to 166%, with indirect and direct costs per lost worker ranging from $951 to $6,368. She estimated a minimum direct cost of $2,500 per lost worker.

It's a vicious cycle: poor quality of worklife begets turnover, which begets poor quality of worklife, which begets more turnover. And, it's not just the CNAs and other aides that are impacted. Once the CNAs are gone, the LPNs will go, then the RNs will be stressed, emotionally burned out, and leave (Kennedy, 2005). Then who will provide the care? The job of the healthcare manager is to improve retention, to slow down or stop turnover by addressing the quality of worklife. The place to start is with a comparable market wage analysis. Are the workers being paid the same, or better, than workers with comparable jobs at other comparable facilities? Nursing home administrators have confided that CNAs will leave one facility to go to another one for a 25-cent per hour pay raise. Is the pay fair? Does the facility pay tuition assistance for CNAs? What kind of benefits package is being offered?

After looking at these basic items the healthcare manager needs to assess the work environment, including employee job burnout and satisfaction, preferably using an outside organization so workers can respond freely without fear of retribution. While not an exhaustive list, some of the items to be included in a worklife analysis include worker perceptions of:

- Job autonomy, variety, and significance;
- Fairness of pay and benefits;
- Opportunities for promotion and advancement;
- Relationships with supervisors;

- Relationships with co-workers;
- Level of job burnout; and,
- Overall job satisfaction.

All healthcare workers, not just nurses, want to be treated as colleagues and with respect. If you conduct a survey of the organizational climate—as seen by the workers—you must be prepared to respond and to intervene. If you do nothing, you will lose employees' trust, and the revolving door of turnover will continue.

MIDLEVEL PRACTITIONERS

Midlevel practitioners include Advanced Practice Nurses (APNs), such as Nurse Practitioners (NPs), Clinical Nurse Specialists (CNS), Nurse Anesthetists, and Nurse Midwives, as well as Physician Assistants (PAs). In 2004, 8.4% (240,461) of the RNs in the United States were APNs (HRSA, 2004). In 2004, PAs held 62,000 jobs in a wide variety of healthcare settings (BLS, 2006c). These healthcare professionals are called **midlevel practitioners** because they work mid-way between the level of an RN and that of an MD. Midlevel practitioners serve in a variety of settings, including: hospital emergency rooms or departments, community health clinics, physician offices, and health maintenance organizations. They may also cover hospital floors for physicians. Midlevel practitioners are usually less expensive than physicians, often replacing MDs at a 2:1 ratio. Although APNs were resisted by many state medical societies early in the 1970s, over time physicians realized that APNs could increase their productivity and ease their workload. Midlevel practitioners are much sought after by healthcare organizations because they can provide many of the same services as physicians, at a lower cost.

Advanced Practice Nurses

There are many organizations and accrediting bodies that certify Advanced Practice Nurses (APNs). The following discussion is not intended to be an exhaustive listing of the specialty certifications that are available. Rather, it is meant to be illustrative of the variety of roles that APNs can assume. In addition to the educational preparation noted below, all APNs must demonstrate continuing competency by obtaining CEUs. APN certification must be renewed every 5 years, either by documenting evidence of practice, or by retaking the examination. Below are some examples of APNs.

Nurse Practitioners (NPs) are prepared in either an NP MSN or in a post-master's certificate program. To become certified by the ANCC, NPs must demonstrate that they have "graduated from a program offered by an accredited institution granting graduate-level academic credit for all course work that includes both didactic and clinical components and a minimum of 500 hours of supervised clinical practice in the specialty area" (ANCC, 2006c). These APNs can become certified in areas of care which include, but are not limited to: acute, adult, adult psychiatric/mental health, advanced diabetes management, family, family psychiatric/mental health, gerontological, and pediatric. They must pass a certification exam and maintain their competency through continuing nursing education, and recertification exams.

Clinical Nurse Specialists (CNSs) have in-depth education in the clinical specialty area at a master's degree level. To be certified as a CNS, the RN must have all of the same educational qualifications as an NP, but in their area of focus, plus a minimum of 500 hours of supervised clinical practice in their specialty area. Areas of certification include, but are not limited to: advanced diabetes, adult health, adult psychiatric/mental health, child/adolescent psychiatric/mental health, gerontological, pediatric, and public/community health. They must pass a certification exam and maintain their competency through continuing nursing education, and recertification exams.

Certified Registered Nurse Anesthetists (CRNAs) are APNs who specialize in providing anesthesia. According to the American Association of Nurse Anesthetists (AANA), nurses have been providing anesthesia care since the U.S. Civil War (AANA, 2006). They work in cooperation with anesthesiologists, surgeons, dentists, and other healthcare professionals. To become a CRNA, in addition to having a BSN and an RN, and having worked at least one year as an RN in an acute care setting, the nurse must graduate from an accredited master's degree nurse anesthesia program. CRNAs must also pass a national certification examination.

Certified Nurse Midwives (CNMs) are licensed as independent practitioners in all states except California, Connecticut, Florida, Illinois, Massachusetts, North Carolina, South Carolina, and Virginia (ACNM, 2006a). Nurse midwives were introduced to the United States in 1925 with the Frontier Nursing Service (FNS), founded by Mary Breckenridge (FNS, 2006). All CNMs must be RNs, with at least 1–2 years of nursing experience, and graduate from a nurse-midwifery education program accredited by the American College of Nurse-Midwives (ACNM) Division of Accreditation (DOA) and pass a national certification examination (ACNM, 2006b).

Physician Assistants

According to the American Academy of Physician Assistants (AAPA), **Physician Assistants (PAs)** were created in the 1960's in response to a primary care physician shortage in the United States. Vietnam veteran medical corpsmen were selected for a "fast-track" training program and trained to assist physicians wherever they practiced (AAPA, 2006a). Since that time, the education and training of PAs has changed dramatically. In 2005, there were 136 accredited PA educational programs, as varied as certificate programs, associate degrees, baccalaureate degrees, and master's degrees (AAPA, 2006b). Only graduates of accredited PA programs are eligible to take the Physician Assistant National Certifying Examination. PAs must demonstrate competency and be recertified every 6 years, and must earn 100 CME hours every 2 years (AAPA, 2006c). PAs are licensed to practice in every state in the U.S. (plus the District of Columbia, the Mariana Islands, Guam, and the U.S. Virgin Islands) and have prescribing authority in every state except Indiana (AAPA, 2006c). PAs practice in every conceivable setting, although the major employers of PAs are single-specialty physician groups, multi-specialty physician groups, solo physician practices, hospitals, community health centers, and HMOs. PAs are versatile and valuable members of the healthcare team and are highly sought after by physician practices, hospitals, and other employers.

ALLIED HEALTH PROFESSIONALS

The term **allied health professionals** refers to more than 2000 programs in over 20 health science occupations (CAAHEP, 2006). Allied health professionals assist physicians and nurses in providing comprehensive care to patients in a variety of settings. Many of the occupations, such as anesthesiologist assistant and surgical assistant, have grown from the unmet demand for help in the highly specialized operating room environment. Other occupations, such as perfusionist and electroneurodiagnostic technician, have grown out of the technological boom and the need for people to operate highly specific equipment. Radiology technologists assist radiographers in imaging technologies, which are changing with dizzying speed.

The following is a list of the occupations described at the CAAHEP website, http://www.caahep.org/, and is not meant to be exhaustive.

- Anesthesiologist assistant;
- Athletic trainer;
- Cardiovascular technologist;
- Cytotechnologist;
- Diagnostic medical sonographer;
- Electroneurodiagnostic technologist;
- EMT—Paramedic;
- Exercise physiologist;
- Exercise scientist;
- Kinesiotherapist;
- Medical assistant;
- Medical illustrator;
- Ophthalmic medical technician/technologist;
- Orthotist/Prosthetist;
- Perfusionist;
- Personal fitness trainer;
- Polysomnographic technologist;
- Respiratory therapist—Advanced level;
- Respiratory therapist—Entry level;
- Specialist in blood banking technology;
- Surgical assistant; and,
- Surgical technologist.

Due to space limitations, this section will address one allied health occupation: respiratory therapists (RTs). In 2004, RTs held about 118,000 jobs, with over 80% in hospital departments of respiratory care, anesthesiology, or pulmonary medicine (BLS, 2006f). RTs evaluate, treat, and care for patients with respiratory disorders, such as asthma, emphysema, pneumonia, and heart disease. An associate's degree is required for entry into the field and more education is required for advancement. RTs are certified by the National Board for Respiratory Care and registration is available only to graduates of CAAHEP accredited programs for Registered Respiratory Therapists (RRTs) and Certified Respiratory Therapists (CRTs). All states (except Hawaii and Alaska), as well as the District of Columbia and Puerto Rico require RTs to obtain a license. In addition, most employers require cardiopulmonary resuscitation (CPR) certification because RTs are usually members of hospital rapid response teams.

Shortages exist in almost all the allied health occupations, but respiratory therapy is particularly affected, along with radiology technologists and certified nursing assistants. Hart (2002) conducted a survey of these three groups and found a disturbing picture of worklife for these healthcare professionals. All three groups were dissatisfied with current worklife, and claimed inadequate staffing was the "number one problem they face." They felt healthcare professional shortages compromised patient care, and that turnover was impacting retention and recruitment. Recommendations from the three groups included: increased salaries, improved staffing ratios, better health benefits, more input into decisions, flexible schedules, increased support staff, and continuing education.

CONCLUSION

This chapter has described the education, training, and credentialing of physicians, nurses, nurses' aides, midlevel practitioners, and allied health professionals, and given an overview of the supply of and demand for healthcare professionals. In addition, some of the reasons for healthcare professional turnover and costs of turnover have been discussed, along with some strategies for increasing retention and preventing turnover. Issues related to the management of the worklife of physicians, nurses, nurses' aides, midlevel practitioners, and allied health professionals have been interwoven through all of these topics. These are issues that can and should be addressed by you, the healthcare manager, with respect for each and every healthcare professional. The challenges await you; there will be no shortage of problems for you to solve.

DISCUSSION QUESTIONS

1. Describe the steps in attaining state licensure for physicians.

2. Describe the steps in attaining state licensure for nurses.

3. What is the difference between licensure and credentialing?

4. What is physician credentialing, and why is it one of the most important jobs in a hospital?

5. What is the National Practitioner Data Base and why was it created?

6. What is an International Medical Graduate and what populations have they traditionally been most likely to serve? Why might we begin to see more foreign-educated nurses in the United States?

7. Define the following terms: job burnout, job satisfaction, retention, and turnover. Why are they of importance in managing healthcare professionals?

8. What is the relationship between nursing education, nursing burnout, job dissatisfaction, and patient mortality?

9. What are the attributes of hospitals with work environments that support professional nursing practice?

10. Distinguish between the following: Advanced Practice Registered Nurse, Certified Registered Nurse, and Physician Assistant.

11. Distinguish between Licensed Practical Nurses and Certified Nurses' Assistants. What are some of the healthcare manager's challenges with these two groups?

12. Who are allied health professionals and what are some of the healthcare management issues in working with them?

REFERENCES

Accreditation Council for Continuing Medical Education (ACCME). *About us.* Retrieved May 20, 2006 from http://www.accme.org/index.cfm/fa/about.home/About.cfm

Accreditation Council for Graduate Medical Education. (2006a). *ACGME fact sheet.* Retrieved April 23, 2006 from http://www.acgme.org/acWebsite/newsRoom/newsRm_factSheet.asp

Accreditation Council for Graduate Medical Education. (2006b). *Resident duty hours and the work environment.* Retrieved April 23, 2006 from http://www.acgme.org/acWebsite/dutyHours/dh_Lang703.pdf

Accreditation Council for Graduate Medical Education. (2006c). *ACGME-Approved specialty specific duty hours language,* effective July 1, 2003. Retrieved April 23, 2006 from http://www.acgme.org/acWebsite/dutyHours/dh_specificDutyHours.pdf

Aiken, L. H., Clarke, S. P., Cheung, R. B., Sloane, D. M., Silber, J. H. (2003). Educational levels of hospital nurses and surgical patient mortality. *Journal of American Medical Association, 290,* 1617–1623.

Aiken, L. H., Clarke, S. P., Sloane, D. M., Sochalski, J., Silber, J. H. (2002). Hospital nurse staffing and patient mortality, nurse burnout, and job dissatisfaction. *Journal of American Medical Association, 288,* 1987–1993.

American Academy of Physician Assistants (AAPA). (2006a). *Information about PAs and the PA profession.* Retrieved May 31, 2006 from http://www.aapa.org/geninfo1 .html

American Academy of Physician Assistants (AAPA). (2006b). *2005 AAPA Physician Assistant census report.* Retrieved May 31, 2006 from http://www.aapa.org/research/ 05census-content.html#1.4

American Academy of Physician Assistants (AAPA). (2006c). *Facts at a glance.* Retrieved May 31, 2006 from http://www.aapa.org/glance.html

American Association of Colleges of Nursing. (2002, January). AACN white paper: *Hallmarks of the professional nursing practice environment.* Retrieved May 27, 2006 from http://www.aacn.nche.edu/Publications/positions/hallmarks.htm

American Association of Colleges of Nursing. (2003, May). AACN white paper: *Faculty shortages in baccalaureate and graduate nursing programs: Scope of the problem and strategies for expanding the supply.* Retrieved May 28, 2006 from http://www .aacn.nche.edu/Publications/WhitePapers/FacultyShortages.htm

American Association of Medical Colleges. (2006). *Making the decision.* Retrieved April 23, 2006 from http://www.aamc.org/students/considering/decision.htm

American Association of Nurse Anesthetists. (2006). *Nurse anesthetists at a glance.* Retrieved May 31, 2006 from http://www.aana.com/aboutaana.aspx?ucNavMenu_ TSMenuTargetID=179&ucNavMenu_TSMenuTargetType=4&ucNavMenu_ TSMenuID=6&id=265

American Board of Medical Specialists. (2006). *What is maintenance of certification?* Retrieved May 1, 2006 from http://www.abms.org/Downloads/Publications/ 1-What%20is%20MOC.pdf

American College of Nurse Midwives (ACNM). (2006a). *Position statement: Principles for credentialing and privileging certified nurse-midwives (CNMs) and Certified Midwives (CMs).* Retrieved May 28, 2006 from http://www.midwife.org/siteFiles/ position/Principles_for_Credentialing_&_Privileging_CNMs_&_CMs_3.06 .pdf?CFID=2187596&CFTOKEN=58530493

American College of Nurse Midwives (ACNM). (2006b). *The credential CNM and CM.* Retrieved May 28, 2006 from http://www.midwife.org/careers.cfm?id=94

American Medical Association (AMA). (1996). American Medical Association Council on Medical Services. *Trends in physician practice consolidation.* CMS Report 9-I-96. Chicago, IL: American Medical Association.

American Medical Association. (2005, October). *Glossary of continuing medical education (CME) related organizations, committees, terms, and credit programs.* Retrieved May 20, 2006 from www.ama-assn.org/ama1/pub/upload/mm/455/ cmeglossary.pdf

American Medical Association. (2006). *Physician credentialing solutions.* Retrieved May 20, 2006 from http://jamacareernet.ama-assn.org/misc/credential.dtl

American Medical Association Medical Students' Section (AMA-MSS). (2004). *Background information.* Retrieved April 23, 2006 from http://www.ama-assn. org/ama/pub/category/print/7570.html

American Nursing Credentialing Center (ANCC). (2006a). *ANCC Magnet Recognition Program®—Recognizing excellence in nursing services.* Retrieved May 28, 2006 from http://nursingworld.org/ancc/magnet/index.html

American Nursing Credentialing Center (ANCC). (2006b). *Accreditation of continuing nursing education providers.* Retrieved May 28, 2006 from http://nursingworld.org/ancc/accred/about.html

American Nursing Credentialing Center (ANCC). (2006c). *ANCC certification.* Retrieved May 28, 2006 from http://nursingworld.org/ancc/cert/index.html

Annotated Code of Maryland (COMAR). (2006). *Licensure—Qualifications for initial licensure.* Retrieved May 20, 2006 from http://www.dsd.state.md.us/comar/10/10.32.01.03.htm

Association of American Medical Colleges. (2005). *Questions and answers about AAMC's new physician workforce position.* Available at http://www.aamc.org/workforce/workforceqa.pdf. Accessed December 13, 2006.

Association of American Medical Colleges. (2006, June). *AAMC position statement on the physician workforce.* Retrieved December 13, 2006 from http://www.aamc.org/workforce/workforce.pdf

Baer L. D. (2004). A proposed framework for analyzing the potential replacement of international medical graduates. *Health & Place, 9*, 291–304.

Baker, D. P., Salas, E., King, H., Battles, J., & Barach, P. (2005, April). The role of teamwork in the professional education of physicians: current status and assessment recommendations. *Journal on Quality and Patient Safety, 31*(4), 185–202.

Bell, J. (2005, October 16) Symptoms of a doctor shortage: Growing population, physicians' desire to cut work weeks add up to a deficit. *The Baltimore Sun.* 1, 6A.

Biviano M., & Makarehchi F. (2002, April 25). *Globalization and the physician workforce in the United States.* Sixth International Medical Workforce Conference, Ottawa, Canada, April 25, 2002. Retrieved December 28, 2005 from ftp://ftp.hrsa.gov/bhpr/nationalcenter/gpw.pdf

Blumenthal, D. (2003). Toil and trouble? Growing the physician supply. *Health Affairs, 22* (4), 85–87.

Boswell, S., Lowry, L. W., & Wilhoit, K. (2004). New nurses' perceptions of nursing practice and quality patient care. *Journal of Nursing Care Quality, 19*(1), 76–81.

Brotherton, S. E., Rockey, P. H., & Etzel, S. (2005). US graduate medical education, 2004–2005: Trends in primary care specialties. *Journal of the American Medical Association, 294*, 1075–1082.

Buchbinder, S. B., Alt, P. M., Eskow, K., Forbes, W., Hester, E., Struck, M., et al. (2005). Creating learning prisms with an interdisciplinary case study workshop. *Innovative Higher Education, 29*(4), 257–274.

Buchbinder, S. B., Wilson, M. H., Melick, C. F., & Powe, N. R. (1999). Estimates of costs of primary care physician turnover. *The American Journal of Managed Care, 5*, 1431–1438.

Buchbinder, S. B., Wilson, M. H., Melick, C. F., & Powe, N. R. (2001). Primary care physician job satisfaction and turnover. *American Journal of Managed Care, 7*(7), 701–713.

Bureau of Health Professions (BHPR). (2003, Spring). *Changing demographics: Implications for physicians, nurses and other health workers.* U.S. Department of Health and Human Services, Health Resources and Services Administration, Bureau of Health Professions, National Center for Health Workforce Analysis. Retrieved May 26, 2006 from http://bhpr.hrsa.gov/healthworkforce/reports/changedemo/content.htm

Bureau of Labor Statistics (BLS). (2006a). *U.S. Department of Labor, career guide to industries, 2006–07 edition.* Health care. Retrieved April 23, 2006 from http://www.bls.gov/oco/cg/cgs035.htm

Bureau of Labor Statistics (BLS). (2006b). *U.S. Department of Labor, career guide to industries, 2006–07 edition.* Registered nurses. Retrieved May 19, 2006 from http://www.bls.gov/oco/ocos083.htm

Bureau of Labor Statistics (BLS). (2006c). *U.S. Department of Labor, career guide to industries, 2006–07 edition.* Physician assistants. Retrieved May 19, 2006 from http://www.bls.gov/oco/ocos081.htm

Bureau of Labor Statistics (BLS). (2006d). *U.S. Department of Labor, career guide to industries, 2006–07 edition.* Licensed Practical and Licensed Vocational Nurses. Retrieved May 31, 2006 from http://www.bls.gov/oco/ocos102.htm

Bureau of Labor Statistics (BLS) (2006e). *U.S. Department of Labor, career guide to industries, 2006–07 edition*, Nursing, psychiatric, and home health aides. Retrieved May 31, 2006 from http://www.bls.gov/oco/ocos165.htm

Bureau of Labor Statistics (BLS). (2006f). *U.S. Department of Labor, career guide to industries, 2006–07 edition*, Respiratory Therapists. Retrieved May 19, 2006 from http://www.bls.gov/oco/ocos084.htm

Cejka Search & American Medical Group Management Association (AMGA). (2005). *2005 physician retention survey.* Retrieved May 31, 2006 from http://www.cejkasearch.com/pdf/2005-Physician-Retention-Survey.pdf

Commission on Accreditation of Allied Health Education Programs (CAAHEP). (2006). *What is CAAHEP?* Retrieved May 27, 2006 from http://www.caahep.org/index.aspx

Commission on Graduates of Foreign Nursing Schools (CGFNS). (2006). *Certification program.* Retrieved May 28, 2006 from http://www.cgfns.org/sections/faqs/cert-prog.shtml#3

Cooper, R. A. (2002). There's a shortage of specialists. Is anyone listening? *Academic Medicine, 77*, 761–766.

Cooper, R. A. (2003). Medical schools and their applicants: An analysis. *Health Affairs, 22*(4), 71–84.

Cooper, R. A., & Aiken, L. H. (2001). Human inputs: The health care workforce and medical markets. *Journal of Health Politics, Policy and Law, 26*, 925–938.

Donabedian, A. (2005). Evaluating the quality of medical care. *The Milbank Quarterly, 83*(4), 691–729.

ECFMG. (2006). Educational Commission for Foreign Medical Graduates 2007 Information Booklet. Retrieved December 13, 2006 from http://www.ecfmg.org/2007ib/ibo/serv.html.

Eiler, M. A. (2006, 2nd Quarter). Helping doctors help patients for 100 years: Happy birthday AMA physician masterfile. *AMA Physician Credentialing Solutions, 9*(2).

Frontier Nursing Service (FNS). (2006). Frontier nursing service. Retrieved May 28, 2006 from http://www.midwives.org/whoweare/fnshistory.shtm

Hagopian, A., Thompson, M. J., Kaltenbach, E., & Hart, L. G. (2003). Health departments' use of international medical graduates in physician shortage areas. *Health Affairs, 22*(5), 241–249.

Hallock, J. A., Seeling, S. S., & Norcini J. J. (2003). The international medical graduate pipeline. *Health Affairs, 22*(4), 64–96.

Hart, P. D. & Associates. (2002, April). *The staffing crisis for health professionals: Perspectives from radiology technologists, respiratory therapists, and certified nursing assistants.* Retrieved May 31, 2006 from http://www.aft.org/pubs-reports/healthcare/HartTechReport2002.pdf

Health Resources and Services Administration (HRSA). (2003, Spring). *Changing demographics: Implications for physicians, nurses and other health workers.* U.S. Department of Health and Human Services, Health Resources and Services Administration, Bureau of Health Professions, National Center for Health Workforce Analysis. Retrieved May 28, 2006 from http://bhpr.hrsa.gov/health workforce/reports/changedemo/content.htm

Health Resources & Services Administration (HRSA). (2004, March). *The registered nurse population: National sample survey of registered nurses, March 2004, preliminary findings.* Retrieved February 20, 2006 from http://bhpr.hrsa.gov/healthwork force/reports/rnpopulation/preliminaryfindings.htm

Herdrich, B. & Lindsay, A. (2006). Nurse residency programs: Redesigning the transition into practice. *Journal for Nurses in Staff Development, 22*(2), 55–62.

Hilliard, F. S. (2004, December 9). POV: Why today's nurses are educated, not trained. *New York Teacher.* Retrieved May 19, 2006 from http://www.nysut.org/newyorkteacher/2004-2005/041209pov.html

Joint Commission on Accreditation of Healthcare Organizations (JCAHO). (2002). *Healthcare at the crossroads: Strategies for addressing the evolving nursing crisis.* Retrieved May 27, 2006 from http://www.jointcommission.org/NR/rdonlyres/5C138711-ED76-4D6F-909F-B06E0309F36D/0/health_care_at_the_crossroads.pdf

Kemski, A. (2002, December). *Market forces, cost Assumptions, and nurse supply: Considerations in determining appropriate nurse to patient ratios in general acute care hospitals R-37-0, SEIU Nurse Alliance.* As cited in Department for Professional Employees AFL-CIO. (2004). Fact Sheet: The costs and benefits of safe staffing ratios Retrieved February 20, 2006 from http://www.dpeaflcio.org/policy/fact sheets/fs_2004_staffratio.htm

Kennedy, B. R. (2005, Fourth Quarter). Stress and burnout of nursing staff working with geriatric clients in long-term care. *Journal of Nursing Scholarship.* Retrieved May 31, 2006 from http://www.blackwell-synergy.com/doi/pdf/10.1111/j.1547-5069.2005.00065.x

Kimball, B. & O'Neil, E. (2002, April). *Health care's human crisis: The American nursing shortage.* Retrieved May 27, 2006 from http://www.rwjf.org/files/publications/other/NursingReport.pdf

Kosel, K. C., & Olivo, T. (2002). The business case for workforce stability. Voluntary Hospitals of America. Retrieved May 27, 2006 from http://www.healthleadersmedia.com/print.cfm?content_id=50603&parent=103

Laschinger, H. K. S. & Finegan, J. (2005). Using empowerment to build trust and respect in the workplace: A strategy for addressing the nursing shortage. *Nursing Economic$, 23*(1), 6–13.

Locke, E. A. (1983). The nature and causes of job satisfaction, In Dunnette, M. (Ed.), *Handbook of industrial and organizational psychology.* New York: John Wiley & Sons, 297–1349.

Maslach, C. (2003, October). Job burnout: New directions in research and intervention. *Current Directions in Psychological Science, 12*(5), 189–190.

McMahon, G. T. (2004). Coming to America—International medical graduates in the United States. *New England Journal of Medicine, 350,* 2435–2437.

Mick, S. S., & Lee, S. D. (1999a). International and US medical graduates in US cities. *Journal of Urban Health: Bulletin of the New York Academy of Medicine, 76*(4), 481–496.

Mick, S. S., & Lee, S. D. (1999b). Are there need-based geographical differences between International Medical Graduates and US Medical Graduates in rural US counties? *The Journal of Rural Health,* Winter, *15*(1), 26–43.

Mick, S. S., Lee, S. D., & Wodchis, W. P. (2000). Variations in geographical distribution of foreign and domestically trained physicians in the United States: 'safety nets' or 'surplus exacerbation'. *Social Science & Medicine, 50,* 185–202.

Mullen F. (2002). The case for more US medical students. *New England Journal of Medicine, 343,* 213–216.

Mullan, F. (2005). The metrics of the physician brain drain. *New England Journal of Medicine, 353,* 1810–1818.

National Commission on Nursing (NCN). (1983). *Summary report and recommendations.* Chicago: Hospital Research and Educational Trust.

National Council of State Boards of Nursing (NCSBN). (2006a). Using criminal background checks to inform licensure decision making. Retrieved June 2, 2006 from http://www.ncsbn.org/pdfs/Criminal_Background_Checks.pdf

National Council of State Boards of Nursing (NCSBN). (2006b). Nurse licensure and certification. Retrieved May 26, 2006 from http://www.ncsbn.org/regulation/nlc.asp

National Council of State Boards of Nursing (NCSBN). (2006c). Quarterly examination statistics: Volume, pass rates & first-time internationally educated candidates' countries. Retrieved May 26, 2006 from http://www.ncsbn.org/pdfs/NCLEX_Stats_Fact_Sheet.pdf

National Institutes of Health (NIH). (2005). *Frequently asked questions.* Retrieved May 20, 2006 from http://www.nih.gov/news/calendar/calendarfaq.htm#cme credit

National Physician Data Bank (NPDB). (2006). *National practitioner data bank: Why the NPDB was created.* Retrieved May 31, 2006 from http://www.npdb-hipdb.com/npdb.html

National Residency Matching Program. (2006). *How the NRMP process works.* Retrieved May 1, 2006 from http://www.nrmp.org/about_nrmp/how.html

New York State Office of the Attorney General (NYSOAG). (2000). Background checks sought for health care workers: New legislation could improve safety in nursing homes. Retrieved June 2, 2006 from http://www.oag.state.ny.us/press/2000/jun/jun05a_00.html

Polsky, D., Kletke, P. R., Wozniak, G. D., & Escarce, J. (2002). Initial practice locations of international medical graduates. *HSR: Health Services Research, 37,* 907–928.

Seavey, D. (2004, October). *The cost of frontline turnover in long-term care.* Retrieved May 31, 2006 from http://www.bjbc.org/content/docs/TOCostReport.pdf

Sexton, J. B., Thomas, E. J., & Helmreich, R. L. (2000). Error, stress, and teamwork in medicine and aviation: cross sectional surveys. *British Medical Journal, 320,* 745–749.

Smart, D. (2006). *Physician characteristics and distribution in the US, 2006 Edition.* Chicago: AMA Press.

Steiger, D. O., Auerbach, D. I., & Buerhaus, P. I. (2000). Expanding career opportunities for women and the declining interest in nursing as a career. *Nursing Economic$, 18*(5), 230–236.

Tamblyn, R., Abrahamowicz, M., Brailovsky, C., Grand'Maison, P., Lescop, et al. (1998). Association between licensing examination scores and resource use and quality of care in primary care practice. *Journal of the American Medical Association, 280*(11), 989–996.

Towson University. (2006). *Admission to the undergraduate nursing major.* Retrieved May 26, 2006 from http://www.new.towson.edu/nursing/admissiontothemajor.html

Weber D. O. (2004, September-October). Poll results: Doctors' disruptive behavior disturbs physician leaders. *The Physician Executive, 30*(5), 6–14.

Whelan, G. P., Gary, N. E., Kostis, J., Boutlet, J. R., & Hallock, J. A. (2000). The changing pool of international medical graduates seeking certification training in US graduate medical education programs. *Journal of the American Medical Association, 288,* 1079–1084.

Williams, T., Sims, J., Burkhead, C., & Ward, P. M. (2002). The creation, implementation, and evaluation of a nurse residency program through a shared leadership model in the intensive care setting. *Dimensions of Critical Care Nursing, 21*(4), 154–161.

Zhang, P., & Thran, S. L. (1999). Physician socioeconomic statistics, 1999–2000 Edition. Chicago: American Medical Association, 124.

CHAPTER 10

The Strategic Management of Human Resources

Jon M. Thompson

LEARNING OBJECTIVES

By the end of this chapter the student will be able to describe:

- Why human resources management includes strategic and administrative actions;
- Current environmental forces influencing human resources management;
- The key role of employees as drivers of organizational performance;
- Major federal legislation affecting human resources management;
- Human resources functions that address employee workforce planning/recruitment, and employee retention;
- The key responsibilities of human resources management staff and line management staff in recruitment and retention;
- Methods of compensating employees;
- Methods of evaluating employees by using employee performance appraisals; and,
- Examples of human resource management issues in healthcare settings.

INTRODUCTION

The management of human resources is one of the most important yet challenging responsibilities within health services organizations. Health services organizations need to be high performing organizations, and human resources are considered the most important factor in creating such organizations (Pfeffer, 1998). A high performing health services organization provides high quality services and excellent customer service, is efficient, has high productivity, and is financially sound.

Human resources management involves both administrative and strategic elements. From a strategic perspective, health services organizations compete for labor. They desire an adequate labor supply and the proper mix of quality and committed healthcare professionals to provide needed services. The strategic perspective acknowledges that organizational performance is contingent on individual human performance. Health services organizations need to view their human resources as a strategic asset that helps create competitive advantage (Becker, Huselid, & Ulrich, 2001). Additionally, organizations must have the capability to understand their current and future manpower needs and develop and implement a clear-cut strategy to meet those needs to achieve the organizational business strategy. Administratively, there are a number of specific functions and action steps that need to be carried out in support of managing the human resources of the health services organization to ensure high levels of performance.

Fundamentally, human resources management addresses the need to ensure that qualified and motivated personnel are available to staff the business units operated by the health services organization (Hernandez, Fottler, & Joiner, 1998). Human resources management encompasses a variety of functions and tasks related to recruiting, retaining, and developing staff in the health services organization. These staff include administrative staff who carry out non-clinical administrative functions such as patient accounting, quality management, and community relations; clinical staff who provide diagnostic, treatment, and rehabilitation services to patients; and support staff who assist in the delivery of clinical, administrative, and other facility services. The human resources activities that support administrative and clinical staff are carried out by dedicated human resources personnel who work in human resources or personnel departments, and are also carried out by line managers who have primary responsibility for directing staff and teams and who are charged with hiring, supervising, evaluating, developing, and when necessary, terminating staff.

Management of human resources is complex, and human resources actions address a variety of issues/situations. Consider the following examples of human resources management in various health services organizations:

- A large physician practice is in need of hiring someone to head up their information management area. The practice has grown from 7 to 23 physicians in the past 5 years, and the practice administrator has realized that the clinical and financial records needs of the practice have outpaced current administrative expertise. The administrator wants to define the job by analyzing job duties and then recruiting personnel to fill the position.
- A large system-affiliated hospital desires to train patient care technicians to assist in direct clinical care of patients. The hospital has experienced a shortage of RNs in the past 3 years, and has found that a multidisciplinary team approach using patient care technicians will help the organization meet patient and manpower needs. The Vice President of Patient Care desires to know the best way to train.
- An assisted living facility is developing a new position for a marketing specialist, who will be tasked with marketing the facility in an effort to increase its census. The facility administrator desires to conduct a job analysis to determine the specific responsibilities of the marketing specialist's job.
- An ambulatory care clinic plans to add new diagnostic imaging equipment in order to compete for more patients in their service area. The purchase of this equipment raises several questions for the organization, including: What are the specific human resources needed to staff the new technology and are they available? How will the addition of new technology and services impact the operating budget and the achievement of the business strategy of the clinic?

Each of these scenarios provides a good illustration of the diverse nature of human resources activities from both strategic and administrative perspectives and suggests how these activities contribute to the effective performance of the organization.

This chapter provides an overview of the specific activities that take place strategically and administratively to manage the human resources of the health services organization. First, environmental forces affecting the management of human resources in health services organizations will be reviewed. Second, the importance of employees as drivers of organizational performance will be addressed. Key functions within human resources management will then be identified and discussed. Finally, conclusions regarding management of human resources in health services organizations will be presented.

ENVIRONMENTAL FORCES AFFECTING HR MANAGEMENT

There are several key environmental forces that impact the availability and performance of human resources within health services organizations (HSOs) (see Table 10-1). The environment for HSOs is the external space beyond the organization that includes other organizations and influences that impact the organization.

First, declining reimbursements from government payers and other third parties have reduced the revenues coming to HSOs. In efforts to contain their expenses, Medicare and Medicaid programs and private insurance and managed care organizations have reduced their payments on behalf of covered beneficiaries. Declining reimbursements for health services organizations have left HSOs with fewer resources to recruit, compensate, and develop their workforces. Because other organizations in local and regional markets are also competing for the same labor, this has made recruitment and retention of staff more difficult for many HSOs.

Second, the low supply of healthcare workers—particularly highly specialized clinical personnel—has made recruitment of needed healthcare personnel very challenging (Fottler, Ford, & Heaton, 2002). Many areas of

TABLE 10-1 Environmental Forces and Impacts on Human Resources Management

Force	Impact
Declining reimbursement	Less resources to recruit, compensate, and develop workforce
Declining supply of workers	Shortage of skilled workers; changes in recruiting and staffing specialized services; lower satisfaction of workers
Increasing population need	Increased volumes of patients and workload for HSOs
Increasing competition among HSOs	Competition for healthcare workers and pressure for higher wages
External pressure on HSOs for accountability and performance	HR must ensure high performance in HSO

the country have experienced shortages of nursing, diagnostic, and treatment personnel, a phenomenon that has left many HSOs understaffed, requiring remaining staff to work longer hours per week (Shanahan, 1993). This has also contributed to lower levels of staff satisfaction and higher rates of turnover in certain staff positions, which has in turn increased human resources costs to the HSOs (Izzo & Withers, 2002; Shanahan). In addition, recruiting staff members who are highly specialized and who are in short supply tends to raise human resources costs as HSOs have to pay these staff members higher wages and provide other incentives to appeal to these potential workers (Shanahan).

Third, competition among health services organizations has increased dramatically in the past 15 years due to an increase in supply of traditional HSOs, such as hospitals and nursing homes, as well as the influence of newly emerging HSOs, such as retirement communities, assisted living facilities, and ambulatory care programs. HSOs have engaged in service competition and to a lesser degree, price competition, in trying to outperform their rivals. Competition in services and competition for labor has contributed to increased demands on human resources management.

Fourth, the population's needs for health and medical care have increased in the past 2 decades and will continue to grow during the next 25 years as the population ages and baby boomers approach retirement and qualify for Medicare. Older adults require more health services, and therefore, HSOs will require more healthcare workers to care for the increasing volumes of patients served at their facilities. This is further complicated by the fact that much of the current healthcare workforce is nearing retirement age themselves (Burt, 2005). Thus, in the future, health services organizations will be faced with declining workforces due to retirements, on the one hand, and expanded demands from the population, on the other hand. Projections of the future number of healthcare workers show significant opportunities for employment (see Table 10-2). However, this puts HSOs in a difficult situation: additional workers are needed to care for the increased patient workload, while the supply of workers in many categories continues to be low. This creates additional challenges for recruiting as well as retaining HSO staff.

Finally, increasing regulation and scrutiny of health services organizations by external organizations have increased pressures for high quality and high performing organizations. While licensing and accrediting organizations monitor HSO conformance to standards, they also make these performance indicators available to the public, legislators, and other stakeholders. In addition,

TABLE 10-2 Projected Growth in Healthcare Occupations Employment, 2002–2012

Occupation	Total Employment (000's)		2002–2012 Change in Total Employment		2002 Self-Employed Percent	2002–2012 Average Annual Job Openings (000's)		2002 Median Annual Earnings (Dollars)
	2002	2012	Number (000's)	Percent		Due to growth & total replacement needs	Due to growth & net replacement needs	
Physician Assistants	63	94	31	48.9	0.8	8	4	64,670
Physical Therapists	137	185	48	35.3	5.7	18	6	57,330
Emergency Medical Technicians and Paramedics	179	238	59	33.1	0.8	36	8	24,030
Nursing Aides, Orderlies, and Attendants	1,375	1,718	343	24.9	1.6	336	52	19,960
Physicians and Surgeons	583	697	114	19.5	16.9	41	19	Over 138,400
Medical and Clinical Laboratory Technicians	147	176	29	19.4	1.6	22	7	29,040
Registered Nurses	2,284	2,908	623	27.3	1.2	236	110	48,090
Medical and Health Services Managers	244	315	71	29.3	5.3	36	12	61,370

Source: U.S. Bureau of Labor Statistics, 2005.

reimbursement organizations and government payers like Medicare and Medicaid are increasing requirements on HSOs for accountability and performance by mandating reports on quality, morbidity, and mortality, as well as efficiency and costs. For HSOs, this means that human resources management must help the HSO become a high performing, high quality organization that can demonstrate quality processes and outcomes to these external stakeholders. Human resources can help accomplish this by hiring staff that are high quality, retaining those that are high quality, and reinforcing the culture of a high performing organization.

In addition to the noted external factors, internal factors also impact human resources management. Increasingly, senior management of HSOs view human resources in terms of its contribution to the success of the HSO, and look to human resources indicators in their assessment of overall organizational performance (Becker, et al., 2001; Galford, 1998; Griffith, 2000; Pieper, 2005). As they do with other departments and services, HSO senior management wants to see a return on their investment in human resources functions and a contribution to the bottom line (Becker et al.). Although a support function to the core focus of delivery of patient care services, human resources activities are evaluated in terms of the contribution to recruitment, training, and development for staff, as well as employee satisfaction and retention. Therefore, human resources strategies and programs to address recruitment and retention needs are being developed and assessed, not in terms of whether they look good or because other organizations are doing them, but rather because they contribute to the organization's mission and goals for the creation of a high performing, high quality organization.

UNDERSTANDING EMPLOYEES AS DRIVERS OF ORGANIZATIONAL PERFORMANCE

The core services provided by HSOs—patient care services—are highly dependent on the capabilities and expertise of the organization's employees. It has been said that successful business strategy is directly connected to having committed, high-performance employees (Ginter, Swayne, & Duncan, 2002). HSOs are only as good as their employees. Why is this so for health services organizations?

There are three primary reasons why this is the case. First, HSOs are service organizations, unlike traditional businesses or manufacturing firms that make and distribute a specific product. Being a service organization means providing a service that is needed and/or desired by a consumer who decides to take advantage of what the HSO has to offer. Providing services involves doing things to help others, and HSOs require employees who have a desire to help others, a "service orientation" (Fottler, et al., 2002). Second, HSOs are highly specialized service organizations that provide a range of specific services that include inpatient, outpatient, surgical, rehabilitation, diagnostic, therapeutic, and wellness services. To provide these specialized services, healthcare workers need to carry out many highly specialized tasks, and they need to have the proper knowledge, training, and experience to do those tasks well. Finally, because of the variety of services provided in HSOs and the fact that specialized staff provide only specific "pieces" of the overall service experience, healthcare workers from different departments and units must work together to provide a comprehensive service that meets all the needs of each patient (Liberman & Rotarius, 2000). Therefore, staff must work together as teams to ensure that all required services are provided, and that the total needs of the patient or health care client are met. Therefore, teamwork is necessary in order for the HSO to provide the high quality, coordinated, and comprehensive services that are required for it to be a high performing organization.

In essence, all HSO employees need to work together to ensure the best service possible, centered on the patient's needs. Managers, therefore, must be able to hire good people with the proper knowledge, skills, and attitudes and provide them the resources and support necessary to do their jobs effectively and efficiently.

KEY FUNCTIONS OF HUMAN RESOURCES MANAGEMENT

In this section, the major functions within human resources management will be reviewed. The primary areas of human resources management activity include: job analysis; manpower planning; establishing position descriptions; recruitment, selection and hiring employees; orienting new employees; providing training and development; managing compensation and benefits; assessing performance; providing employee assistance services; and offering employee suggestion programs. Typically, these key functions can be collapsed into two major domains called workforce planning/recruitment and employee retention (see Table 10-3). In the discussion below, the reader should note that activities in these two domains are typically car-

TABLE 10-3 Human Resources Functions

Function	Related Tasks
Workforce Planning/Recruitment	Job Analysis Manpower Planning Recruitment, Selection, Negotiation, and Hiring Orientation
Employee Retention	Training and Development Compensation and Development Assessing Performance Labor Relations Employee Assistance Programs Employee Suggestion Programs

ried out by human resources staff professionals who are under the supervision of a Vice President, Director, or Manager of Human Resources. In some HSOs, this office may be called "personnel," but most health services organizations—particularly large HSOs—now have a department or office of human resources which reflects both a strategic and administrative focus.

The human resources department or office develops and maintains all employee policies and procedures that reflect hiring, evaluating, promoting, disciplining, and terminating employees. In addition, policies and procedures related to assessing employee satisfaction, giving employee awards, compensating employees, and providing benefits are also developed and managed by the human resources staff. Furthermore, all employee records are maintained in the human resources office and in the human resources information system.

It should be noted that many federal and state laws impact human resources management in HSOs. There is a lengthy history of federal legislation that has been enacted to protect the rights of individual employees and to ensure non-discrimination in the hiring, disciplining, promoting, compensating, and terminating of employees on the basis of age, sex, religion, color, national origin, or disability. Many states have also enacted specific laws that protect employees. Other employment issues such as sexual harassment, whistleblowing (identifying wrong-doing), and workplace harassment are also addressed under federal and state law and offer employees protection. The legal environment for HSOs related to human resources management is constantly changing, and employers must carry out their activities with full knowledge of applicable laws and emerging rulings from court cases. Table 10-4 provides a summary of key federal legislation impacting human resources management in HSOs.

TABLE 10-4 Key Federal Legislation Affecting Human Resources Management

---

1935	**National Labor Relations Act** (as amended in 1974). Provides for bargaining units and collective bargaining in hospitals and health services organizations.
1938	**Fair Labor Standards Act** (as amended many times). Employees who are non-exempt from minimum wage and overtime provisions must be paid minimum wage and time and a half for hours beyond 40 hours per week. Special provisions for health services organizations.
1963	**Equal Pay Act.** Prohibits discrepancies in pay between men and women who perform the same job.
1964	**Civil Rights Act** (as amended many times). Prohibits discrimination in screening, hiring, and promotion of individuals based on gender, color, religion, or national origin (Title VII).
1967	**Age Discrimination in Employment Act.** Prohibits employment discrimination against employees age 40 and older.
1970	**Occupational Safety and Health Act.** Requires employers to maintain a safe workplace and adhere to standards specific to healthcare employers.
1973	**Rehabilitation Act.** Protects the rights of handicapped people (physically or mentally impaired) and protects them from discrimination.
1973	**Employee Retirement Income Security Act (ERISA).** Grants protection to employees for retirement benefits to which they are entitled.
1978	**Pregnancy Discrimination Act.** Requires employers to consider pregnancy a "medical condition" and prohibits exclusion of pregnancy in benefits and leave policies.
1986	**Consolidated Omnibus Budget Reconciliation Act (COBRA).** Gives employees and their families the right to continue health insurance coverage for a limited time due to various circumstances such as termination, layoff, death, reduction in hours worked per week, and divorce.
1986	**Immigration Reform and Control Act.** Establishes penalties for employers who knowingly hire illegal aliens.
1986	**Worker Adjustment and Retraining Notification Act.** Requires employers who will make a mass layoff or plant closing to give 60 days advance notice to affected employees.
1990	**Americans With Disabilities Act (ADA).** Gives people with physical and mental disabilities access to public services and requires employers to provide reasonable accommodation for applicants and employees.
1993	**Family Medical and Leave Act (FMLA).** Permits employees in organizations to take up to 12 weeks of unpaid leave each year for family or medical reasons.
2003	**Health Insurance Portability and Accountability Act (HIPAA).** Affords employee protection from outside access to personal health information and limits employers' ability to use employee health information under health insurance plans.

Sources: Lehr, McLean & Smith, 1998; and Busse, 2005.

WORKFORCE PLANNING/RECRUITMENT

Human resources functions carried out within the workforce planning/recruitment domain are directed to analyzing jobs needed within the HSO; identifying current and future staffing needs; establishing position descriptions; recruiting, selecting, negotiating, and hiring employees; and orienting new employees.

Job Analysis

One of the fundamental tasks of human resources is to conduct an analysis of all jobs or positions that are a part of the HSO. Every position in the HSO—whether administrative, support, or clinical—needs to be justified in terms of its specific responsibilities and day-to-day activities. **Job analysis** involves identifying those unique responsibilities, duties, and activities specific to every position in the HSO. This is necessary to clarify individual responsibilities, but is also critical to avoid duplication of tasks and responsibilities across positions. The outcome of job analysis is to clearly state the responsibilities, duties, and tasks of every position within the HSO.

Recent human resources experts have suggested that HSOs should focus on those positions that contribute most directly to the completion of the organization's business objectives (Huselid, Beatty, & Becker, 2005). This is important because filling these critical positions with the best personnel—"A" players—will then increase the organization's ability to perform.

Manpower Planning

For every position established for the HSO, there needs to be an estimate of the number of staff members needed to carry out those responsibilities at the present time, as well as projections of the number of staff members needed at some future target date. For example, how many RNs does our hospital currently need for all the various services that we currently offer, and how many will we need in 5 years? This is a very complex decision process, and must be based on consideration of many factors. For example, consider a hospital. Will the hospital be downsizing or eliminating any services in the next 5 years? Will the facility be adding any new services that are not presently offered? How will the addition of new technology, or the addition of nursing assistants, affect the need for RNs in the future, across all services of the hospital?

Identifying current numbers of staff is based on volume statistics that reflect the current performance of the HSO. The need for clinical staff is based typically on patient care statistics, such as the number of patients admitted, number of outpatient visits, or the number of patients receiving a specific service. In some cases, need will be determined by licensure standards that govern the minimum number of staff for certain services. For non-patient care areas, including such support functions as medical records, information technology, and financial services, the number of staff needed is contingent on the current volume of records and patient accounts that must be processed. Each support person in these areas can handle a minimum number of accounts or records per day, which becomes the basis for estimating current need. This is a called a **ratio method of determining needs**. The managers in various units calculate these estimates and forward them to human resources for the development of aggregate estimates of staffing needs for the total facility.

Projections of staffing needs for a future target date are based on a similar method. Projections of future service volumes are made and associated staffing requirements are projected as well to serve that anticipated volume. Again, line managers usually develop these projections. Future volumes are typically determined through a consensus-based strategic planning process where there is agreement on **future service volumes**. In this process, consideration is also made for retiring staff, transfers, and service changes (such as eliminations or expansions of beds and services) to arrive at the needed number of staff to recruit or to acquire on a temporary basis from outside staffing firms. Once the projected staffing needs are identified for the total facility, strategies and timeframes are established for recruiting. Projections of staffing needs are revisited every year as annual performance is assessed to see if projections remain accurate.

Accuracy of projections has important implications for preparing budgets and evaluating financial performance of the HSO. For example, future staffing levels may be unrealistic if forecast revenues don't match projected expenses. Therefore, planned positions may remain unfilled and flexible staffing arrangements used as necessary. In addition, if demand shifts occur, some services may not realize projected patient volumes and cutbacks in staffing arrangements may be necessary. In conclusion, projections of future staffing requirements are just that—projections that may or may not hold up given the uncertain and dynamic nature of the health services environment. Many factors affect these projections and a thorough and periodic assessment is needed to ensure projections are realistic and revised as appropriate.

Establishing Job Descriptions

Position descriptions or job descriptions are required for every position within the HSO. Job descriptions are necessary to define the required knowledge, skills, responsibilities, training, experience, certification or licensure, and line of reporting for a specific job within the HSO. Such descriptions are important to both the organization and employee. The position description elaborates on the findings from the job analysis and provides a means by which the organization clarifies each position in terms of expectations, locus within the organizational structure, and how it contributes to the organization's overall performance. For the employee, the position description clarifies expectations and duties and allows prospective employees a means to evaluate the "fit" between a position and their own individual knowledge, skills, and experience.

Position descriptions are developed through joint efforts of line managers and human resources staff. Line managers specify job requirements; human resources staff keep job descriptions in a consistent format and ensure accuracy of the positions as they are included in the HSO's Human Resources Information System. An example of a position description for a hospital is shown in Figure 10-1.

Recruitment, Selection, Negotiation and Hiring of New Employees

A key principle of human resources recruitment is making sure that HSO positions are filled with competent and highly skilled personnel. Once recruitment needs are made known by line managers, it is the responsibility of human resources to follow the appropriate procedures to fill those positions. In some cases, existing employees will have an interest in a new position for which they are qualified, and internal candidates will be considered. Human resources recruitment personnel use a standard process for external recruiting. These steps include advertising, screening applicants, determining those to be interviewed, conducting interviews, selecting the candidate, negotiating, and hiring. Activities for both human resources staff and line managers related to recruitment are identified in Table 10-5.

BON SECOURS HEALTH CORPORATION
St. Francis Medical Center

POSITION DESCRIPTION

TITLE:	Environmental Services Aide	JOB CODE: 950
DEPARTMENT:	Environmental Services	
REPORTS TO:		FLSA: Non-exempt

I. GENERAL PURPOSE OF POSITION:

The primary responsibility of this position is to perform cleaning tasks to maintain designated areas in a clean, safe, orderly and attractive manner. The employee is expected to follow detailed instructions and/or written task schedules to accomplish assigned duties. This position serves all populations of visitors, employees, physicians and patients.

II. EMPLOYMENT QUALIFICATIONS:

1. Ability to communicate and interpret assignments issued through a computerized paging system.
2. Dependability and flexibility demonstrated through previous work or school history.
3. Previous housekeeping work experience preferred.

III. ESSENTIAL JOB FUNCTIONS:

1. Communicates all hospital-related issues to Supervisor.
2. Performs the duties necessary to maintain the sanitary conditions of the hospital, including routine cleaning and maintenance of all floor types.
3. Prepares patient rooms for new admissions through the proper utilization of the Bedtracking® system. (LoginlLogout)
4. Cleans and sanitizes isolation rooms and other contaminated areas following written techniques appropriate for that type of isolation (i.e., tuberculosis, HIV, hepatitis).
5. Performs general cleaning tasks using the 7 Steps process.
6. Follows hospital policy regarding storage and security of housekeeping chemicals.
7. Accurately uses Bedtracking® system to meet departmental response and cleaning time standards.
8. Responsible for the use and care of equipment and other hospital property. Maintains equipment by proper cleaning and storage; reports dangerous or broken equipment to team leader. Makes sure EVS cart is clean, box locks, and wringer free of lint.
9. Understands basic safety procedures. (RACE, PASS, MSDS, etc.)

IV. OTHER JOB EXPECTATIONS:

1. Actively participates in the hospital's Continuing Educational Improvement programs (i.e., Essential Skills, Safety Fairs, etc.)
2. Assists in the orientation of new employees in departmental methods and procedures.
3. Responds to unusual occurrences such as flood, spillage, etc.

V. WORKING CONDITIONS:

Works in all areas of the hospital and off-site properties. May be exposed to hazardous chemicals, but potential for harm is limited, if safety precautions are followed.

The individual performing this job may reasonably come into contact with human blood and other potentially infectious materials. The individual in this position is required to exercise universal precautions, use personal protective equipment and devices, when necessary, and learn the policies concerning infection control.

VI. BON SECOURS MISSION, VALUES, CUSTOMER ORIENTATION AND CONTINUOUS QUALITY IMPROVEMENT FOCUS:

It is the responsibility of all employees to learn and utilize continous quality improvement principles in their daily work.

All employees are responsible for extending the mission and values of the Sisters of Bon Secours by understanding each customer, treating each patient, staff member, and community member in a dignified manner with respect, kindness, and understanding, and subscribing to the organization's commitment to quality and service.

VII. APPROVALS   DATE

Department Manager

Administration _____

Human Resources

The above statements are intended to describe the nature and level of work being done by individuals assigned to this classification and are not to be construed as an exhaustive list of all job duties. This document does not create an employment contract, and employment with Bon Secours Richmond Health System is "at will".

_____

Source: Reprinted with permission from Bon Secours St. Francis Medical Center, Midlothian, Virginia.

FIGURE 10-1 Position Description

TABLE 10-5 Responsibilities of HR Staff and Line Managers in Recruitment

HR Staff Person
Prepares Position Description
Does job pricing
Prepares advertisements/recruitment materials
Keeps track of applicants/maintains HR Information System
Checks applicant references
Maintains personnel files
Narrows candidate pool
Line Manager
Clarifies job function/provides input into Position Description
Interviews candidates
Ranks candidates
Selects candidate
Negotiates with candidate
Hires candidate

Advertising

Different modes of advertising are used to target candidates and generate interest. These sources include local newspapers and electronic media including radio and television, organizational web sites, and Internet job search engines, e.g., www.monster.com and CareerBuilder.com. The human resources department uses standards for communication that address the position, required degrees, training and/or certification, experience, functional line of reporting and general expectations of the position. Applicants submit information in response to the advertising and submit their credentials that are reviewed and evaluated by human resources staff.

Candidates are recruited also through private recruitment or "headhunter" firms, and these may include firms that engage in general staff recruiting or firms that specialize in health services organization staff by recruiting nurses, technicians, financial analysts, or office personnel. Arrangements with recruiters usually involve paying a percentage of the first year salary to the recruiter if the candidate referred by the recruitment firm is selected for the position. This method of recruiting will result in costs that exceed the normal expected costs of filling position vacancies. However, this technique may be a necessary option when recruiting for highly specialized positions where the candidate pool is limited.

Another frequently used option in recruiting is to work with educational programs that prepare specialized health personnel, such as nurses, physical therapists, and diagnostic technicians (Shanahan, 1993). Sending announcements of positions to these educational programs, attending recruitment open houses, and developing important referral relationships with faculty and staff of these programs are helpful in building interest and identifying candidates. Other sources include placing ads in targeted professional journals that are read by healthcare professionals, disseminating recruitment materials to healthcare workers identified through association membership listings, and attending regional or annual meetings of professionals where human resources representatives can meet with interested candidates. A final option to identify interested candidates is for human resources staff to attend healthcare recruitment or job fairs held locally or regionally, or for the HSO to hold its own.

Some observers have suggested that HSOs use a pre-employment assessment by the candidate of the fit between their credentials and the job (Liberman & Rotarius, 2000). This is recommended to ensure that only appropriate, well-qualified applicants apply.

Interviewing, Selection, Negotiation, and Hiring

Human resources staff complete the preliminary review and analysis of candidates based on their applications, check candidate references, and identify past employers' satisfaction with the candidates. As a result, human resources staff narrow the pool down to those candidates that provide the best fit for the position based on training, experience, and other factors such as motivation and attitude. These applicants are then discussed with the line manager to select those to be interviewed. The candidates are invited to come to the organization and interview and spend some time with management, staff, and others. From the HSO's perspective, this is important for two reasons. It enables the HSO to assess first-hand the candidates and verify their knowledge and skills; also, it enables the assessment of the candidates' fit and compatibility with the organization and staff with whom they would be working. From the candidate's perspective, an interview is important to get a close look at the organization and staff, and to assess their fit and interest in the position and the organization.

Depending on the position, human resources staff may participate in candidate interviews, and line managers will definitely participate in interviews with candidates. Structured interviews with clearly defined questions are thought to be best for assessing candidates (Foster & Godkin, 1998). Subsequent to the interviews, the staff who have interviewed candidates meet to review the candidates, determine how the candidates match with position requirements and rank order candidates. Once the staff agree on the applicant they would like to hire, an offer is extended.

An offer of employment is made in writing and the offer letter must specify the position for which the offer is made, start date, associated salary/compensation and benefits, and any other key information regarding the offer. Although an offer has been extended, the recruitment process is not complete. Depending on the position, there may be a period of negotiation over salary, benefits, start time, flexible scheduling, and other issues. Once agreement is reached, the position is assumed filled and the candidate responds with a formal letter of acceptance agreeing to the position and conditions of acceptance. Completion of hiring paperwork is necessary at the time that the person starts the job. It should be noted that if agreement is not reached with the first choice candidate, then the offer would be extended to the next best candidate, and then the next, until agreement with a suitable candidate is reached.

Orientation

One of the key requirements of a new staff member is to attend an orientation program coordinated by human resources. This program is important for several reasons. An orientation program informs the new employee of policies, procedures, and requirements, and it offers an opportunity for the new employee to ask questions and clarify understanding about the organization. The **Employee Staff Manual** is provided to each new employee. During orientation, various policies and procedures are highlighted, including expectations for the work day, proper attire and behavior, employee assessment, disciplinary actions and grievances, probationary period, and opportunities for training and development. The organization's values, mission, vision, and goals are reviewed, as are strategic and long-range plans. Specific employee benefits are identified and reviewed, and employees are informed about options concerning benefits and associated costs. Safety and security policies and practices are reviewed, and in large HSOs such as hospitals and nursing homes, special codes are revealed so that employees know when and how to respond to emergency situations such as fires, patient medical emergencies, patient problems, intruders, and chemical and environmental emergencies. With the passage of the Health Insurance Portability and Accountability Act (HIPAA) in 1996, training in the requirements of this law regarding confidentiality of health information has been incorporated into many HSO's employee orientation sessions. Training in compliance with Medicare rules and regulations, along with the dissemination of Whistleblower Protection Act information is also becoming a part of new employee orientation in many HSOs.

Orientation is usually held once a month to coincide with the start date for new employees. Part-time, full-time, and short-term temporary employees are typically required to attend orientation. New employees have an opportunity to meet the senior management team, who typically provide an overview of their respective management domains during orientation. This helps new staff gain an understanding of their respective roles in the HSO.

EMPLOYEE RETENTION

Employee retention functions include all of those key activities that address care, support, and development of employees to facilitate their long-term commitment to the organization. The key functions under employee retention include training and development, managing compensation and benefits, assessing performance, providing employee assistance programs, and offering employee suggestion programs.

Training and Development

Training and development of the workforce are extremely important human resources functions for several reasons. First, the organization's need for specific knowledge and skills is always changing because of the rapid changes being experienced by HSOs. For example, HSOs frequently add new medical technologies that require different technical skills of employees. Another example of additional skills needed is in the information technology area, where new computer information systems, electronic medical records, databases, and integrated patient and financial data systems are being acquired to generate, store, and retrieve patient-level and organizational information. Second, training is necessary to provide for continuing education of some staff. For clinical staff that require continuing education as part of their licensure and/or certification, HSOs may coordinate the provision of training that is provided either on site or at remote locations. While it is clear that not all the training and development needs of staff can be met due to resource limitations, the human resources staff determines priorities for annual training and education efforts and implements and manages those programs. Human resources staff typically accomplish this through organization-wide needs assessments or through identification of specific training needs that are made known to human resources staff by managers. Typically, the cost of training and development programs is provided for in the human resources budget; in some cases, other departments or services within the HSOs may cover the cost of training that is coordinated by human resources.

The goal of any training or development effort is to provide value for the organization by returning benefits, such as increased productivity, greater effectiveness, higher quality, greater coordination of care, and enhanced patient or customer service. Therefore, training and development programs are evaluated by human resources for cost-effectiveness to ensure that training was effective in terms of return on investment, and that methods of training were appropriate (Phillips, 1996). Training programs cover a range of topics, including technical training on equipment and software programs, customer service training, and training to improve inter-personal communications and leadership, among others. Training and development of teams within HSOs are also increasingly common, as HSO staff work frequently in teams to coordinate the delivery of care. The effectiveness of team leaders has been shown to influence team learning, development, and performance (Edmonson, Bohmer, & Pisano, 2004).

Managing Compensation and Benefits

The following sections describe the management of employee compensation and benefits in healthcare organizations and how it can contribute to a high-performing organization.

Compensation

The human resources department has the specific responsibility of managing the pay or compensation and benefits associated with all positions held within the HSO. This is no easy task, as specific pay ranges and benefits must be established for each position, which in the hospital industry includes over 300 distinct jobs or major job classifications (Metzger, 2004). The management of compensation begins with a clear definition of the HSO's compensation philosophy, which reflects the organization's mission, values, and strategy regarding human resources, as well as consideration of internal (e.g., equity) and external (e.g., competitive) factors (Gering & Conner, 2002; Joiner, Jones, & Dye, 1998).

Determining compensation refers to the establishing of a specific financial value for a job. Compensation for each position is set based on the consideration of a number of factors, including the specialized knowledge and skills associated with the position, the experience required for the position, the relative availability of skilled individuals to fill the position, and average wages that are specific to the local labor market. This is called "job pricing" (Joiner et al., 1998). Some positions are **hourly rated** (i.e., nonexempt, and eligible for overtime pay), where a compensation rate per hour of work is established (e.g., for maintenance staff and floor nurses), and some positions are salaried (i.e, exempt and not paid overtime), where an annual salary is paid the employee (e.g., nurse managers and other managerial staff). In short, compensation is set to account for the special skills and experiences required of employees and to enable the organization to be competitive in the market in securing and retaining needed employees. Pay ranges will vary by type of position, but within a position class there must be equity. However, HSOs typically account for differences in training, experience and special considerations of the job (working weekends or evenings) by allowing for pay/shift differentials. Also, some jobs are subject to significant external market pricing, because the skill set is unique and the market is national or international.

The typical large HSO, such as a hospital or hospital system, has a separate, designated staff to handle the administration of compensation, on the one hand, and benefits, on the other. Human resources staff responsible for compensation keep records of wages and salaries, compensation adjustments, and the basis for compensation adjustments in individual employee personnel files and in the Human Resources Information System. Every few years, human resources administers a compensation or salary survey for positions within the HSO in order to **benchmark** current compensation to local and regional market trend (i.e., a comparative market analysis of wages), and adjust salary ranges for positions as appropriate to remain competitive.

Job pricing is used to establish equitable pay scales by position within HSOs, but reward systems beyond base pay are frequently considered of greater importance to employees (Joiner et al., 1998). In addition to base compensation tied to expectations for a specific job, many HSOs have embraced incentive compensation. While compensation plans focus on individual performance and allocating rewards such as raises to high performers based on individual performance, incentive plans are designed to improve organizational performance (Gibson, 1995). In an **incentive** or **pay-for-performance plan**, the purpose of the plan is to stimulate employees to higher levels of achievement and performance that benefits the organization. Meaningful measures such as profits (return on investments), productivity, attendance, safety, quality, and customer satisfaction are a few examples of financial, as well as non-financial organization-wide, performance indicators that can be used in developing incentive plans. The incentive plan would work in the following way. The organization would set target goals for performance in a specific time period. At the end of that time period, the organization would collect and review relevant information to measure the status of performance. If the measurement of performance on specific indicators met the target goals, the organization would then reward employees for the "organization-wide" performance. These programs are also known as **gainsharing** or **goal-sharing programs**, and payouts (revenues derived from savings, increased productivity or volumes, increased customer retention, and quality) would be shared with employees as a bonus for their contributions to high performance within the HSO (Gomez-Mejia, Welbourne, & Wiseman, 2000).

Incentive compensation plans have long been thought to be associated with higher levels of organizational performance (Bonner & Sprinkle, 2002). The theory behind this approach is that use of incentives such as compensation bonuses positively affects motivation which leads to higher performance (Gibson, 2002). Many health services organizations have begun to follow the lead of business and industry who pioneered these programs, but published literature addressing the impact of incentive compensation on organizational performance in healthcare is limited (Griffith & White, 2002). There is some recent evidence to show that more HSOs are using incentive programs for executives that are tied to organizational performance (HMFA, 2001). However, recent research in the business literature has shown that the relationship between incentive pay and performance may not hold up.

Beer and Katz (2003) found in their survey of senior executives from among many firms that bonuses have little to no positive effect on performance, and that their real function may be to attract and retain executives. They looked at firms that had implemented executive bonus compensation systems and assessed relationships to performance, but found that the only key explanatory factor was that the incentive system promoted *teamwork*. Similarly, Luthans and Stajkovic (1999) found in their analysis of research on pay-for-performance that social recognition and administrative feedback to employees on performance were just as influential as pay-for-performance in achieving higher levels of performance in a manufacturing setting. Moreover, Beer and Cannon (2004) found that many senior managers view incentive compensation programs with concern, and question whether the benefits outweigh the costs. However, none of the studies cited above were specific to health services organizations.

Benefits

The human resources staff is responsible for managing benefits provided to employees working in an HSO. A benefit is defined as any type of compensation provided in a form other than salary or direct wages, that is paid for totally or in part by an employer (Jenks & Zevnik, 1993). As benefits extended to workers in general have increased over the past two decades, the number and type of benefits made available to HSO employees have increased as well (Griffith & White, 2002; Runy, 2003). However, the HSO is faced with a dilemma. On the one hand, HSOs are under pressure to manage costs, and employee benefits have been a high cost item for HSOs, which directly affects the HSO's cost management strategy, financial status, and competitive position. On the other hand, benefits as a portion of total compensation have increased in importance, as more and more employees indicate that benefits are important in their choice of an employer (Runy).

Benefits may differ by level within the organization, as management may receive one set of benefits to offset the higher level of skill needed to complete the job, versus lower level employees who may receive fewer benefits due to a lower level of skills required for the job. The availability of benefits, as well as the percentage of employee cost sharing, varies widely by HSO. However, typical benefits offered by HSOs include the following:

Sick leave. A certain number of days per year are allocated for the employee being unable to be on the job due to illness or injury.

Vacation. A certain number of vacation days are allocated to employees for them to use as free time. In many HSOs, this is combined under a **Paid-time-off (PTO)** plan with sick leave days and holidays.

Holidays. Designated national holidays are given to employees with pay as part of their benefits.

Health insurance. Medical coverage for the employee and optional coverage for dependents are typically made available. Depending on the type of health insurance plan offered to employees (and there may be one or more plans offered by the HSO), the total plan cost for the employee may be shared by the employer and employee. HSOs, like other organizations, have turned to managed care plans as a way to reduce health benefits expense for the HSO. Typical plan features include greater cost-sharing and out-of-pocket expenses for employees, along with the trend of increased access to out-of-network and specialty care. In addition, much of the coverage by health insurers today focuses on the management of certain chronic clinical conditions, such as cardiovascular problems and diabetes. These **disease management programs** are offered in an attempt to help the employee and dependent manage their conditions to promote better quality of life and reduce cost.

Life Insurance. Coverage is provided that will help offset the loss of earnings for a limited time and to cover burial and other expenses related to the death of an employee. The employee is typically provided a base amount of life insurance with an option to increase coverage for an additional cost.

Flexible health benefits. Flexible or "cafeteria" benefits are increasing in popularity as they are offered to employees as options. Flexible benefits most often include health insurance, dental insurance, eye coverage, and other health benefits such as disability insurance and long-term care insurance, where the employee is granted a choice in benefits for specific costs. Flexible benefits offer advantages to the employee in that the employee can tailor benefits to meet individual needs at varying costs (Joiner et al., 1998). For the HSO, overall benefit costs can be reduced under flexible benefit plans due to the fact that the employer is no longer paying for a specific base package of benefits for all employees (Joiner et al.).

Retirement benefits. Many HSOs have retirement plans in place where employees are granted a certain percentage of their compensation over and above their compensation that is put into a retirement fund. This fund can be a pension fund that is set up specific to the HSO or more likely, a 401(k) or 403(b) plan where employees can manage their retirement dollars in mutual fund investments (Jenks & Zevnik, 1993). Many HSOs also have included the option in the retirement plan of offering to "match" employees' contribution to the plan with employer-paid funds up to a maximum amount. Retirement funds can only be accessed at the age of retirement or fund withdrawals are subject to penalties.

Flexible Spending Accounts. These are also called reimbursement accounts, and are offered by the HSO to help the employee and their dependents by allowing pre-tax dollars to be placed into a healthcare or dependent care account. These accounts are then used to pay for costs incurred by the employee and dependents that are not covered under other benefits plans or for the care of a child or dependent, disabled parent (Jenks & Zevnik, 1993).

Other benefits. Several other categories of benefits are also made available to HSO employees, although the degree to which they are offered and the scope of coverage will vary considerably. These benefits may include personal health benefits (complementary and alternative healthcare, yoga and pilates classes, wellness/fitness center memberships, health education programs, and personal health risk appraisals); transportation (use of a van pool); educational reimbursement (tuition for employee or dependent's college); employee incentives (profit sharing, stock options); flexible work scheduling, job-sharing and telecommuting; child care assistance and on-site child care; and savings programs (matched savings plans), among many others (Jenks & Zevnik, 1993).

Occupational safety and health. The Human Resource Department contributes to the organization's efforts to maintain a safe and healthy work environment. Responsibilities are carried out in several ways to address this concern. First, **workers' compensation coverage** is required for organizations under state law, in order to protect workers who may get sick due to the job or become injured or incapacitated due to working conditions. This coverage is separate from any health insurance provided. Second, the HSO monitors federal and state regulations for occupational safety and monitors risk in the organization and works to eliminate safety risks. Sometimes these human resources staff activities are conducted in conjunction with the risk management activities within the HSO.

Employee Assistance Programs

Employee Assistance Programs (EAPs) are HSO-sponsored programs that are made available to employees, and in many cases their dependents, to assist with personal or family problems that also affect the employee's job performance (Howard & Szczerbacki, 1998). Such problems include stress and mental health problems, family dysfunction and divorce, alcohol and substance abuse problems, financial problems, legal issues, and adjustment issues stemming from a death in the family, loss of a job, or severe illness. In addition, the patient care services provided in an HSO are often challenging and stressful, and providing care to individuals who are sick, injured, and in some cases dying or near death, is very trying and stress inducing for employees (Blair, 1985). This may lead to feelings of helplessness, guilt, or grief that negatively impact attendance and threaten the employee's focus, effectiveness, and productivity. Workplace stress may also be exacerbated by personal and family stress outside the HSO. As a result, HSOs have recognized the value of EAPs to help employees in their times of need, by making available counseling, stress reduction programs, health education programs, and other interventions based on need to lessen the impact of these problems. A problem-free, happy employee is an employee who is more likely to be focused and productive on the job. This results in positive performance for the individual employee as well as the HSO. The cost of services to the employee will vary depending on how the EAP is structured; some of the needed EAP services may be covered under other current employee benefits. EAP services can be offered on-site at the HSO or offered at remote locations under contract with other providers, which facilitates greater confidentiality for users. Employees are also afforded protection from harassment and job loss due to use of the EAP.

In summary, the benefit package has become more important to employees in recent years as employees balance tradeoffs between compensation and an appropriate array of benefits that are important to the employee and dependents. For example, many employees with young families may be more interested in a broad range of benefits, such as those discussed above, rather than the highest salary possible. Such benefits help employees meet their own unique needs, and become a significant factor in employee recruitment and retention. In the end, benefits may be one of

Management Summary Form	Development Level:	_____ Annual Review
	1 = Performs below standard	_____ Other
	2 = Inconsistently meets the standard	
Confidential	3 = Consistently meets the standard	(For the initial review, please
	4 = Frequently exceeds the standard	use the "Introductory
	5 = Consistently exceeds the standard	Performance Review" Form)

Instructions: The Performance Improvement Plan is a tool designed to assist in managing, developing and reviewing an employee's effectiveness and efficiency. It also provides a common understanding of job expectations for present and future performance review periods. ***Please note all supporting comments on the Development Plan.***

I. Values (includes integration of Quest for Excellence Behaviors) *(see page 6-7 of the Process Guide)*

Developmental Level

		1	2	3	4	5
A.	Respect - commitment to treat people well (e.g., responsive - returns calls/emails).	1	2	3	4	5
	Justice - supporting and protecting the rights of all people.					
	Integrity - honest in dealings (e.g., honors commitments, keeps promises).					
	Compassion - experiencing empathy with another's life situation.					
B.	Stewardship - responsible use of Bon Secours resources (e.g., consistently on time).	1	2	3	4	5
	Innovation - creating or managing new ideas, methods, processes and/or technologies.					
	Quality - continuous improvement of service; involved in Gallup/Quest planning.					
	Growth - developing and improving services and promoting self-renewal; completion of previous year's Development Plan. (e.g., thinks "Big Picture").					

Average Developmental Level for Section I (A + B/2):

II. Leadership Competencies (see page 10-14 of the Process Guide)

Developmental Level

	1	2	3	4	5
Change Management & Organization Development - planning & designing change strategies as needed; integrating individual dev. & organizational dev. into strategies.	1	2	3	4	5
Communication & Interpersonal Skills - listening & responding in constructive manner; promoting understanding while building productive working relationships.	1	2	3	4	5
Critical Thinking - examining underlying causes & determining best course of action.	1	2	3	4	5
Human Resource Development - facilitating others to achieve professional dev. goals.	1	2	3	4	5
Planning & Strategic Direction Setting - determining shape of present & future job environment; efficiently maintaining & improving practices; setting direction for dept./org.; **developing Gallup Impact, PRC, Quest for Excellence Plans.**	1	2	3	4	5
Promotion of Mission & Values - setting an example by integrating org. standards into day-to-day functions; guiding others to a common Mission & Vision.	1	2	3	4	5
Self-Knowledge & Insight - using personal understanding to promote positive self-change.	1	2	3	4	5
Team Building - promoting teamwork to accomplish dept./org. objectives.	1	2	3	4	5
Proficiency in Field - subject matter expert in field; resource to others.	1	2	3	4	5

Average Developmental Level for Section II (Sum of 9 Leadership Competency Dev. Levels/9):

III. Essential Job Functions
(This section is determined by the Job Description and will vary with the Position being evaluated)

Average Developmental Level for Section III:

Overall Average: *(Average Level for Section I x .5) + (Average Level for Section II x .25) + (Average Level for Section III x .25)*

FIGURE 10-2 Performance Evaluation

Development Plan

Name: _____

Facility & Dept.: _____

The Purpose of the Development Plan is to aid in the process of developing specific skills and behaviors. The Plan is reviewed and finalized during the performance review meeting. At a minimum, progress towards reaching agreed upon goals should be discussed once during the year. *This form must be completed by each employee and returned prior to the performance review.*

1 Previous Objectives, Goals and Accomplishments. Review learning and development objectives, goals and accomplishments achieved since last performance review; include knowledge and skill strengths used to accomplish objectives and goals.

_____

_____

_____

_____

_____

_____

2 New Objectives and Goals. Identify new learning and development objectives and goals for he coming year, which include addressing opportunities for growth. Include issues, which may need to be addressed and opportunities needed to successfully implement, including implementation of Quest/Team Player improvements.

_____

_____

_____

_____

_____

_____

3 Employee and/or Manager's Comments. Additional comments may be made on a separate sheet of paper and attached to this form.

_____

_____

_____

_____

_____

_____

_____

FIGURE 10-2 (continued) Performance Evaluation

the most critical factors in making the HSO competitive in attracting and retaining staff.

Assessing Employee Performance

The human resources department is charged with developing and maintaining a system for measuring employee performance for all employees of the HSO. The central theme of this chapter is that organizational performance is paramount and that individual employee performance in an HSO is highly contributory to organization-wide performance. Therefore, assessing individual employee performance is critical to understanding and achieving high levels of organizational performance.

Under human resources department leadership, a **Performance Appraisal System** is established for the HSO. **Performance appraisal** means assessing the performance of an individual employee. In order for the HSO to know how individuals are performing and to develop a plan and program for employees to improve performance, an annual performance assessment is required. The assessment form includes several criteria that are determined to be important for the HSO in evaluating performance. These criteria may include measures of both quality and quantity of the work as specified in the position description and include technical skill assessment, as well as other criteria that address the employee's motivation, attitude, and interpersonal skills in carrying out their respective work. Human resources, in conjunction with senior management of the HSO, will determine what specific criteria are included in the performance appraisal. Performance appraisals also include an assessment of the degree to which an individual's annual goals and objectives have been achieved as spelled out in the yearly management plan. See Figure 10-2 for an example of a Performance Appraisal used by Bon Secours-St. Francis Hospital.

Kirkpatrick (2006) argues that a performance appraisal system must be part of the organization's efforts for continuously improving performance. Performance assessment is conducted by line managers for their subordinates on an annual basis, at the time of the employee's anniversary date or more commonly, at a standard time to coincide with the budget development process for the upcoming year. Using the agreed upon form, the manager will complete an assessment of each subordinate's performance for the assessment period. The manager then will sit down with the employee and review the appraisal and discuss areas of favorable performance, as well as areas of improvement opportunity. This will also give the subordinate an opportunity to express any concerns and/or seek clarification as to the basis for the evaluation ratings. Many managers also ask subordinates to complete a self-evaluation for the performance period under review, using the same criteria, for discussion at the meeting. It should be noted that good managers communicate with their subordinates about employee performance regularly throughout the year, with an interest in monitoring, correcting, and improving performance on an on-going basis.

At the designated annual performance appraisal meeting between a manager and a subordinate, a meaningful exchange can be carried out in order to frankly discuss performance, identify opportunities for improving performance, and developing a specific plan for achieving higher levels of performance. A two-way discussion of these matters is the most fruitful for both parties, as the employee will understand the manager's concern and interest in the employee and the sincere desire for improving performance. In addition, the employee can express likes and dislikes about the job, which the manager needs to know (Butler & Waldroop, 2005). However, it is essential that clarity be provided in communicating performance as perceived by the supervisor, so that there is no confusion as to the intent of the evaluation (Timmreck, 1998). A key outcome of the performance evaluation is the setting of **performance improvement goals**, actions to achieve the improvements, and priorities for action (Kirkpatrick, 2006). In addition to an annual performance appraisal, the HSO may require some or all employees to be reviewed for satisfactory performance at the end of their first 90 days of employment (often referred to as the **probationary period**), and at other times as specifically requested by a manager or if conditions warrant.

Performance appraisals are helpful to management and employees in the following ways (Longest, Rakich, & Darr, 2000):

- The manager can compare absolute as well as relative performance of staff;
- Together, the manager and employee can determine a plan for improving performance if such improvement is needed;
- Together, the manager and employee can determine what additional training and development activities are needed to boost employee performance;
- The manager can use the findings to clarify employee desires to move up to higher level positions and/or expand responsibilities;

- The manager can document performance in those cases where termination or reassignment is necessary;
- The manager can determine adjustments to compensation based on performance; and,
- The manager can determine promotional or other advancement opportunities for the employee.

In addition to the traditional method of assessing performance described above, many HSOs are now employing **360-degree performance appraisal systems**. While this method also includes a manager-subordinate evaluation, it provides for multisource feedback on employee performance from a number of other stakeholders—including peers, the employee's subordinates and internal and external customers, if applicable. Feedback is aggregated and communicated to the employee through a neutral third party such as a human resources staff member. The advantages to using the 360-degree evaluation are reduction of fear of repercussion from evaluative comments and a greater range of feedback from a larger number of observers of the employee/manager (Garman, Tyler, & Darnall, 2004). However, there are some disadvantages as well. These include the higher cost of administration of a 360-degree evaluation compared to a traditional evaluation, and the lack of an instrument suitable for health services managers (Garman et al.). In addition, peer feedback included in 360-degreee evaluation may also be biased or inaccurately given, due to difficulties in determining an individual's contribution to the unit or service, or fear of providing negative feedback to a colleague (Peiperl, 2005).

One of the most challenging outcomes of the performance appraisal process is the need to terminate an employee. Although the goal of human resources management is to retain high performing staff, not all employees will be retained. There are many reasons why an employee can be discharged, but in every case the primary reason must relate to performance deficiency. Terminating an employee is not easy and is uncomfortable at times for managers who have the authority to discharge an employee. However, failure to act decisively will jeopardize the HSO's performance and will certainly reflect negatively on the manager's ability as a leader (Hoffman, 2005). In situations where an employee is not likely to be retained, it is essential that the manager not wait until the appraisal to assess the employee's performance. In fact, ongoing monitoring of performance, efforts to correct performance problems, and documentation of the steps taken in any corrective processes are all typically required prior to discharge. This process should be done by the line manager in close consultation with the human resources manager. The HSO policies and procedures must be adhered to carefully to prevent subsequent allegations of wrongful discharge, and potentially avert a lawsuit against the HSO and/or the line manager.

Managing Labor Relations

Labor relations is a general term that addresses the relationships between staff (labor) and management within HSOs. Labor relations is associated with **collective bargaining** where a union, if certified (i.e, voted in by the workers), represents the interests of employees who become members of that union. Nationally, about 20% of HSOs have at least one union represented in their organizations (Longest et al., 2000). In the period 1980–1994, there were 4,224 certification elections held in health services organizations: 31% of these were in hospitals, 40% in nursing homes, and 29% were in other healthcare facilities (Scott & Lowery, 1994). Union elections in health services organizations vary by type of healthcare setting, but overall about 60% of elections result in a union being approved (Deshpande, 2002). Unions have a higher than average win rate in hospitals, and hospitals have been the focus of increased union organizing efforts in recent years (Deshpande, 2003).

Why do unions get involved in HSOs? As seen in manufacturing, the fundamental reason for unionization in health care is that employees are dissatisfied with some aspects of the work and/or the work environment, and feel that management is insensitive to their needs. Unions often step in where management has failed to do its job. If staff are strongly dissatisfied with various aspects of the HSO, view senior management as poor communicators, and/or perceive that management is insensitive to staff issues, they may believe that a union is the only way to have their voice heard and needs met. If elected to represent employees in an HSO, a union is then authorized to engage in collective bargaining with management of the HSO regarding wages, working conditions, promotion policies, and many other aspects of work (Longest et al., 2000).

The National Labor Relations Act of 1935, as amended, enables union organizing and collective bargaining in health services organizations. The Act also created **The National Labor Relations Board (NLRB)**, which recognizes several bargaining units for healthcare employees, including nurses, physicians, other professional employees, and non-professional employees, among others. The NLRB has the authority to oversee and certify the results of union elections. There are many rules and regulations that must be followed in unionization activity, and there are certain restrictions placed on management as well as staff that govern what can and cannot happen regarding union discussions, organizing and elections.

The presence of a union creates significant challenges for management of an HSO. From management's perspective, unions create an unnecessary third party in decisions that affect the employment relationship and work of the HSO's staff, which raises potential for conflict. Union requirements may restrict the administrator's ability to use the number and type of staff in desired ways, and compensation negotiated by the union may reduce management's ability to directly control staffing expenses. Labor unions can also limit an HSO's discretionary authority to make changes in the workplace and in workplace practices (Holley, Jennings, & Wolters, 2001). Also, some research has shown that productivity may be negatively affected after unionization (Holley et al.).

Beyond general impact on administration, unionization has been shown to significantly affect the human resources function in HSOs. Deshpande (2002) found in a study of hospital unionization activity that the presence of unions resulted in higher numbers of employees who were screened, a higher number of employee training programs, a greater number of job classifications, greater use of employee performance appraisal methods, and lower productivity, as reported by CEOs of hospitals.

Various strategies have been discussed with respect to the administrative stance vis-a-vis unions (Deshpande, 2003). To reduce the possibility of union discussions and union organizing, administrators are encouraged to keep communication open and fluid, provide competitive salaries and benefits, establish grievance policies and procedures, and ensure staff participation and involvement in decision-making as much as possible. In all respects, administrators and human resources staff should continuously assess staff satisfaction and needs, as well as opportunities for staff and management to work together for the better of the organization and larger community. There are many challenging issues that affect HSOs, including lowered reimbursements from managed care and government payers, cost reduction practices, and lower staffing ratios. These can lead to employee dissatisfaction, and management needs to be cognizant of the negative impact of some of their decisions on staff motivation, satisfaction, and commitment.

If one or more unions are certified to represent employees in an HSO, then much of the time and effort of the human resources staff will be spent in addressing unionization issues. These include negotiating (bargaining) aspects of the union contract, ensuring that specific aspects of the contract are met, communicating with union representatives, and being the focal party in carrying out all union discussion and negotiation under the auspices of federal labor law (Longest et al., 2000).

Employee Suggestion Programs

Employee suggestion programs (ESPs) are increasingly being considered by HSOs in an effort to encourage creativity on the part of employees and to identify needed improvements in processes and outcomes. Employee suggestion programs have been in existence for quite some time (Carrier, 1998), but the primary locus has been in manufacturing and other business enterprises as opposed to HSOs.

An ESP works simplistically by soliciting employee suggestions for change and acknowledging and rewarding those suggestions that offer the most potential to meet organizational goals and implementing those suggestions. These programs usually are formally structured, widely communicated throughout the organization, and managed by human resources staff. Current ESPs have gone far beyond the old suggestion box model and include elements of electronic submission and web-based applications, as well as formal recognition and reward (Fairbank, Spangler, & Williams, 2003).

ESPs are part of an overall effort by HSOs to stimulate innovation and creativity for ideas that will help the HSO. The underlying rationale for the program is that employees of HSOs, as key providers of its services and activities, are in the best position to know what can be improved and may have good ideas as to how such improvements can be made. ESPs are built on the premise that innovation in organizations can be understood from a problem-solving approach (Fairbank et al., 2003). Goals of ESPs can include organizational improvements, such as reducing costs, improving methods and procedures, improving productivity, improving equipment, and cutting waste, as well as increasing job satisfaction and organizational commitment on the part of employees (Carrier, 1998). This second goal of ESPs is very important and should not be overlooked by the human resources staff. Part of the overall satisfaction in working in an HSO is the belief that management understands and appreciates its employees, and is interested in their input. ESPs are not, however, without their limitations. Drawbacks to the program include difficulties in designing a program, effectively administering it, and sustaining the program over several years. (Kim, 2005).

CONCLUSION

The management of human resources is an important function within HSOs because the performance of HSOs is tied directly to the motivation, commitment, knowledge, and skills of clinical, administrative, and support staff. Human resources actions of HSOs are undertaken for both strategic and administrative purposes. A variety of human resources activities are included within the human resources area, and these activities typically fall within the domains of workforce planning/recruitment and employee retention. While human resources serves as a support function for line managers within HSOs, line managers and staff managers carry out human resources management roles as well, because they are involved in hiring, supervising, evaluating, promoting, and terminating staff. Therefore, human resources staff and other managers work closely to ensure that HSOs perform well. The contribution of the human resources management function is increasingly being evaluated by senior management, similar to other organizational functions, to determine the net contribution of human resources staff to organizational success. It is likely that management of human resources will increase in importance in the future, as HSOs face heightened external and internal pressures to recruit and retain committed and high performing staff.

DISCUSSION QUESTIONS

1. Describe why human resources management is comprised of strategic and administrative actions.

2. For each human resources scenario described in the introduction to the chapter, identify the steps you would take to address the specific human resources issue being faced. From your perspective, which is the most challenging issue, and why?

3. Two key domains of human resources management are workforce planning/recruitment and employee retention. Describe several human resources functions that fall under each and describe their importance to human resources management.

4. Identify and describe some environmental forces that affect human resources functions in health services organizations.

5. Define and contrast "Employee Assistance Programs" and "Employee Suggestion Programs."

6. Why do HSOs offer incentive compensation programs? How do these programs differ from base compensation programs?

REFERENCES

Becker, B. E., Huselid, M. A., & Ulrich, D. (2001). *The HR scorecard.* Boston: Harvard Business School Press, 2001.

Beer, M., & Cannon, M. D. (2004, Spring). Promise and peril in implementing pay-for-performance. *Human Resources Management, 43*(1), 3–48.

Beer, M., & Katz, N. (2003). Do incentives work? The perceptions of a worldwide sample of senior executives. *Human Resource Planning, 26*(3), 30–44.

Blair, B. (1985). *Hospital Employee Assistance Programs.* Chicago: American Hospital Publishing, Inc.

Bonner, S. E., & Sprinkle, G. B. (2002). The effects of monetary incentives on effort and task performance: Theories, evidence and a framework for research. *Accounting, Organizations and Society, 27,* 303–345.

Burt, T. (2005, November/December). Leadership development as corporate strategy: Using talent reviews to improve senior management. *Healthcare Executive, 20*(6), 14–18.

Busse, R. C. (2005). *Your rights at work.* Naperville, IL: Sphinx Publishing.

Butler, T., & Waldroop, J. (2005). Job sculpting: The art of retaining your best people. In *Appraising employee performance* (pp. 111–136). Boston: Harvard Business School Press.

Carrier, C. (1998, June). Employee creativity and suggestion programs: An empirical study. *Creativity and Innovation Management, 7*(2), 162–72.

Deshpande, S. P. (2002). The impact of union elections on human resources management practices in hospitals. *Health Care Manager, 20*(4), 27–35.

Deshpande, S. P. (2003). Labor relations strategies and tactics in hospital elections. *Health Care Manager, 22*(1), 52–55.

Edmondson, A., Bohmer, R., & Pisano, G. (2004). Speeding Up Team Learning. In Harvard Business Review on *Teams that Succeed* (pp. 77–97). Boston: Harvard Business School Publishing Corporation.

Fairbank, J. F., Spangler, W. E., & Williams, S. D. (2003, Sept/Oct). Motivating creativity through a computer-mediated employee suggestion management system. *Behavior and Information Technology, 22*(5), 305–314.

Foster, C., & Godkin, L. (1998, Winter). Employment selection in health care: The case for structured interviewing. *Health Care Management Review, 23*(1), 46–51.

Fottler, M. D., Ford, R. C., & Heaton, C. (2002). *Achieving Service Excellence: Strategies for Healthcare*. Chicago: Health Administration Press.

Galford, R. (1998, March/April). Why doesn't this HR department get any respect? *Harvard Business Review, 76*(2), 24–32.

Garman, A. N., Tyler, J. L., & Darnall, J. S. (2004, Sept/Oct). Development and validation of a 360-degree-feedback instrument for healthcare administrators. *Journal of Healthcare Management, 49*(5), 307–322.

Gering, J., & Conner, J. (2002, November). A strategic approach to employee retention. *Healthcare Financial Management, 56*(11), 40–44.

Gibson, V. M. (1995, February). The new employee reward system. *Management Review, 84*(2), 13–18.

Ginter, P. M., Swayne, L. E., & Duncan, W. J. (2002). *Strategic management of health care organizations* (4th ed). Malden, MA: Blackwell Publishers, Inc.

Gomez-Mejia, L. R., Welbourne, T. M., & Wiseman, R. M. (2000). The role of risk sharing and risk taking under gainsharing. *Academy of Management Review, 25*(3), 492–507.

Griffith, J. R. (2000, Jan/Feb). Championship management for healthcare organizations. *Journal of Healthcare Management, 45*(1), 17–31.

Griffith, J. R., & White, K. R. (2002). *The well-managed healthcare organization* (5th ed). Chicago: Health Administration Press/AUPHA Press.

Healthcare Financial Management Association (HFMA). (2001, August). More healthcare organizations using quality measures to reward executives. *Healthcare Financial Management Association, 55*(8), 22–25.

Hernandez, S. R., Fottler, M. D., & Joiner, C. L. (1998). Integrating management and human resources. In Fottler, M. D., Hernandez, S. R., & Joiner, C. L. (Eds). *Essentials of Human Resources Management in Health Services Organizations*. Albany, NY: Delmar Publishers.

Hoffman, P. B. (2005, Nov/Dec). Confronting management incompetence. *Healthcare Executive, 20*(6), 28–30.

Holley, W. H. Jr., Jennings, K.M., & Wolters, R. S. (2001). *The labor relations process* (7th ed.). Orlando, FL: Harcourt College Publishers.

Howard, J. C., & Szczerbacki, D. (1998). Employee assistance programs in the hospital industry. *Health Care Management Review, 13*(2), 73–79.

Huselid, M. A., Beatty, R. W., & Becker, B. E. (2005, Dec). 'A Players' or 'A Positions'? The logic of workforce management. *Harvard Business Review*, 110–117.

Izzo, J. B., & Withers, P. (2002). Winning employee-retention strategies for today's healthcare organizations. *Healthcare Financial Management, 56*(6), 52–57.

Jenks, J. M., & Zevnik, B. L. P. (1993). *Employee benefits*. New York: Collier Books/Macmillan Publishing Company.

Joiner, C. L., Jones, K. N., & Dye, C. F. (1998). Compensation management. In Fottler, M. D., Hernandez, S. R., & Joiner, C. L. (Eds) *Essentials of human resources management in health services organizations*. Albany, NY: Delmar Publishers.

Kim, Dong-One. (2005, July). The benefits and costs of employee suggestions under gainsharing. *Industrial and Labor Relations Review, 58*(4), 631–652.

Kirkpatrick, D. L. (2006). *Improving employee performance through appraisal and coaching* (2nd ed.). New York: American Management Association/AMACOM.

Lehr, R. I., McLean, R. A., & Smith, G. L. (1998). The legal and economic environment. In Fottler, M. D., Hernandez, S. R., & Joiner, C. L. (Eds). *Essentials of human resources management in health services organizations*. Albany, NY: Delmar Publishers.

Liberman, A., & Rotarius, T. (2000, June). Pre-employment decision-trees: Jobs applicant self-election. *The Health Care Manager, 18*(4), 48–54.

Longest, B. B., Rakich, J. S., & Darr, K. (2000). *Managing health services organizations and systems*. Baltimore: Health Professions Press.

Luthans, F., & Stajkovic, A. D. (1999, May). Reinforce for performance: The need to go beyond pay and even rewards. *The Academy of Management Executive, 13*(2), 49–57.

Metzger, N. (2004). Human resources management in organized delivery systems. In Wolper, L. F. (Ed) *Health care administration* (4th ed.). Sudbury, MA: Jones and Bartlett Publishers.

Peiperl, M. A. (2005). Getting 360-degree feedback right. In *Appraising employee performance* (pp. 69–109). Boston: Harvard Business School Press.

Pieper, S. K. (2005, May/June). Reading the right signals: How to strategically manage with scorecards. *Healthcare Executive, 20*(3), 9–14.

Pfeffer, J. (1998). *The human equation*. Boston: Harvard Business School Press.

Phillips, J. (1996, Apr). How much is the training worth? *Training and Development, 50*(4), 20–24.

Runy, L. A. (2003, Aug). Retirement benefits as a recruitment tool. *Hospitals and Health Networks, 77*(8), 43–49.

Scott, C., & Lowery, C. M. (1994, Winter).Union election activity in the health care industry. *Health Care Management Review, 19*(1), 18–27.

Shanahan, M. (1993). A comparative analysis of recruitment and retention of health care professionals. *Health Care Management Review, 18*(3), 41–51.

Timmreck, T. C. (1998, Summer). Developing successful performance appraisals through choosing appropriate words to effectively describe work. *Health Care Management Review, 23*(3), 48–57.

U.S. Department of Labor, Bureau of Labor Statistics. (2005). 2002 Employment and Wage Estimates and Projections Between 2002 and 2012. Retrieved April 27, 2005 from www.bls.gov

Teamwork

Sharon B. Buchbinder
Jon M. Thompson

LEARNING OBJECTIVES

By the end of this chapter the student will be able to describe:

- What a team is versus a task force or committee;
- Challenges associated with teamwork in healthcare organizations;
- Current trends among and techniques used by teams in healthcare;
- Benefits of teamwork, as well as costs;
- How to fit into a team and how to select team members;
- The importance of communication on teams;
- Methods of managing teams of healthcare professionals; and,
- Examples of teams in healthcare settings.

INTRODUCTION

Unless you've lived alone your entire life, by the time you obtain your first job in the healthcare arena, you will have been on a team. Family teams organize chores, vacations, and household projects. In school, students are assigned tasks—almost from the sandbox—that require small group work and cooperation. Extra-curricular activities—Girl Scouts, Boy Scouts, Junior Achievement, Habitat for Humanity—all require young people to work in cooperative groups. And, let us not forget the soccer moms and dads, who chauffeur their offspring from pre-school through high school to participate in sports teams. So, why does the thought of teamwork assignments make entire classes of students cringe? Despite years of team-work experiences, few students in any discipline are actually educated and trained in the "how-to" of working in teams. Yet, in healthcare management, from the day you enter the door of your first job, you will be part of an interdisciplinary team. Teamwork requires leadership, strategic thinking, diverse groups of people with different perspectives and disciplines, excellent organizational and interpersonal skills, and a good sense of humor. The purpose of this chapter is to help you learn how to navigate the sometimes tricky waters of teamwork.

WHAT IS A TEAM?

Most simply, a team is a group of people, working together to achieve a common goal (Grumbach & Bodenheimer, 2004). Teams typically include individuals with complementary skills who are committed to a common approach for which they hold themselves mutually accountable (Katzenbach & Smith, 2004). In healthcare organizations, teams can be composed of one or more disciplines, e.g., the nursing team, the physician leader team, the management team, or the quality improvement team. Because the healthcare needs of patients cut across an organization's different disciplines or functions, it is important that interdisciplinary clinical teams be set up to ensure the delivery of safe, effective, and timely care. In addition, teams can be organized to address a short-term, quality assurance problem, such as "Why did Mrs. Jones fall out of bed?" or long-term problems, such as preventing harm to all patients in all aspects of care (Ball, 2005). (See the sidebar "Quality Improvement Teams in a Hospital.")

QUALITY IMPROVEMENT TEAMS IN A HOSPITAL

The West Florida Regional Medical Center established a Continuous Quality Improvement (CQI) process for its hospital in Pensacola, Florida. The purpose of the CQI process was to improve the way that services were provided to patients. The approach the hospital took was to place employees into teams of individuals that analyzed the clinical (e.g., patient care) and non-clinical processes (e.g., support services) that were in need of improvement. For example, teams were formed that examined the labor/delivery/recovery/postpartum (LDRP) services, and the distribution and use of medications within the hospital. The teams critically reviewed these processes and came up with suggestions for improving quality. For LDRP, changes were identified to develop packaged pricing for having a baby, as well as ensuring the LDRP met the needs of consumers. The team examining the use of medications found that listing medications for physicians in order of increasing costs per average daily dose rather than alphabetically resulted in an annual savings of about $200,000. This illustrates the impact of team decision-making through a CQI process on reducing costs and improving quality of operations in a hospital.

Source: McLaughlin, 2004.

Task forces require teamwork, but don't have the life of a **committee**. A blue-ribbon task force may be commissioned for several years by a professional association or instituted to examine issues in healthcare services delivery, such as medical errors and patient safety (Institute of Medicine, 2001). These groups focus on a specific agenda, have a limited term of tenure, and disband when a report or book is issued. At the intra-organizational level, a quality assurance **committee** may have people appointed to 3-year terms. At the end of that time, a person whose term has expired steps down, but the committee and the work of the committee lives on. Committees such as these usually have a person for whom this area is her full-time job, but representatives of multiple disciplines and areas of the organization are required to examine problems and to implement organizational policy decisions.

THE CHALLENGE OF TEAMWORK IN HEALTHCARE ORGANIZATIONS

Originally hospitals grew out of religious orders, and nuns and monks provided healthcare to the poor. If you were wealthy, uneducated nurses tended to you at home, and physicians made house calls. Prior to the late 1700s and early 1800s, medical training was an apprenticeship and there were no university-trained nurses. The U.S. Civil War and the Crimean War fueled the development of the nursing profession (Wilson, 2004). The First Nurse Training School in the United States was created in 1798 at New York Hospital, by a physician. Florence Nightingale, a nurse, founded the first training school for nurses at St. Thomas Hospital in England in 1860 after the Crimean War and published her landmark book, *Notes on Nursing*, in 1890 (Donahue, 1985). Over time and as the field of nursing evolved, nursing education moved out of strictly hospital training programs into university-based settings (Donahue).

The American Medical Association (AMA) was formed in 1842 and its first meeting was to discuss the appalling lack of quality in U.S. medical schools and their products—physicians. The AMA Council on Medical Education was formed in 1847. Abraham Flexner, working at the Carnegie Foundation, traveled around the United States and Canada to examine the structure, processes, and outcomes of the over 300 medical schools that existed at that time. His 1910 report, *Medical Education in the United States and Canada*, often referred to as "The Flexner Report," called for dramatic re-organization in the medical education system. Those schools that were at the "A" level (such as the Johns Hopkins School of Medicine) were the standards by which all other schools were evaluated. The report recommended that "B" level schools either get the resources to become "A" level schools, or go out of business. Flexner urged all "C" level schools, which were considered sub-standard (some had no books!) to cease production of physicians (Flexner, 1910).

Compared to medicine and nursing, healthcare management is a young discipline. The University of Chicago founded the first program in health administration in 1934 under the leadership of Michael M. Davis, who had a PhD in sociology. Davis recognized that there was no formal training for hospital managers and that an interdisciplinary program of education was needed. Envisioning the role of the healthcare manager as both a business and social role, he utilized the expertise of medical, social service administration, and business faculty to create an interdisciplinary model that has been replicated repeatedly across the United States and throughout the world (University of Chicago, n.d.). Schools with a degree in healthcare management or administration originally all offered only master's degrees, geared to preparing hospital administrators. Now, in addition to master's degrees, there are baccalaureate and doctoral programs in healthcare management. More jobs in healthcare management are being created outside of hospital settings than within. Increasing specialization of healthcare, burgeoning allied healthcare disciplines, a diversity of healthcare organizations, greater variety in jobs, higher expectations for healthcare outcomes, and demanding consumers mean that healthcare organizations must be able to respond appropriately, effectively, and efficiently. Interdisciplinary teams and teamwork provide the mechanism for improved responses to these demands.

Despite the demonstrated need for and effectiveness of interdisciplinarity, formal education and training in teamwork for physicians and nurses is rare (Baker, Salas, King, Battles & Arach, 2005; Buchbinder, Alt, Eskow, Forbes, Hester, Struck & Taylor, 2005). A poll conducted in 2004 by the American College of Physician Executives (ACPE) revealed that about one quarter of the physician executive respondents were seeing problem physician behaviors almost weekly (Weber, 2004). Thirty-six percent of the respondents reported conflicts between physicians and staff members (including nurses) and 25% reported physicians refused to embrace teamwork. The Institute of Medicine has recommended that healthcare organizations develop effective teams (Institute of Medicine, 2001). Physicians and nurses work from a clinical framework of advocating at the individual level for patients and families. Healthcare managers, on the other hand, are trained to look at population-level and organization-wide issues. Sometimes, clinicians and managers have head-on collisions due to these contrasting world views (Edwards, Marshall, McLellan & Abbasi, 2004).

Healthcare executives recommend that to engage medical staff, managers need to promote alignment between hospitals and physicians. This alignment can be accomplished through the use of shared goals, especially patient safety (Sherman, 2006). Understanding physicians is key to getting them on board with teamwork and reducing medical errors. Physicians are pulled in multiple directions by multiple demands and their time is at a premium. Valuing a physician's time means organizations must have competent team members in place who can take on some of the physician's tasks. Promoting interdependence on trustworthy teammates is critical in achieving safe, effective patient care. As a healthcare manager, you will be responsible for working with and encouraging all healthcare professionals to become good team members. It will not always be an easy task, but in the long run, it will be rewarding.

THE BENEFITS OF EFFECTIVE HEALTHCARE TEAMS

One of the best ways to convince clinicians that interdisciplinary teamwork is important is to show them the relationship to patient care. According to Mickan (2005), some of the benefits of effective teams include improved coordination of care, efficient use of healthcare services, increased job satisfaction among team members, and higher patient satisfaction. Ruddy and Rhee (2005) echoed these findings in their literature review of primary care for the underserved. Roblin, Vogt, and Fireman (2003) demonstrated that primary healthcare teams in ambulatory care settings could improve quality of care and corporate productivity when employees are empowered to be innovative and rewarded for performance. In addition, it has been shown that specialized hospital services can benefit from "service line" team approaches that show increased trust among staff, shared goals and greater patient satisfaction (Liedtka, Whitten, & Sorrells-Jones, 1998). (See sidebar "Collaboration of Staff in a Service Line Approach.)

COLLABORATION OF STAFF IN A SERVICE LINE APPROACH

The existing literature suggests that collaboration should make possible simultaneous improvement in both quality and cost-effectiveness of care. Collaboration supports on-going learning for providing good care, and can assist with effective redesign of care processes. An academic medical center, with a capacity of 500 beds, reorganized from a traditional departmental structure to a service line approach, which included 12 service centers. The service line structure used "focused teams." Focused teams, in contrast to functional or coordinated teams, are distinguished by the fact that non-nursing professionals report to unit or service managers rather than to a central department.

The medical center staff designed a questionnaire to assess perceptions of effectiveness of the service line model in promoting collaboration and improving care outcomes. Overall, respondents—including administrators, physicians, and nurses—indicated that the successful service line collaboration was associated with a sense of greater ownership, a high level of trust, realistic expectations, and shared goals. However, there were differences in perceptions of effectiveness of the service line approach as viewed by administrators, physicians, and nurses. This showed that staff may have different views of the value of service line models. For example, nurses expressed feelings of being left out of decision-making processes and believed that unrealistic expectations were placed on them. Physicians viewed the need for important input into the decision-making process as well, and expressed the need to have a clear sense of strategic direction. Outcome data, in terms of patient satisfaction, cost per case, and length of stay, remained consistent for the period of time studied. The authors note that the lack of positive change in these indicators may be due to the newness of the implementation of the service line model, and the possibility that chosen measures may not be sensitive enough to capture positive outcomes associated with service line collaboration. The authors concluded that the diversity of staff perspectives and experiences with service line management models created significant challenges for leaders of healthcare institutions, and that successful collaboration can result only when these professional differences are understood and addressed.

Source: Liedtka, Whitten & Sorrells-Jones, 1998.

Clinicians are not always the reluctant team builders. Sometimes higher level management is uncertain that teamwork is worth the effort and short-term costs. For this audience, the answer lies in the bottom line: improved communication, increased productivity, increased job satisfaction, and decreased nursing turnover (Amos, Hu, & Herrick, 2005; Institute for Healthcare Improvement, 2004). In an era when nurses are retiring faster than new ones are coming into the field, healthcare managers cannot afford to ignore the loss of nurses from the workforce (Health Resources & Services Administration, 2004). Nursing turnover costs have been estimated to be around $65,000 per lost nurse (Kemski, 2002). Multiply that by the number of nurses who quit their jobs, and the costs can be in the millions of dollars for healthcare organizations. Any strategy that improves the retention of nursing staff saves the organization the costs of using agency or traveler nurses, replacing lost nurses and training new ones, as well as the loss of productivity from burdening the remaining staff. In a large system, like the Veterans Health Administration, High Involvement Work Systems that include teamwork can mean lower service costs in the millions of dollars (Harmon, Scotti, Behson, Petzel, Neuman, & Keashly, 2003). Show higher level management the money to be saved in the long run with effective teamwork, and their approvals will follow.

THE COSTS OF TEAMWORK

Despite all the benefits of teamwork noted above, there can be a downside with its associated costs. The costs of teamwork include:

- the costs of actually having meetings (e.g., the money spent on facilities, travel, and food);
- the costs involved with planning and setting up meetings (including the time spent trying to arrange a time that's convenient for most of the participants);
- the costs of the time spent in meeting, including the related **opportunity costs** (i.e., how that time might have been better spent); and,
- the hard-to-measure interpersonal costs associated with having to work with other people, develop mutually respectful behaviors and trust, risk-taking associated with letting go of one's turf, and the potential embarrassment of looking bad in a group.

In 1995, Lucente, Rea, Vorce, and Yancey reported on the impact of creating a patient-focused care delivery model. (See the sidebar on the "Use of Teams in a Patient-Focused Care Model in a Community Hospital.")

USE OF TEAMS IN A PATIENT-FOCUSED CARE MODEL IN A COMMUNITY HOSPITAL

In 1994, Augusta Medical Center, Fishersville, Virginia, opened its new facility and instituted a redesign of its patient care delivery system. The redesign project embodied the "future care model," which is a patient-focused care delivery system that focuses on the value for the patient through a continuous quality improvement process. The "Patient-Focused Care Model" is based on the following assumptions:

1) Services at the point of delivery will reduce wait times and improve patient services.
2) Patients will be grouped according to resources needed.
3) High volume and low risk services will be decentralized.
4) For all patient services, professional staff will be assisted by cross-trained, multi-disciplinary, non-licensed extenders, which will result in improved cost-effectiveness and efficiency.
5) Physician-nurse communication and collaboration are essential for appropriate care, resource utilization, and preventing patient problems.

Implementation of the model began in 1992 in the existing facility on a pilot basis with the formation of patient care teams, including a case manger (an RN), an RN Team Leader, an LPN, a patient care technician, and a patient care assistant. The latter two team members were unlicensed assistive personnel used by the hospital to address the shortage of RNs and to reduce the non-nursing time being experienced by RNs. The Patient Care Teams were assigned to care for a defined group of patients in particular clinical units within the hospital. In addition, certain non-nursing clinical and support services—such as selected respiratory therapy activities, phlebotomy, patient transport, and specimen collection, patient registration and environmental services—were decentralized to the care unit levels.

Evaluation of the pilot project was conducted in the period 1992–1993 to assess quality, patient satisfaction, and cost-related outcomes in a 22-bed medical unit. Findings from interviews with 400 medical-surgical patients indicated a 6% increase in the number of patients demonstrating patient education knowledge upon discharge, and a record review of 100 medical-surgical patients indicated a 50% increase in the number of medical records of discharged patients with patient educational interventions documented. In addition, the hospital experienced an average hourly wage reduction of 26 cents per hour as a result of using unlicensed, multi-skilled extenders. Length of stay decreased by 12% for all patients in the pilot project unit, and, for those patients who were actively case managed, length of stay decreased by 17% during the study period. Patient satisfaction levels did not change considerably during the pilot project. However, physicians reported that the patient-focused care model improved the quality of care that the patient received, and that the new roles of nurses in the team approach also enhanced the quality of patient care.

Source: Lucente et al., 1995.

Due to the merger of two acute care facilities, the hospital decided to create a patient-focused care model and a new team organization for case management to streamline care and reduce costs. A multidisciplinary steering group developed the model and nurse managers, physicians, and patient care technicians implemented it. The authors found that patient education and quality of care improved; overtime decreased with a savings of $112,000; and patient satisfaction was unchanged. However, when they attempted to survey 500 employees to obtain staff satisfaction levels in

1992 and 1993, only four questionnaires were returned. The poor initial response to the staff satisfaction survey could have been due to methodology—or the fact that people dislike change. Resistance to organizational change is always a potential cost in teamwork, and one that shouldn't be readily discounted.

Tuckman (1965) conducted a comprehensive literature review of small group behavior in therapy groups, t-group studies, natural groups, and laboratory group studies. After examining the literature, he devised a classification scheme for small group dynamics. In this classic article, Tuckman provided the following five stages that teams go through: **forming**, **storming**, **norming**, **performing**, and **adjourning**. When teams are **forming**, they are getting oriented to the team goals and each other, finding out what the tasks are and who they will be working with. Then the **storming** begins. With storming, there is intragroup conflict. Individuals may vie for dominance and exhibit passive-aggressive behaviors, along with information withholding, and other forms of resistance to team tasks and goals. Peace breaks out when the storming stage passes, and team members actually begin **performing** the work at hand, have open dialogue with one another, and share information to accomplish the team's goals. Winding down and **adjourning** brings its own emotional turbulence. Team members who may have disliked each other at the start, have worked together over a long period of time, and have developed respect for one another. They've grown to like each other as individuals and the team as a whole and become sad that they are disbanding (Tuckman).

When teams don't work well together, there are significant costs to the organization in terms of human resources and opportunity costs. These costs mean that teamwork may not always be as efficient as other forms of problem-solving and decision-making. According to Drinka and Clark (2000), "To become efficient . . . the team members must learn to define the scope of the problem . . . and select the least disciplines needed to address the problem well." The more is not always the merrier. Teams function efficiently only when each carefully selected team member knows the goal(s) of the team. It takes less time (usually) for one person to decide on a potential strategy than a group of people. However, without having team advocates in each of the areas affected by the decision, implementing a unilateral decision can become a healthcare manager's worst nightmare.

WHO'S ON THE TEAM?

When you first start out in healthcare management, it is unlikely that you will be able to choose your teammates. It will be your job to learn the culture of the organization and to determine how best to fit into a team. Some of the questions that you can ask when you are assigned to a team are:

- What are the goals of the team?
- How will they be measured?
- What are the short-term and long-term deadlines?
- When and where does the team meet?
- To whom do I report? (Sometimes staff members are loaned to teams, so this is an important issue to resolve.)
- What is my role on the team?
- What are my responsibilities in that role?

Good managers don't mind if a new staff member makes a list of questions and asks for clarification and direction. Coaching, mentoring, and guiding are all part of the manager's role, and healthcare management is a continuous learning experience. Managers *do* mind, however, if you don't ask questions, and go off and do the wrong thing. Additionally, good managers want thoughtful observations from a new perspective—yours.

Over time, as you assume more responsibilities and learn the organization, you may be asked to recommend team members or to convene a team to address a specific organizational issue. Getting the right people on a team is one of the most critical tasks a healthcare manager can have. When this opportunity comes, ask for counsel and advice from your manager and your co-workers. The last thing you want to do is exclude the Chairman of Surgery on a team that is addressing Operating Room productivity.

Real world healthcare management problems are complex, complicated, and messy. Drinka and Clark (2000, p. 37) talk about "tame versus wicked problems." Tame problems can be defined; wicked problems are difficult to define and not easily resolved. You need to have every involved area's input to analyze a wicked problem, because it won't be solved by one person—or one discipline. Most problems fall along the continuum of tame to wicked, with many levels of messiness along the way. As a healthcare manager, you will need to assess the strengths and weaknesses of each potential team member before inviting him or her onto your team. You will need to ask the following questions.

Does this person . . .

- Belong to an area that's affected by the problem at hand?
- Have the knowledge, skills, and disposition to do the tasks at hand?
- Understand and agree with the role he or she will play on the team?
- Have the authority to make decisions and implement recommendations?
- Follow through on assignments and tasks and meet deadlines?
- Think beyond the confines of a department or discipline?
- Work collaboratively and respectfully with other disciplines?
- Have the ability to defuse tensions and de-escalate conflict?
- Have a sense of humor?
- Have a good reputation within the organization as a team player?

One tool that is sometimes used for understanding differences in team members' personalities is the Myers-Briggs Type Indicator (MBTI), a personality inventory based on Jung's theory of psychological types (Rideout & Richardson, 1989). The MBTI assesses four domains and four subsets within those domains on a four-by-four grid (Wideman, 2003). On the vertical axis of this grid is the Introvert-Extrovert scale; on the horizontal axis is the Sensing-Intuitive scale. Within each of the four quadrants of this grid are two more axes—the Perceiving-Judging axis and the Thinking-Feeling axis. After taking this paper-and-pencil, self-administered inventory, the individual finds her "Myers-Briggs Type" on a large square. The types are designated by letters, so when a search firm is looking for a strong executive, they would want an "ESTJ," someone who is "responsible, dependable, highly organized, likes to see things done correctly, tends to judge in terms of standard operating procedures, realistic, matter-of-fact, and loyal to institutions" (Wideman, p. 11).

When building a team, you may not want everyone to be a leader. You also need good followers, i.e., people who are willing to bring their strengths to the group process, who may be more on the end of the sensing, introverted, intuitive end of the axis on the MBTI, rather than the extroverted end. Wideman (2003) suggests that while project management and teamwork are becoming mandatory in most employment settings, not everyone in the workforce population is suited, by their personality type, to function well on a team. He suggests judicious use of the MBTI to see where people fit in the leadership versus followership mode and to be cautious about who is placed on a team.

Many healthcare recruiters utilize the MBTI to help them select candidates for healthcare placements. In addition, many healthcare management professional organizations offer seminars and workshops for individuals to learn about their personality styles. The key thing to know about this popular tool is that it is one of many ways to understand healthcare team members, but it is not the only way. Oftentimes, experience and the oral history of the healthcare organization where you work are the best predictors of selecting good team members.

TEAM COMMUNICATION

Frequent, positive communications improve team interactions and increase trust. Organizations that empower their employees promote employee job satisfaction. Laschinger and Finegan (2005) found that nurses who felt they had access to opportunity, honest relationships, open communication with peers and managers, and trusted their managers were more likely to be attached to their organizations and have higher job satisfaction.

Dreachslin, Hunt, and Sprainer (1999) conducted research to assess how diversity affected patient-centered team communication and whether it improved communication and patient care. Focus groups were convened to elicit key issues and to develop recommendations. They found that more training was needed for team members and nurse managers in the clinical and relationship management arenas. The authors concluded that healthcare managers should facilitate open and honest dialogue between management and care production teams and within the teams themselves. They should also involve care production team members in process improvement. The patient-centered care model must emphasize caring for patients, include 360-degree feedback where nurses and technicians evaluate each other, be implemented for assessment, be communicated to team members, and be used as a management tool for continuous quality improvement. This article underscores the need for diversity training as part of team and leadership training.

In a classic article on management teams, Eisenhardt, Kahwajy and Bourgeois (1997) observed teams in twelve technology companies. Much like healthcare today, these companies operated in a high-stakes, fast-paced environment, where today's technology is tomorrow's dinosaur. Teams had to be lightning fast in their responses and almost precognitive to stay ahead of the competition. The authors found that teams with minimal interpersonal conflict had the same six strategies. "Team members: worked with more, rather than less information, and debated facts; developed multiple alternatives to enrich the level of debate; shared commonly agreed upon goals; injected humor into the decision process; maintained a balanced power structure; and resolved issues without forcing consensus" (Eisenhardt, Kahwajy, & Bourgeois, p. 78). By keeping the focus on the facts and not on personalities, and communicating in an open, honest, and safe forum, the teams were able to have fun and be productive.

Recently, the airline industry has become a team building model for hospitals and other healthcare organizations. Pilots are trained to be team players because a plane full of people may die if they don't pay attention to their teammates' observations. **Crew resource management** has been developed to address attitudes, change behavior, and improve performance. Sexton, Thomas, and Helmreich (2000) have applied crew resource management research to the hospitals, where stakes are also high, and lives depend on the smooth functioning of the healthcare team. Senior surgeons were least likely in favor of teamwork and flat hierarchies. Medical staff responded that teamwork was imperative, but that they were not encouraged to report safety concerns. Doctors and nurses differed widely in their opinions regarding teamwork. Almost three quarters of surveyed intensive care physicians reported high levels of teamwork with nurses, but less than half of the nurses felt the same way. These results point to the need for a more realistic appraisal of safety concerns, improved communication between team members, and enhanced team training for healthcare professionals, in all disciplines and specialties. These studies suggest that managers should work to understand the need for and invest in providing ongoing team training for their healthcare workers as a strategy for creating high performing teams.

METHODS OF MANAGING TEAMS OF HEALTHCARE PROFESSIONALS

Koeck (1998) observed that, while healthcare delivery demands extensive teamwork, the reality is that healthcare teams often fail due to resistance to organizational change and lack of effective leadership. Effective leadership, addressed in the first chapter of this book, is needed at every level of the healthcare organization, but especially in teamwork. Because, by definition, interdisciplinary health teams are made up of people from different fields, it's the healthcare manager's job to take the lead and to establish team guidelines and foster good communication. It's the responsibility of the team leader to establish communication networks. At the first meeting, the leader should obtain names, all phone numbers, email addresses, and any other way the team members can be contacted. One of the things a team leader can do to facilitate good communication early in the life of the team, is to establish guidelines for expected behaviors, processes, and outcomes in a written document.

As can be seen in Figure 11-1, *Guidelines for Teamwork*, the document does not have to be complicated. This tool can be used to evaluate the performance of individual members of the team, thus avoiding the **social loafer** or **free-rider syndrome**, where a member of the team does nothing, but gets credit for the work done by others. Managing social loafers and other problem teammates can be the biggest part of managing a team. As an effective team leader, your job is to get the best out of each team member. Attaining top performance requires understanding who your teammates are, what they need, and what it will take to build consensus, being aware that you may not have 100% agreement on every decision.

After introductions, and establishing the purpose of the team in a written document, Maginn (1995) recommends that the team leader go around the table and ask each person his or her ideas about the problem. As a leader, you should acknowledge each idea, recording it as the team member speaks. Be sure to wait for people to respond to the question—and to each other. Don't interrupt, and don't let others interrupt a person when he/she has the floor. Ask critics for ideas and suggestions, getting those negative comments out on the table so they can be addressed. Remain calm, open-minded, and non-defensive. At the end of each meeting, thank everyone for their thoughtful comments, summarizing what you thought you heard and asking for clarification.

Before the meeting ends, ask people to do some homework. Who is willing to do what task? Will there be research needed? What process should be used for reporting to each other? Send a summary of the meeting to everyone on the team, and include a list of steps that need to be taken before the next meeting. Communication that includes everyone is key. Establish an email list and be sure all correspondence regarding the project goes through it. The more information team members have, the more buy-in and cooperation will occur.

The purpose of Team XYZ is to _____**<goals>**_____.
Our deadline for solving this problem is _____**<date>**_____.
The team will meet __**<number of times or frequency of meetings>**__.
Representatives from each affected area have been asked to serve on Team XYZ.
Those representatives are: _____**<List names of team members>**_____

Team members will

- Attend all team sessions, unless there is an emergency;
- Prepare for each session;
- Listen to each other with respect;
- Work collaboratively to identify and meet session goals;
- Be an active participant in group discussions;
- Keep an open mind; be willing to modify opinions or conclusions to keep the project moving forward;
- Present ideas concisely;
- Be considerate and tactful when participating in group discussions;
- Submit delegated work on time and fulfill responsibilities as agreed; and,
- Work actively to achieve group consensus on issues and problems.

By __**<deadline>**__, Team XYZ will have achieved the goals listed above, documented in the following:*

- Reports of proceedings, data analyses, recommendations, and an evaluation plan for implementation of the recommendations.

Note: The Leader of Team XYZ is responsible for presentation of this report, with all team members present, if possible, to the administration for review and approval.

Interim deadlines may be needed, so consider those as you discuss these guidelines.

FIGURE 11-1 Guidelines for Teamwork

To build trust, meet commitments and do what you say you are going to do. Bring reliable information to the team. Accurate data and demonstrated skill at your work inform the team members that you are competent—and trustworthy (Maginn, 1995). Even when team members trust each other, conflict happens. At some point in time, there will be a disagreement about which choices and decisions the team should make. Maginn recommends five potential strategies for conflict resolution in teams:

bargaining, problem solving, voting, research, and **third-party mediation**.

Bargaining is when someone says, "If you go along with me this time, I'll back you up next time." If the choices are equally good, then bargaining can be a good tool; if the choices aren't equal, then it may not be a good tool. **Voting** is democratic, but also bears the weight of potentially taking a team to the incorrect choice. **Problem solving** may be the better way to go. This means taking time to answer the "what if" scenarios of each alternative. "If we do this, then what might happen?" "How will we assess if we've chosen the right option?" The team may not know until it picks an approach and tries it. Doing more **research** is safe, but the team may have time pressures that preclude it from doing an in-depth study. When all else fails, **third-party mediation** is probably a win-win situation, especially if the third-party is the boss. Oftentimes, the team presentation to the boss will include choices that have been laid out, like a menu, for an upper level manager to select from. The alternatives are listed, the pros and cons of each alternative are provided, and the assessment plan for each alternative is in place. You win, your team wins, and your organization wins.

CONCLUSION

This chapter has described what a team is and some of the challenges associated with teamwork in healthcare organizations. Some current trends in using teams, and the benefits of teamwork, as well as costs, have been described. Fitting into a team and selecting team members were discussed, along with the Myers-Briggs Type Indicator personality inventory. The importance of communication on teams and some methods of managing teams of healthcare professionals have been reviewed. In addition, some examples of teams in healthcare settings have been presented. You have the background and tools—now you can begin to build your team.

DISCUSSION QUESTIONS

1. What are the differences between a team, a task force and a committee? What are some of the potential differences in dynamics between people in these different groups?

2. What are some of the unique challenges associated with teamwork in health care? Describe three benefits and three costs of teamwork in healthcare organizations.

3. After working in a hospital for 6 months, you have been selected to head up the team to conduct hand washing audits on all the nursing units. Who do you want on your team and why?

4. A member of the hand washing audit team comes to you and complains that another team member is not pulling her weight. This individual is not your employee, but she is on your team. What should you do?

5. List and describe five potential strategies for conflict resolution in teams. Which method is likely to be most successful if your manager likes to be involved in every decision?

6. What are the five stages of team development? Describe each stage and how that might appear in a healthcare setting.

7. What is the Myers-Briggs Type Indicator personality inventory and why is it a useful tool for healthcare executives?

REFERENCES

Amos, M. A., Hu, J., & Herrick, C. A. (2005, January/February). The impact of team building on communication and job satisfaction of nursing staff. *Journal for Nurses in Staff Development, 21*(1), 10–16.

Baker, D. P., Salas, E., King, H., Battles, J., & Barach, P. (2005, April). The role of teamwork in the professional education of physicians: current status and assessment recommendations. *Journal on Quality and Patient Safety, 31*(4), 185–202.

Ball, M. J. (2005, October 25). Culture of safety. *Advance for Nurses, 7*(23), 31–32.

Buchbinder, S. B., Alt, P. M., Eskow, K., Forbes, W., Hester, E., Struck, M., et al. (2005). Creating learning prisms with an interdisciplinary case study workshop. *Innovative Higher Education, 29*(4), 257–274.

Cuthbert, H. (2006). Group dynamics: Unwelcome group members. Retrieved March 14, 2006 from http://home.snu.edu/~hculbert/groupmem.htm#slacky

Donahue, M. P. (1985). *Nursing, The finest art: An Illustrated History*. St. Louis, MO: CV Mosby.

Dreachslin, J. L., Hunt, P. L., & Sprainer, E. (1999). Communication patterns and group composition: implications for patient-centered care team effectiveness. *Journal of Healthcare Management, 44*(4), 252–268.

Drinka, T. J. K., & Clark, P. G. (2000). *Health care teamwork: Interdisciplinary practice and teaching.* Westport, CT: Auburn House.

Edwards, N., Marshall, M., McLellan, A., & Abbasi, K. (2003, March 22). Doctors and managers: a problem without a solution? *British Medical Journal, 326*(7390), 609–610.

Eisenhardt, K. M., Kahwajy, J. L., & Bourgeois, L. F. (1997). How management teams can have a good fight. *Harvard Business Review, 75*(5), 77–85.

Flexner, A. (1910). *Medical education in the United States and Canada.* New York: Carnegie Foundation for the Advancement of Teaching.

Grumbach, K., & Bodenheimer, T. (2004). Can primary health care teams improve primary care practice? *Journal of the American Medical Association, 291*(10), 1246–1251.

Harmon, J., Scotti, D. J., Behson, S., Petzel, R., Neuman, J. H., & Keashly, L. (2003, November/December). Effects of high-involvement work systems on employee satisfaction and service costs in veterans healthcare. *Journal of Healthcare Management, 48*(6), 393–406.

Health Resources & Services Administration. (2004, March). *The Registered Nurse population: National sample survey of registered nurses, March 2004, preliminary findings.* Retrieved February 20, 2006 from http://bhpr.hrsa.gov/healthworkforce/reports/rnpopulation/preliminaryfindings.htm

Institute for Healthcare Improvement. (2004). *Transforming care at the bedside.* Retrieved February 20, 2006 from http://deltarhpi.ruralhealth.hrsa.gov/documents/IHITCAB%20paper037_TCAB5a.pdf

Institute of Medicine. (2001). *Crossing the quality chasm: A new health system for the 21st century.* Washington, DC: National Academy Press.

Katzenbach, J. R., & Smith, D. K. (2004). The discipline of teams. In *Teams that succeed.* Boston: Harvard Business School Press.

Kemski, A. (2002, December). *Market forces, cost assumptions, and nurse supply: Considerations in determining appropriate nurse to patient ratios in general acute care hospitals, R-37-01,* SEIU Nurse Alliance. As cited in Department for Professional Employees AFL-CIO. (2004). Fact Sheet: The costs and benefits of safe staffing ratios. Retrieved February 20, 2006 from http://www.dpeaflcio.org/policy/factsheets/fs_2004_staffratio.htm

Koeck, C. (1998, November 7). Time for organizational development in healthcare organisations: Improving quality for patients means changing the organisation. *British Medical Journal, 317*(7168), 1267–1268. Retrieved March 16, 2006 from http://www.pubmedcentral.nih.gov/articlerender.fcgi?artid=1114203

Laschinger, H. K. S., & Finegan, J. (2005). Using empowerment to build trust and respect in the workplace: A strategy for addressing the nursing shortage. *Nursing Economic$, 23*(1), 6–13.

Liedtka, J. M., Whitten, E., & Sorrells-Jones, J. (1998). Enhancing care delivery through cross-disciplinary collaboration: A case study. *Journal of Healthcare Management, 43*(2), 185–206.

Lucente, B., Rea, M. R., Vorce, S. H., & Yancey, T. (1995). Redesigning care delivery in the community hospital. [Electronic version]. *Nursing Economic$, 13*(4), 242–247.

Maginn, M. (1995). *Effective teamwork*. West Des Moines, IL: American Media Publishing.

McLaughlin, C. P. (2004). West Florida regional medical center. In Rakich, J. S., Longest, B. B. & Darr, K. (Eds.). *Cases in health services management* (4th ed.). Baltimore: Health Professions Press, Inc.

Mickan, S. M. (2005). Evaluating the effectiveness of health care teams. *Australian Health Review, 29*(2), 211–217.

Rideout, C. A., & Richardson, S. A. (1989, May). A teambuilding model: Appreciating differences using the Myers-Briggs Type Indicator with developmental theory. *Journal of Counseling and Development, 67*(9), 529–533.

Roblin, D. W., Vogt, T. M., & Fireman, B. (2003, January-March). Primary health care teams: Opportunities and challenges in evaluation of service delivery innovations. *Journal of Ambulatory Care Management, 26*(1), 22–35.

Ruddy, G., & Rhee, K. (2005). Transdisciplinary teams in primary care for the underserved: A literature review. *Journal of Health Care for the Poor and Underserved, 16*, 248–256.

Sexton, J. B., Thomas, E. J., & Helmreich, R. L. (2000). Error, stress, and teamwork in medicine and aviation: cross sectional surveys. *British Medical Journal, 320*, 745–749.

Sherman, J. (2006, Mar/Apr). Patient safety: Engaging medical staff. *Healthcare Executive, 21*(2), 20–23.

Tuckman, B. W. (1965). Developmental sequence in small groups. *Psychological Bulletin, 63*, 384–399. Reprinted in *Group facilitation: A research and applications journal*, Number 3, Spring 2001. Available at http://dennislearningcenter.osu.edu/references/GROUP%20DEV%20ARTICLE.doc. Retrieved March 7, 2006 from http://en.wikipedia.org/wiki/Forming-storming-norming-performing

University of Chicago. (n.d.). *About GPHAP*. School of Social Service Administration, Chicago, IL, The Graduate Program in Health Administration and Policy. Retrieved March 7, 2006 from http://gphap.uchicago.edu/aboutgphap.shtml

Weber, D. O. (2004, September-October). Poll results: Doctors' disruptive behavior disturbs physician leaders. *The Physician Executive, 30*(5), 6–14.

Wideman, M. (2003). *Project teamwork, personality profiles and the population at large: Do we have enough of the right kind of people?* Retrieved March 14, 2006 from http://www.maxwideman.com/papers/profiles/profiles.pdf

Wilson, B. (2004). *Men in American nursing history*. Retrieved February 20, 2006 from http://www.geocities.com/Athens/Forum/6011/index.html

CHAPTER 12

Cultural Competency and Diversity

Joanna Basuray

LEARNING OBJECTIVES

By the end of this chapter the student will be able to describe:

- The impact of changing demographics on patients and providers;

- Cultural dimensions in varied healthcare settings and contexts;

- Systems and processes of cultural competency; and,

- The essential steps for building cultural awareness.

INTRODUCTION

With an ever increasing emphasis on cultural competency in management and leadership, it is obvious that cultural diversity is an emerging horizon in the discipline and requires careful study, research, and new strategies in healthcare management. For the past 30 years, we have seen rapid population changes in the United States. The U.S. Census Bureau (2000 & 2005) showed that 30% of the overall U.S. population composition is comprised of racial and ethnic minorities, as compared to the 17% reported in 1970. Large-scale immigration from Latin America and Asia in the 1980s accounted for a high growth in minority populations. The U.S. Census Bureau (2004) projects that by 2050 nearly 50% of the overall U.S. population will be composed of minority groups. Also, in 2000, the census form was revised, designating 15 different race categories and 3 options for specifying one's own race (Grieco & Cassidy, 2001). This change of the census form reveals important sociological implications, and also reinforces the importance of a multicultural perspective to healthcare. This complex, multicultural perspective must be integrated into the traditional framework of healthcare management, which has historically been based primarily on European and Western industrial managerial styles and workforce ideologies.

The United States is a pluralistic country. Multicultural groups exist, and have been previously identified as "ethnic groups," such as Irish, Italian, German, Jewish, British, African American, and Native American. A multicultural perspective to healthcare management must also recognize new immigrant groups, such as those representing several countries in Asia, Africa, and Latin America. These minority ethnic populations reside in many cities and rural communities of this country (Morrison & Donnelly, 2002). Reports on migration flows in the U.S. for immigrants and domestic migrants affect metropolitan populations. Frey (2005) reported how immigrant minorities who are low skilled, as well as those who are educationally highly prepared, are affecting a changing demographic landscape shaped by a distinct racial, ethnic, and educational profile in each area. The census data of 1990 and 2000 were analyzed in Frey's report, indicating a high growth in large metropolitan cites such as Atlanta, Phoenix, and Charlotte, as well as slow growing cities such as Detroit and Cleveland. Frey suggested that a rapid domestic migration of the middle-class, well-educated population to the suburbs creates demand for immigrant groups for employment in new services, retail, and construction work. These and other reports on economic integration of immigrants suggest that the reader must also look into how immigration policies are tied into the labor market and economy of the host country (Cornelius, Martin, & Hollifield, 1994; Frey, 2005; Lynch & Simon, 2003; Portes & Rumbaut, 2001).

Not only must we revise the definition of a multicultural United States, but also consider and redefine our notion of **diversity**. Diversity has been historically defined by broad categorical markers such as age, sexual orientation, religion, and ethnicity. The latter category further narrows our understanding of diversity as ethnicity encompasses many other factors including economic status and marginalization. Therefore, not only must we consider the prolific numbers of ethnic groups in the United States, we must also consider factors relevant to their minority status, such as whether they are migrants, uninsured, poor, or refugees. Rapid global changes to the economy have brought attention to our national borders, especially in policy concerning trade and the migration of people. Movement of labor across borders has influenced organizations and businesses to re-establish management policies for their diverse clients *and* their workforce. Currently, global economic changes show an intense shift toward geographical diversification of labor (Connerley & Pederson, 2005). In addition to ethnic differences among patients and clients, health industries in large cities also face language barriers and cultural differences in recruitment and retention of employees (Pamies, Hill, Watkins, McNamee, & Colbur, 2006). An ethnic ethnic match is not always possible between the caregiver and the receiver of healthcare services. An example of this is the recent trend in hiring newly arrived immigrant workers and temporary staff (particularly those from Southeast Asia and the Phillipines), by numerous hospitals, rehabilitation centers, and nursing homes (Andrews & Boyle, 2003; Satcher & Pamies, 2006).

Diversity is often used to explain differences among people, such as their particular lifestyles, economic status, race, or gender, as well as how legal, political, and social policies apply to affirmative action laws. Management of healthcare systems in the 21st century requires the student to recognize difference as "normal" rather than holding onto pre-established standards of management that apply to homogenous population groups. This expanded concept of "normal" also means re-evaluating leadership styles and management strategies. Thus, by becoming *aware* of difference—be it geographical, linguistic, or religious—the healthcare manager places staff performance and client needs in a cultural context. It is important for the healthcare organization's managers and employees to be effective communicators and interpreters. Part of this includes learning and teaching appropriate behaviors for addressing diversity in employee and client populations.

CULTURAL FRAMEWORKS IN HEALTHCARE MANAGEMENT

Management functions may be unique to each individual organization, but the most commonly practiced functions are leading, planning, organizing, staffing, directing, controlling, coordinating, and representing (Goldsmith, 2005). Healthcare systems face cultural diversity across the spectrum of these managerial functions. Several functional items are managed daily at healthcare systems in local, national, or international markets. The essential processes in managing diversity are communicating the institution's policies and practices in clear language, establishing and running effective interdisciplinary teams, obtaining cultural knowledge about employees and clients, and utilizing cultural competency as a benchmark for evaluating healthcare services. While the universal focus of management, especially healthcare management, is to keep track of the articulated organizational purpose, the infusion of culture-related elements make the interest in human affairs an organizational priority. Managers are concerned about creating a workplace that demonstrates effectiveness and productivity and focuses on behavior and functionality. Healthcare institutions are establishing behavioral and cultural norms that are observable and measurable. Connerley and Pederson (2005) emphasize focusing on behaviors "because behaviors have no meaning outside their own cultural context" (p. 16). Thus, observation of behaviors is irrelevant unless one also considers culture. Healthcare management needs to be culturally conscious and develop a culturally integrated workplace.

One widely used model of managing diversity in the workplace is called the "Four Layers of Diversity" (Gardenswartz, Rowe, Digh, & Bennett, 2003). The layers of this model involve four dimensions: **personality**, **internal dimensions**, **external dimensions**, and **organizational dimensions**. This multidimensional model allows the manager to understand the workforce by using a cultural lens that focuses on race and gender. It also attempts to address management through four tiers beginning with the individual's personality. **Personality** is identified as the first layer—the intrinsic or inherent set of characteristics within a person. The second layer involves the **internal dimensions** of an individual, including that person's age, race, gender, sexual orientation, physical ability, and ethnicity. The third layer considers the **external dimension** of an individual, which consist of his or her income, personal habits, recreational habits, work experience, appearance, parental status, marital status, and geographic location. Finally, the fourth layer examines the individual's **placement within the organization** or workplace. This layer examines such factors as the individual's functional level or classification, division or field of work, work location, seniority, management status, and union affiliation. Gardenswartz and Rowe (1998) reported that this four dimensional model allows for a better understanding of the worldviews of organizations' managers, employees, and clients.

The corporate culture may be viewed as a microcosm of the larger societal cultural values and traditions, which promotes a collection of beliefs, habits, value systems, behaviors, or communication patterns—traditions and customs of conducting business that both reflect and depart from the larger system. Culture, in this context, is defined as a patterned way of thinking, feeling, and reacting that is acquired and transmitted mainly by symbols (Kroeber & Kluckhohn, 1952).

So, how does culture influence the healthcare organization, especially with respect to the relationship of cultural symbols to thinking and feeling? **Organizational culture** is best understood by using a multi-tiered model (Morgan, 1997). The most difficult aspect is to clearly define how values and beliefs are manifested in the workplace. Many studies have provided vague descriptions of values as they relate to culture. **Organizational culture** is often described as a set of social rules that guide perceptions and thinking. Edgard Schein (2004) describes three levels of organizational culture: **artifacts, espoused beliefs and values**, and **basic underlying assumptions. Artifacts** are "visible organizational structures and processes," **espoused beliefs and values** are "strategies, goals, and philosophies, espoused justifications," and **underlying assumptions** are "unconscious, taken-for-granted beliefs, perceptions, thoughts, and feelings, the ultimate source of values and actions." (p. 26). **Artifacts** can range from the architecture of the building to the use of technology. **Espoused values and beliefs** are usually found in organizational mission, vision, and value statements. Schein notes that sometimes these can be at odds with each other when the mission statement indicates that it will give maximum value to stockholders, employees, *and* clients. **Basic underlying assumptions** are cognitive maps i.e., the way things are done in an organization and are taken for granted. If someone violates a basic underlying assumption by using a different process to achieve an outcome, coworkers may respond with surprise, even shock, and say things like, "But we've always done it *this* way!" These basic underlying assumptions are key to organizational change and must be addressed when managers think about becoming more responsive to racial and ethnic diversity.

Assumptions about the way culture works and its dimensions are continuously discussed and debated in the literature (Morgan, 1997; Sackmann, 1991). However, the most widely discussed framework on the assumptions that occur in organizations is based on the work of Kluckhohn and Strodtbeck (1961). The authors postulated five basic assumptions of culture in their "**values orientation culture model**." These assumptions focus on (a) **people's relationship with nature**; (b) the **temporal focus of human life**; (c) the **innate character of human nature**; (d) the **modality of human activity**; and (e) the **modality of a person's relationships to other persons**. Cultural values of the respective group or society are identified as each question is addressed. When applied to healthcare management, one may differentiate one's own values from another's. As future healthcare managers, it is important to understand how different cultural groups function with patients, as well as healthcare providers. For example, a person's relationships with other people may be categorized as individualistic or group-based. Thus, strategies and activities related to decision making on hiring, rewarding, and promoting varies between cultures. Likewise, a person's temporal orientation may be posited in the past, present, or future. Physical space, meeting rooms for executives, use of cubicles and offices with door and windows, or use of secretaries to assure privacy, are based on the unique cultural interpretations in our society. To Glastra (2004), the way that different cultures approach life and human behaviors speaks to the particular cultural perspective. In the workplace, these cultural orientations translate into behaviors and decision-making abilities for healthcare managers.

Similar to the values orientation culture model, other models exist that are based on the acknowledgment of human needs as well as our understanding and ability to solve cultural issues and dilemmas. For example, Hofstede (1991) examined cultural difference as a concept that is distinguishable, especially when one examines human nature and the individual's personality. Emphasizing that culture is learned, human nature, or the "software of the mind," as Hofstede defined it, carries emotions, such as fear, anger, or love, while the personality is unique to each person's set of mental programming. Based on a large study of employees in 40 countries, Hofstede identified culture's strong influence on relationships within and outside the employees' workplace or organization divisions. He asserted that cultural dimensions, which address societal problems, are critical to the knowledge base and practice of managers and leaders. Hofstede (1980; 1991) defined these cultural dimensions as (a) **relationships between the individual and the group**; (b) **social inequality**; (c) **social implications of gender**; and (d) **handling of uncertainty inherent in economic and social processes**. For example, in many cultures of Africa, Asia, and Latin America, there is strong commitment to family (immediate or extended) and it is not at all uncommon to see employees leave work sites to tend to their families' needs and to be absent for days while tending to their families in sickness and mourning of the dead. Gender issues in a multicultural society have critical implications for the roles of females and males, given their respective cultural orientations. For example, gender clashes are not uncommon in hospital situations when Caucasian-American female nurses work alongside African, Mediterranean, Asian, or Indian male physicians (Mor-Barak, 2005; Kavanagh & Kennedy, 1992).

CULTURAL COMPETENCY AND DIVERSITY STAFF TRAINING

Cultural knowledge, cultural awareness, and cultural skill building are common terms defining **cultural competency** in the workplace. Lewis (1996) observed that many people mistakenly believe that common sense will enable people to cope in another culture. Common sense is basic and unsophisticated, but not neutral. The ability to communicate verbally does not necessarily indicate cultural awareness and sensitivity. Lewis pointed out that common sense is derived from experience, but that experience is culturally bound. Moreover, sharing a profession is not sufficient experience to override cultural differences.

Other discrepancies persist beyond that of common sense, and although several models of managing diversity in the workplace are available, these often emphasize communication and skill-building techniques useful for the advancement of transnational corporations and outsourcing (Mor-Barak, 2005; Gardenswartz, Rowe, Digh, & Bennet, 2003; Kavanagh &

Kennedy, 1992; Pederson & Ivey, 1993). Many institutions in the United States have instituted specific polices and programs to enhance recruitment, inclusion, promotion, and retention of employees who are minorities or immigrants. Mor-Barak indicates that the present focus on *diversity* differs from the 1964 equal rights legislation and affirmative action programs of the 1972 Executive Order 11246. The new emphasis on diversity utilizes the concept to create culturally competent strategies that provide advantages to businesses.

In nursing management, Conway-Welch, Rasch, Watkins, McNamee & Colburn (2006) describe a paradigm of cultural relativism in diversity management. This model addresses cultural conflicts by building a complementary set of cross-cultural policies and behavioral activities that acknowledge each individual's point of view as it relates to his or her cultural environment. In this model, emphasis is placed on the emotional intelligence of the individuals.

Goleman (1998) described four abilities that underlie **emotional intelligence**: self awareness, self management, social awareness, and relationship management. Gardner's (1983, 1999) theory of multiple intelligences is useful in diverse work environments. Gardner (1983) identified eight types of intelligences in people: linguistic-verbal, logical-mathematical, visual-spatial, bodily-kinesthetic, musical-rhythmic, interpersonal, and naturalistic. In multicultural work environments, understanding the different abilities and talents of people is beneficial to the organization. As noted in the chapters on teamwork and leadership, as healthcare managers we need to learn to identify and utilize the strengths of all employees and coworkers to achieve our healthcare organization's goals. Diversity management works when all participants are encouraged to achieve their full potential.

Cox (1994) preferred a **multicultural organization** that is characterized by a culture that fosters and values cultural differences of the membership. The organization is inclusive to all members within an acculturation process context rather than one concerned with assimilation. According to Cox, this form of organization is effective in managing diversity since it is focused on integration. In all instances, it is important that cultural competency building starts with becoming aware of one's own culture, worldview, and skills. Self awareness is the key to developing effective, competent work teams and services.

CULTURAL COMPETENCY AT THE WORKPLACE

Beyond self awareness, healthcare workers and managers need to address language and communication within a multicultural healthcare organization. Spoken American English varies regionally in the United States and, although mutually intelligible with an assumed English standard, these dialects can create communication barriers. Among the varied ethnic groups that make up the multicultural demography of this country, workplace culture coupled with cultural heritage guides communication patterns and styles of speech. In a conversation with the author, an African-American healthcare provider stated that in the south, when a person enters a room of people in a work setting or gathering, he or she exchanges greetings with familiar and unknown people—simply to arrive without acknowledging the presence of others is considered impolite. This exemplifies a cultural rule understood within southern African-American cultures. In this manner, language is an expression of cultural thought and values.

As future healthcare managers, students would greatly benefit from reading some of the classic works of Edward T. Hall on cross-cultural communication and the use of space (Hall, 1959, 1966; Hall & Hall, 1989). As an anthropologist who studied nonverbal communication, Hall was one of the first researchers to note cultural differences in "personal space" distances, an area of research called "proximic theory." One of the most famous episodes of *Seinfeld*, the long-running television sitcom, was about a "close talker," a man who got into everyone's personal space, and face, when he talked. In the show, everyone kept backing away from the "close talker," bumping into walls, stumbling over furniture, in an attempt to put distance between them. Viewers who saw that episode still cringe when they talk about it, because personal space is highly valued in the American culture. However, Mediterranean, Latin American, Arab, and Italian cultures have much smaller personal spaces and are offended when too much space is between people who are speaking (Rosenbloom, 2006).

In addition to personal space, other cultures also have different expectations regarding touching. Americans, as Rosenbloom reported (2006) "hate to be touched." For other cultures, however, touching is a way of being friendly, or intensifying communication. This can be perceived as inappropriate body contact by a female American employee if she is touched by a Latin-American male. Complaints of sexual harassment could ensue. Eye contact is another important nonverbal communication. Too much eye contact can be perceived as threatening, and a "staring contest" can lead to violence in some cultures. For Americans, too little eye contact during a job interview can make the applicant appear too shy or passive. If a person's eyes are looking all over the room and not at the interviewer, the applicant risks being perceived as "shifty-eyed" or dishonest.

Touch, personal space, and proximity during communication are essential components of interaction in cultures. Different cultures have their own unique styles, rules, and taboos regarding proximity and touch (Hall, 1966). For example, during diversity workshops conducted by the author, many African Americans and Anglo Americans said that proximity of one foot to three feet with another person during work-related conversation is acceptable, but that a further closing of space is deeply frustrating and provokes anxiety. Through discussions, the participants proposed ways to resolve the problem by asking their clients or staff members to sit down or to directly let them know how they feel about personal space. Becoming acquainted with cultural differences in expectations regarding personal space, eye contact, and touching is an important and valuable interpersonal skill for healthcare managers.

A large percentage of the global population's beliefs regarding illness and wellness are not based on germ theory or other principles of allopathic medicine. In fact, terms used to describe the intensity of an illness episode or the symptoms and associated cause and effect of an illness vary from culture to culture, and the cause or reason for an illness may be ascribed to natural as well as supernatural conditions (Murdock, 1980). These variations in language are often observed in healthcare providers who practice in the United States, but were trained or worked in foreign countries.

Communication styles and patterns in a multicultural workplace are therefore widely varied, despite the cultural adaptations between the newly arrived and tenured staff. In a healthcare system, minority managers who lead teams comprised of non-minority employees are inevitably going to face issues related to different language and communication patterns, as well as the implications of hegemony, or the predominance of influence, in the greater culture. Depending on the preparation of the staff in diversity issues, a minority manager may experience either a negative or a positive relationship with his or her team. Several cultural factors influence work-related interactions in groups. One factor is how employees or clients view authority and the line of command in the decision-making process. For example, the author was invited to assist a large urban hospital that was preparing to employ a few hundred nurses from the Philippines. During a workshop discussion with hospital healthcare providers a particular cultural value was highlighted, specifically that Philippino nurses value the importance of group decisions over individual decisions in the group. For example, if asked by their manager or a physician, they will accept or take difficult assignments or work overtime, and will do so without complaint or discussions of their personal preferences.

Likewise, as in many Asian cultures, individuals do not make direct eye contact if conversing with, or receiving instructions from, a person in authority or of greater age or status. This is a common way to show respect and deference for the aged and the experienced (Reynolds & Valentine, 2003). The frequent breaks in eye contact observed in many other cultures are essential in demonstrating respect and non-aggression towards the speaker (Spector, 2004). In contrast, in European and Anglo-American cultures sustained eye contact during a conversation conveys honesty and attentiveness.

While age is revered in many Asian cultures, in the United States there is a tendency to view aging as a degradation of health, awareness, and beauty, a phenomenon referred to as gerontophobia, which can affect interactions between older clients and their physicians, nurses, hospital staff, and family members (Ronch, 2006). This phenomenon is obviously a greater cause of concern in the context of cross-cultural communication.

Standard communication practices also differ between cultures. Communication in a hierarchal culture, as seen in Asian cultures such as the Philippines, Japan, Korea, or India, is also displayed through language. Persons of authority are addressed using formal speech, including titles, and are often greeted by standing. Many Asian, Mediterranean, Latin American, and African cultures are concerned with relationship building in job tasks. In these cultures, building connections is a legitimate and respectable way of conducting business. Asking about family, children, occupation, or hobbies is practiced as an affiliative process before approaching a task.

Secondly, time orientation often becomes a primary cause of frustration and miscommunication between different cultural groups in the workplace, since many management functions have a temporal dimension—schedules and deadlines that apply to daily tasks, meetings, and projects.

Not all cultures describe or experience "time" in the same manner. Some cultures view time as cyclical—sunrise to sundown, or season to season (Leininger & McFarland, 2002; Hall & Hall, 1989). In certain cultures, while work is accomplished and many tasks undertaken, priorities such as relationship building take precedence over "saving time." Measuring performance in terms of efficient, productive output is contrary to the temporal values of such cultures (Spector, 2004).

Cultural competency means that sometimes healthcare managers must make adjustments in their behavior. A manager in a busy urban health clinic near an American Indian reservation allowed his secretary to give a 1-hour leeway on appointments, especially to Native American clients to allow for temporal differences across cultures. This worked effectively, as the secretary was able to accommodate all the clients. In another example, a social worker who regularly worked with refugees and new immigrants from Africa and the West Indies often found that clients would arrive without an appointment to see him, especially as he was leaving his office to attend meetings. Initially, he denied them appointments because of his tight schedule. Shortly afterward, he realized that his behavior had deeply hurt his clients: they took his actions as a personal rejection. He successfully changed his strategy by telling those clients who arrived without an appointment to see him after his scheduled meetings.

As the U.S. demography becomes more pluralized, healthcare organizations are encouraged to increase the number of minority health professionals. Satcher & Pamies (2006) recommend increasing minority students in health professions. All healthcare managers must be cognizant of the impact of social, political, and economic factors that influence relationships in a diverse healthcare workforce. One may expect problems and clashes in values between foreign healthcare providers and those schooled in the United States. Furthermore, language differences can create misunderstandings and misconceptions among team members. Prejudices, cultural stereotypes, and bigotry negatively affect relationships among the staff and client services. Andrews and Boyle (2003) note that prejudices in the workplace, in addition to black-white conflicts, may include those against women, older workers, individuals with disabilities, foreign-born workers, and white workers.

Models for how to provide culturally-sensitive services and care exist. Practitioners include a few trainers and consultants, who offer conflict resolution or conflict mediation models to solve issues related to a multicultural and diverse work environment (Gardenswartz & Rowe, 1998; Kavanagh & Kennedy, 1992; Leininger & McFarland, 2002; and Munoz & Luckmann, 2005). In today's multicultural healthcare workforce, managers need to address all managerial functions through lenses that promote a healthy, multicultural work environment. Focusing this lens begins with preparing the existing staff with diversity training, and recruiting, interviewing, and orienting new staff to the diverse workplace. Campinha-Bacote (2003) emphasizes cultural competency in healthcare services because, "everyone needs a cultural assessment; not just people who look like they need one" (p. 35). Reviewing and revising existing forms of documentation and records are essential to include the multicultural and diverse populations being served in the healthcare system, as well as assuring accurate measurement/benchmarks for the evaluation of employee performance.

Diversity training, while well-intended, can often go awry. Diversity training includes learning new skills that should be provided as a proactive measure rather than a retroactive solution. The author, while exploring efficacy of diversity training, interviewed senior partners and a manager of a large nursing unit in an East Coast metropolitan hospital. She learned that their entire hospital staff received two 4-hour sessions on diversity training. A diversity council at the organization focuses on how diversity is introduced into everyday conversation. The hospital has a large and very diverse workforce; however, nursing as a field overall is still largely composed of Caucasian employees. The hospital website includes multicultural educational information on cultural and religious preference in nutrition and spiritual practices.

When asked if the workshops showed changes among staff in how they relate to differences, slow and gradual changes were noted, especially in the treatment of foreign-born nurses. For example, when a foreign-born nurse started work, the staff initially complained to the manager about the new nurse not taking her 'full and complete' responsibility during work hours. They thought she was not pulling her weight on the team. The staff was asked, in turn, if they had done anything to help the new nurse accept her tasks. In addition, the senior partners and the manager agreed that the best way to promote integration in a diverse workplace (and nursing unit) was to be culturally sensitive role models themselves. One of the senior partners had worked for more than 15 years in the unit and offered suggestions to address diversity issues at work, as well as including how to prepare the staff before a new individual is hired, with special concern for how to communicate with a new staff member who may have an accent or pronounce words differently from the norm. She also suggested that when change is instituted in the unit, a manager needs to be in close communication with the staff. Despite the new aggressive initiatives of healthcare managers, it can take a long while before preset stereotypes, cultural blindness, and prejudices are diminished.

The author conducted diversity training for a healthcare organization of nearly 1000 professionals, managers, bus drivers, janitors, dietary staff, secretaries, and clergy. The organization showed serious commitment to promoting cultural competency. Several sessions were held with the intent to portray diversity training as a two-way street. Just as the administration wanted the staff to attend the session, the administration also had a responsibility to listen to the needs and goals of the staff. During each session, the consultant asked all participants to complete a "Diversity Accountability Questionnaire" (Gardenswartz & Rowe, 1998), a tool that asked participants if their workplace addresses diversity and cultural sensitivity in service, environment, and treatment of staff. In addition to a discussion of the questionnaire, the consultant also asked each participant to brainstorm individual goals or activities that would promote diversity in their respective units. Participant responses were collected and shared with the administration. The participants' overall impressions of the agency were positive. It was also noted that during the exercise several participants doubted that the administration would be interested in their suggestions or that these suggestions actually would be considered and implemented, while others eagerly provided goals for addressing change on their units.

Outside of the hospital or nursing home setting, healthcare management must address the most persistent and difficult health problems in the following communities: namely, the homeless, the poverty-stricken, Medicaid/Medicare recipients, refugees, and immigrants. While the Healthy People 2010 campaign strongly emphasizes reducing health disparities, health problems continue to rise. Vulnerable population groups' categories have increased and include prevalent chronic diseases in children and the aged, addiction in adolescents, and particular health problems in women and minority populations (Sebastian & Bushy, 1999). Healthcare managers can effectively utilize collaborative and integration-oriented models for care services. Aside from the programs instituted by healthcare and small non-governmental organizations and the funded projects located in research-based hospitals or universities, there is little coordination of services for marginalized population groups. Public health education and prevention of illness/disease is the usual modus operandi of most institutions. Therefore, building cultural competency remains an untapped area for further study and strategy building in healthcare management for local, regional, and global communities.

CONCLUSION

Cultural diversity in the management of health care is both a challenge and an imperative given our increasingly multicultural population. Language and cultural differences are faced everyday with the growing diversity of the healthcare workforce, especially in large cities. Such differences affect the recruitment and retention of employees and require ongoing reviews of the institution's policies and practices. In order to establish effective workplace teams, relevant cultural frameworks and models were discussed. One widely used model of managing diversity in the workplace is called the "Four Layers of Diversity" and provides a guideline for understanding cultural dimensions in the workforce. An all encompassing understanding comes from looking beyond just measurement benchmarks and mono-cultural standards and finding models that allow managers to understand human behavior within its cultural context. Cultural knowledge, cultural awareness, and cultural skill-building are critical for multicultural work environments, and cultural competency skills require awareness-building in the organization. Cultural dimensions, such as perceptions of time, space, and relationships, can be built into staff training to improve communication and work relationships among and between employees of an organization.

DISCUSSION QUESTIONS

1. How has the definition of diversity changed over the last decade? How do these changing definitions impact healthcare management and the delivery of healthcare services?

2. How do immigration trends impact the provision of healthcare services? Where might the brunt of these effects be felt in a hospital setting?

3. A nursing home that employs a large number of CNAs from the Caribbean is having a turnover problem. Over 75% of the facility's CNAs left last year and it looks like the same number or more might leave this year. How might the "Four Layers of Diversity" model assist the managers of this organization in addressing their turnover problem?

4. What is organizational culture and how does it impact cultural competency in healthcare organizations?

5. A female American nurse comes to you to complain that a Latin American male physician stands too close to her and keeps touching her inappropriately. She wants to file a sexual harassment complaint. What should you do?

6. Two foreign-educated nurses from the Philippines come to you to complain that their American-educated coworkers are treating them badly. The Americans aren't friendly, don't ask them to join them at meals, and haven't invited them out after work. When you meet with the four American-educated coworkers, they look at each other in astonishment and say, "Those nurses talk to each other all the time in their own language and barely speak to us, except when they have to. What are we supposed to do?" What's going on here and what are your next steps?

REFERENCES

Andrews, M. M., & Boyle, J. S. (2003). *Transcultural concepts in nursing care* (4th ed.). NJ: Prentice Hall.

Campinha-Bacote, J. (2003). *The process of cultural competence in the delivery of healthcare services: A culturally competent model of care.* Cincinnati, OH: Transcultural C.A.R.E. Associates.

Connerley, M. L., & Pederson, P. B. (2005). *Leadership in a diverse and multicultural environment: Developing awareness, knowledge, and skills.* Thousand Oaks, CA: Sage Publications.

Conway-Welch, C., Rasch, F. R., Watkins, L., McNamee, M. J., & Colburn, L. (2006). Diversity management in nursing. In D. Satcher & R. J. Pamies (Eds.). *Multicultural medicine and health disparities* (pp. 427–436). New York: McGraw-Hill Publishers.

Cornelius, W. A., Martin, P. L., & Hollifield, J. F. (1994). *Controlling immigration: A global perspective* (2nd ed.). Stanford, CA: Stanford University Press.

Cox, T. (1994). *Cultural diversity in organizations: Theory, research and practice.* San Francisco: Barrett-Koehler.

Frey, W. H. (2005, April). *Immigration and domestic migration in US metro areas: 2000 and 1990 census findings by education and race* (Report No. 05-572). Ann Arbor, MI: University Of Michigan Population Studies Center, Institute for Social Research.

Gardenswartz, L., & Rowe, A. (1998). *Managing diversity in health care*. San Francisco: Jossey-Bass Publishers.

Gardenswartz, L., Rowe, A., Digh, P., & Bennett, M. F. (2003). *The global diversity desk reference: Managing an international workforce*. San Francisco: Pfeiffer Publishers.

Gardner, H. (1983). *Frames of mind: The theory of multiple intelligences*. New York: Basic Books.

Gardner, H. (1999). *Intelligence reframed: Multiple intelligences for the 21st century*. New York: Basic Books.

Glastra, F. (2004, October). *When Diversity matters: Frames of reference and everyday practice of social workers*. Paper presented at the conference entitled "Professionals: Between People and Policy, Care and Welfare in Europe," Amsterdam/Utrecht.

Goldsmith, S. B. (2005). *Principles of health care management: Compliance, consumerism, and accountability in the 21st century*. Sudbury, MA: Jones and Bartlett Publishers.

Goleman, D. (1998). *Working with emotional intelligence*. New York: Bantam.

Grieco, E. M., & Cassidy, R. C. (2001, March). Overview of race and Hispanic origin: Census 2000 Brief. Retrieved on November 23, 2006 from http://www.census.gov/prod/2001pubs/c2kbr01-1.pdf

Hall, E. T. (1959). *The silent language*. Garden City, NY: Doubleday & Company, Inc.

Hall, E. T. (1966). *The hidden dimension*. Garden City, NY: Doubleday & Company, Inc.

Hall, E. T., & Hall, M. R. (1989). *Understanding cultural differences*. Yarmouth, ME: Intercultural Press.

Hofstede, G. (1980). *Culture's Consequences*. Beverly Hills, CA: Sage Publications.

Hofstede, G. (1991). *Cultures and organizations: Software of the mind*. London: McGraw-Hill Publishers.

Kavanagh K. H., & Kennedy, P. H. (1992). *Promoting cultural diversity: Strategies for health care professionals*. Newbury Park, CA: Sage Publications.

Kluckhohn, F., & Strodtbeck, F. K. (1961). *Variations in value orientation*. Evanston, IL: Row, Peterson & Company.

Kroeber, A., & Kluckhohn, C. (1952). *Culture*. New York: Meridian Books.

Leininger, M., & McFarland, M. R. (2002). *Transcultural nursing: Concepts, theories, research and practice* (3rd ed.). St. Louis, MO: Mosby Publications.

Lewis, R. D. (1996). *When cultures collide: Managing successfully across cultures*. Boston: Nicholas Brealey Publishing.

Lynch, J. P., & Simon, R. J. (2003). *Immigration the world over*. Lanham, MD: Rowman & Littlefield.

Mor-Barak, M. E. (2005). *Managing diversity*. Thousand Oaks, CA: Sage Publications.

Morgan, G. (1997). *Images of organization* (2nd ed.). Thousand Oaks, CA: Sage Publications.

Morrison, B. A., & Donnelly, P. (2002, December). Attracting new Americans into Baltimore's neighborhoods: Immigration is the key to reversing Baltimore population decline. Retrieved November 24, 2006 from The Abell Foundation http://www.abell.org/pubsitems/cd_attracting_new_1202.pdf

Munoz, C., & Luckmann, J. (2005). *Transcultural communication in nursing* (2nd ed.). London: Thomson Learning.

Murdock, G. P. (1980). *Theories of illness: A world survey.* Pittsburgh, PA: University of Pittsburgh Press.

Pamies, R. J., Hill, G. C., Watkins, L., McNamee, M. J., & Colbur, L. (2006). Diversity and the health-care workforce. In D. Satcher and R. J. Pamies (Eds.), *Multicultural medicine and health disparities* (pp. 405–426). New York: McGraw-Hill Publishers.

Pederson, P. B., & Ivey, A. E. (1993). *Culture-centered counseling and interviewing skills: A practical guide.* Westport, CT: Praeger.

Portes, A., & Rumbaut, R. G. (2001). *Legacies: the story of immigrant second generation.* Berkeley, CA: University of California Press.

Reynolds, S., & Valentine, D. (2003). *Guide to cross-cultural communication.* Upper Saddle River, NJ: Prentice Hall.

Ronch, J. L. (2006). Changing institutional culture: Can we revalue the nursing home? *Journal of Gerontological Social Work, 43*(1), 61–82.

Rosenbloom, S. (2006, November 16). In certain circles, two is a crowd. *The New York Times.* Retrieved on November 24, 2006 from http://www.nytimes.com/2006/11/16/fashion/16space.html?ex=1164517200&en=b297909a77c1286c&ei=5070

Sackmann, S. A. (1991). *Cultural knowledge in organizations: Exploring the collective mind.* Newbury Park, CA: Sage Publications.

Satcher, D., & Pamies, R. J. (2006). *Multicultural medicine and health disparities.* New York: McGraw-Hill Publishers.

Schein, E. (2004). *Organizational culture and leadership* (3rd ed.). San Francisco: Jossey Bass Publishers.

Sebastian, J. G., & Bushy, A. (1999). *Special populations in the community: Advances in reducing health problems.* Gaithersburg, MD: Aspen Publications.

Spector, R. E. (2004). *Cultural diversity in health and illness* (6th ed.). Upper Saddle River, NJ: Pearson Prentice Hall.

United States Census Bureau. (2000). Census 2000 Demographic Profile Highlights. Retrieved November 23, 2006 from http://factfinder.census.gov/servlet/ACSSA FFFacts?_event=&geo_id=01000US&_geoContext=01000US&_street=&_county=&_cityTown=&_state=&_zip=&_lang=en&_sse=on&ActiveGeo Div=&_useEV=&pctxt=fph&pgsl=010&_submenuId=factsheet_1&ds_name= DEC_2000_SAFF&_ci_nbr=null&qr_name=null&reg=null%3Anull&_key word=&_industry=

United States Census Bureau. (2004). Census bureau projects tripling of Hispanic and Asian populations in 50 Years; Non-Hispanic Whites may drop to half of

total population. Retrieved November 23, 2006 from http://www.census.gov/
Press-Release/www/releases/archives/population/001720.html

United States Census Bureau. (2005). 2005 American Community Survey Data Profile Highlights. Retrieved November 23, 2006 from http://factfinder.census.gov/
servlet/ACSSAFFFacts?_event=&geo_id=01000US&_geoContext=01000US&
_street=&_county=&_cityTown=&_state=&_zip=&_lang=en&_sse=on&
ActiveGeoDiv=&_useEV=&pctxt=fph&pgsl=010&_submenuId=fact
sheet_1&ds_name=DEC_2000_SAFF&_ci_nbr=null&qr_name=null&reg=null
%3Anull&_keyword=&_industry=

CHAPTER 13

Ethics and Law

Patricia M. Alt

LEARNING OBJECTIVES

By the end of this chapter the student will be able to:

- Describe the distinctions and overlaps between ethics and law;
- Define the concepts of respect for persons, beneficence, nonmaleficence, and justice;
- Define common law, statutes, rules, regulations, and executive orders;
- Distinguish between civil and criminal law;
- List the elements of a contract and describe the relationship to torts;
- Identify the types of torts;
- Define malpractice;
- Provide an overview of patient and provider rights and responsibilities; and,
- Identify some of the legal issues in managed care, biomedical care, and beginning and end-of-life care.

INTRODUCTION

In order to discuss legal and ethical issues in healthcare management, we must first examine what we mean by "ethics" and "law." The two categories overlap, with ethical principles underlying the development of laws, but they approach the world of health care from somewhat differing perspectives. In America, laws are publicly-enforced standards and rules that are created by courts, legislatures, executive orders, and administrative agencies. Each of those bodies has a unique process, creating laws in varying ways.

TABLE 13-1 Overlap of Legal and Ethical Activities

	Is It Legal?		
Is It Ethical?	Yes	Uncertain	No
Yes			
Uncertain			
No			

There are also differences between the authority of federal and state law-making entities. Ethical viewpoints, on the other hand, stem primarily from family, community, and religious traditions. Of course, those creating or challenging laws often operate at least partly from their own ethical beliefs. As we have seen in such cases as that of Terri Schiavo, clashes between and among individuals' deeply-held ethical principles and legal interpretations can cause major disruptions in the healthcare system (Dresser, 2004). This chapter will begin by defining ethics and law as they apply to healthcare, then discuss patient, provider, and organizational rights and responsibilities. Ethical management will be examined, with a particular focus on managed care settings. Finally, we will discuss some biomedical areas of ethical and legal concern, and provide an overview of a few key beginning and end-of-life issues affecting the administration of healthcare services. Table 13-1 illustrates the overlap of perspectives on what is legal and ethical in healthcare settings. There is very little absolute agreement about what actions belong in each cell, but in healthcare, choices must be made on a daily basis.

ETHICAL CONCEPTS

"Ethics" is a term that has been used in many different (sometimes contradictory) ways. We talk of ethical behavior, meaning the ability to tell the difference between right and wrong. But where does one's "sense of right and wrong" come from? At an individual level, ethical perspectives generally come from family upbringing and/or religion. We are also members of communities (ethnic, residential, national) and of professions that have codes, traditions, and practices setting out standards of ethical behavior. At the organizational level, we speak of similar standards, which may vary depending on the type of organization under examination (public/private;

for-profit/non-profit; religiously based/non-sectarian). In all these settings, we must also distinguish between "normative" ethics, which set a standard of what ought to be done, and "descriptive" ethics, illustrating what is actually done.

On the theoretical level, ethics discussions in health care hark back to moral philosophies such as utilitarianism, deontology, natural law, and the hybrid philosophy of John Rawls, among others. As crises in human subject research came to the public's attention in the 20th century, a whole new field of "bioethics" emerged, examining not just the physician-patient relationship, but also areas such as the allocation of scarce resources, genetics, transplantation, and end-of-life care.

In documents including the World Medical Association's 1964 Declaration of Helsinki, and the 1978 report of the National Commission for the Protection of Human Subjects of Biomedical and Behavioral Research, a simplified listing of key ethical principles for healthcare research was created and widely circulated. Callahan and Jennings (2002) (and many others) make a persuasive argument for the application of those same ethical principles to a much wider array of healthcare settings. These central principles are: **respect for persons**, **beneficence**, **nonmaleficence**, and **justice**.

Respect for Persons

A number of key aspects of medical ethics fall under this heading, including **autonomy**, **truth-telling**, **confidentiality**, and **fidelity**. Individuals have the right to make informed decisions about their care, when they are competent to do so, and to have respectful guardianship when they cannot be self-determining. The principle of **truth-telling** indicates that those involved in health care are to be honest with patients/clients as much as possible. **Confidentiality**, which requires keeping information about others involved in the healthcare interaction private, has taken on a heightened meaning with the passage of the 1996 Health Insurance Portability and Accountability Act (HIPAA). **Fidelity**, the fourth element of the respect for persons concept, requires keeping one's word. This includes practitioners' and administrators' responsibility to provide care as promised whether a formal contract exists or not.

Beneficence

Beneficence requires doing the best one can for the recipient of one's services. Stemming from the Hippocratic tradition, it requires a positive duty to care. Beauchamp and Childress (2001), in their groundbreaking bioethics work, divided beneficence into 1) providing benefits and 2) balancing benefits and harms (utility). For a health administrator, this would mean approaching cost-benefit analysis carefully, and always with the requirement of putting the patient's welfare first. Under this standard, practitioners are to use the full array of their skills for all patients, regardless of demographic or cultural factors that might separate them, and (as much as possible) regardless of the ability to pay.

Nonmaleficence

The parallel concept to beneficence, in many ways, is the "do no harm" or at least "don't make it worse" principle behind **nonmaleficence**. Healthcare workers and administrators are admonished to not increase patients' difficulties by their actions (or inactions). Of course, this principle can't always be followed to the letter, as some risks and harms may be inevitable in the attempt to make the situation better. Such trade-offs are acceptable only with patient understanding and consent. Where possible, practitioners and organizations are to minimize risk, and they are to always protect against active, intentional harm to patients.

Justice

As a healthcare principle, **justice** is a bit harder to pin down than the preceding three. It implies fairness, but authors and policymakers have defined "fairness" according to a range of definitions, ranging from exactly equal treatment for all, to having individuals receive the treatment they "deserve." Also included in the policy mix under this heading are issues such as having extra protections for certain classes of patients and/or workers (children, the disabled, racial minorities). Another aspect of justice can be an organization's choices in the allocation of resources among patients, employees, or care settings.

LEGAL CONCEPTS

The law is a body of official rules of conduct, subject to interpretation and change over time. In most cases, federal laws take precedence over state laws, although the U.S. Constitution in the Tenth Amendment does reserve some areas specifically for state decisions, and states can always be more stringent than the federal government. In addition to the U.S. Constitution, each state also has a constitution, setting the basic principles for its legal system. As the judiciary interprets previous precedents for each particular case, they create what is known as **common law**. Legislatures create law by passing **statutes**, which will be able to overrule common law findings for a given jurisdiction unless the judiciary finds the statutes to be unconstitutional. Another way in which laws are created is by administrative agencies, which establish the necessary **rules** and **regulations** to carry out statutes. **Executive orders** are also used on occasion to establish a binding policy, rather than waiting for the legislature or courts to act.

As if the above variants on the law weren't confusing enough, we must also keep in mind the distinction between **civil** and **criminal** laws. **Criminal law** is concerned with wrongs against society as a whole, even if only a particular individual is harmed. There appears to be a growing willingness to use criminal law charges in the healthcare field, including in cases of malpractice, Medicare fraud, abortions, and the unlicensed practice of medicine. **Civil law**, on the other hand, is concerned with wrongs against a particular person or organization. It encompasses **contractual** violations, involving voluntary agreements between two or more parties. **Torts** also fall under civil law, as a category of "wrongful acts" committed against another person without a preexisting contract, for which courts seek to determine and apply remedies.

ELEMENTS OF A CONTRACT

In order for a contract to exist, there must be four key elements: 1) the agreement must be between two or more parties; 2) the parties must both be competent to consent to such an agreement; 3) the agreement must be for something of value; and 4) the agreement must be lawful. If any of these elements are missing, the parties are not bound by their agreement. Even in situations where there is no formal written contract, a "contract" can exist. For instance, if a provider agrees to take on a new patient, they have an implicit contractual agreement that will constrain the provider's ability to refuse to care for that person in the future.

TYPES OF TORTS

Under tort law, there are several key categories of violation that can apply to healthcare organizations. Usually enforced at the state level, these include: 1) **negligence**, which involves the unintentional commission or omission of an act that a reasonably prudent person would or would not do under the same circumstances; 2) **intentional torts**, such as assault and battery, false imprisonment, defamation of character, and invasion of privacy; and 3) the infliction of **mental distress**.

In order for **negligence** to be proven, there must be four key factors involved: 1) the negligent party must have a **duty** toward the harmed party. In health care, this includes the practitioner exercising the level of skill expected in routine practice while treating a person with whom he/she has a patient-provider relationship; 2) there must have been a **breach of duty**, by failing to meet the appropriate standard of care; 3) the plaintiff must prove that he or she suffered **injury** or **damages** from the interaction; and 4) **causation** must be proved. In other words, the breach of duty has to have been directly connected to the harm that occurred. Negligence charges are usually brought against the practitioner involved, but they can also be brought against an organization under the doctrine of *respondeat superior* (meaning that organizations can be liable for harm caused by their employees or agents). There are various types of negligent acts: misfeasance, or performing the correct action incorrectly and causing injury; malfeasance, or performing an unlawful act (such as abortion in states where it is illegal); and nonfeasance, or failing to act where there is a duty that a reasonably prudent person would have fulfilled (perhaps failing to test for an obvious cause of a person's symptoms).

Intentional tort cases depend on proving that the harm was committed deliberately. In **assault and battery** cases, for example, there must be a deliberate threat on one person by another for **assault** to apply, and actual physical contact for the situation to be considered **battery**. One example in the healthcare field would be surgery mistakenly performed on an unconscious patient without his/her consent. **False imprisonment** is another form of intentional tort. This could include inappropriately restraining a patient, or keeping someone in a more restrictive level of care than necessary. **Defamation of character** can be slander or libel—oral or written false representations of a person's character that will hold that person up to shame or ridicule. Another important aspect of intentional torts in healthcare settings is **invasion of privacy**, which violates the right to privacy implicit in the Constitution. Confidentiality of patient records constitutes a major concern under this heading, as does the need to evaluate when a "need to know" overrides privacy, as in the legal requirement to report child or elder abuse, sexually transmitted diseases, or other public health concerns.

MALPRACTICE

Malpractice, or the negligence or carelessness of a professional person, can be either a civil concern or a criminal one, depending on whether it involved "reckless disregard" for the safety of another (criminal) or simple carelessness (civil). The legal dictionary definition includes: "negligence, misconduct, lack of ordinary skill, or a breach of duty in the performance of a professional service (as in medicine) resulting in injury or loss" (Merriam-Webster, 1996). For a healthcare administrator, this is a central concern in hiring, training, and monitoring the performance of employees and those with admitting privileges, both in order to protect the patients from harm and out of concern for the reputation and financial stability of the organization itself.

PATIENT AND PROVIDER RIGHTS AND RESPONSIBILITIES

Both the healthcare provider and the patient have rights and responsibilities in a host of different areas relating to the provision of care, compliance, respect, and numerous other areas, as discussed further below.

Responsibilities

Of course, one key provider responsibility is to avoid harming patients and to use one's skills to (ideally) better their situation. This has both legal and ethical underpinnings and is directly connected to concerns about malpractice. The legal notion of "duty" is critical, as it flows both from the provider's training and professional oath and from the existence of a relationship (contractual or implied) with the patient. In the case of people seeking emergency care, for instance, the federal **Emergency Medical Treatment and Active Labor Act (EMTALA)** of 1985 requires that hospitals participating in Medicare must provide screening examinations and treatment in their emergency departments unless they can prove that a patient requested a transfer (having been fully informed about EMTALA) and/or that the hospital cannot provide the necessary care for the patient's condition.

Another critical responsibility of the healthcare organization itself is its fiduciary duty to the patient. **Fiduciary duty** means that people or organizations have an obligation to those who have placed their trust in them. The healthcare organization, its board of trustees, and its staff are in a position of relative power with the patients. This entails fiduciary duties to protect the organization's assets, abide by its articles of incorporation, and refrain from personal gain at the organization's or patients' expense.

Along with fiduciary duty to their patients, healthcare organizations have an obligation to balance the responsibility to meet the need for their services against the urge to create unnecessary demand for them. Marketing can be a particularly sticky ethical area for any organization or practitioner. How far is it acceptable to go in convincing potential patients that they "need" your services? When does providing public information cross over into creating demand in order to increase your own income? And is it ethical to attract or keep patients in your institution or professional practice when they might be served better elsewhere?

In addition to their responsibilities to patients, healthcare organizations have the responsibility to ensure that all employees and attending staff are treated fairly and with dignity. Providers are to be protected from sexual or other harassment, and have been generally allowed to excuse themselves from patient care with which they disagree, although this is an area under litigation and pressure for legislative change (Stein, 2006).

Individual medical providers are obliged to abide by the requirements of their licenses, living up to the standards of their professions. This includes protecting patient information, providing the best quality of care, serving as advocates for their patients within the healthcare organization, keeping their own training up to date, and reporting any unethical behavior by their co-workers. For their part, patients have the responsibility to ask questions of their care providers, to provide accurate information to them (including insurance information), and to attempt to follow the directions and prescriptions given for their care.

Rights

In America, legal and ethical standards support the notion of patient self-determination as a central aspect of health care. Closely linked to this concept is the requirement for confidentiality of patient information. The federal **Health Insurance Portability and Accountability Act (HIPAA)** of 1996 is one effort to protect patient information in the modern hospital. According to the U.S. Department of Health and Human Services (DHHS, 2003), a portion of the HIPAA was designed to protect patient privacy and confidentiality in secure environments, particularly through electronic transactions. The regulations protect medical records and other individually identifiable health information, whether on paper or in electronic or oral communications. Key provisions of these new standards include rules and regulations regarding: access to medical records; notice of privacy practices; limits on the use of personal and medical information; prohibitions on marketing; stronger state laws; confidential communications; and provisions for patient complaints in case they feel their rights have been violated.

Long before HIPAA, however, there was an acknowledged legal right of patients to make informed decisions about their own care. If a patient is not mentally competent to make such decisions, he/she is entitled to a **surrogate decision maker**, usually a family member or a close friend. Whether it is the patient or the surrogate making a decision, the key element here is "informed consent." Consent cannot be considered valid if the person giving it did not fully understand the situation, including the potential benefits and risks involved. Adult patients (or their surrogates) also have an absolute right to refuse care, even if medical practitioners disagree.

LEGAL/ETHICAL CONCERNS IN MANAGED CARE

By definition, "managed" care imposes limits on patient and provider choices. When it was originally developed, the goal was to avoid "unnecessary" care, and to encourage the use of preventive care as much as possible. However, the more recent concerns are that care is being "rationed," that doctors' hands are tied, and/or that managed care disproportionately harms those dependent on public funding for their care (hence unable to pay higher premiums to ensure a wider range of choices). As most employers have moved to requiring some version of managed care for their employees, the last concern (of unfair treatment of recipients of medical assistance) has waned somewhat. But the issues of rationing and physicians' divided loyalties remain.

In order to be able to treat patients in a managed care plan, the physician must be found acceptable to the plan because of his/her treatment record and charges. Once in the plan, a physician is constantly pressured to use only approved medications, treatments, and referrals in order to save money and to maintain him- or herself in the plan's good graces. Such cases as *Wickline v. California* (1986) established that physicians are obliged to act as advocates for their patients and resist inappropriate care determinations made by managed care organizations. Other cases have reiterated the point that both the physician and the managed care organization are legally liable for harm caused to the patient by inadequate care due to cost-containment. Managed care organizations are also obliged to hire and retain competent physicians, and to ensure that they remain qualified to practice (Perry, 2002).

One approach to improving patient choice in managed care settings that has been tried in many states ever since the 1980s is the use of "**Any Willing Provider**" **(AWP)** laws. These laws "require managed care plans using provider networks to permit all providers to participate in the network if they agree to accept the plan's contract terms, such as payment rates, quality monitoring, and other conditions" (Butler, 2003). As of 2003, two thirds of these laws apply only to pharmacies. AWP laws have been strenuously opposed by managed care organizations as limiting their ability to control costs and to restrict their networks to the "best" providers (Butler).

The federal law which is most frequently cited in the struggles over state laws regulating managed care is **ERISA, the Employee Retirement and Income Security Act of 1974**. ERISA was created to protect employees' pensions and benefits by asserting the preeminence of federal law over state regulation of pensions and other private sector employee benefit plans. It aimed to provide a national standard for benefit plans and to provide a federal remedy for employees denied their pensions, health insurance, or other benefits. However, it only applies to private-sector, employer-sponsored plans. While it contains a clause guaranteeing that states can retain their power to regulate "insurance providers," it still leaves states unable to regulate "self insured" entities, and managed care organizations can exist under either label. Healthcare organizations are in the somewhat unique situation of choosing which managed care plans to belong to as providers, as well as choosing which to offer to employees in their own health benefits packages. This can bring home rather bluntly the cost-benefit decisions involved.

BIOMEDICAL CONCERNS

While healthcare managers do not have to personally make life and death medical decisions, the organization's policies can strongly influence what happens under its supervision. In briefly examining several key issues in the field, this chapter provides a backdrop for further exploration. One area of ongoing concern is the question of resource allocation implicit in most healthcare decisions, and explicit in managed care settings. As long as equal access to particular levels of care and/or treatments is not available, this will continue to occur. How do we decide which patient will receive an organ transplant? Can we be positive that a particular combination of genetics, age, demographics, and lifestyle factors will enable one person to have a longer and more productive life than another? Should we be influenced by the available level of family support, or by the family's need to be involved in a relative's care? How can a healthcare organization best reflect the ethical preferences of its community, while abiding by the law? And should the ability to have care reimbursed affect the decision to provide it?

Another overarching issue is that of consent. As mentioned above, informed consent is a keystone of medical practice, requiring the practitioner to provide the patient with sufficient information to participate in decisions about his/her care. With laws such as the Americans with Disabilities Act, this responsibility has been expanded to require providing information that is understandable to the patient or, if the patient is not able to decide, to a surrogate decision maker. Particularly in highly emotional settings, such as beginning and end-of-life care decisions, this process needs to occur. Most hospitals have patient advocate offices for the specific purpose of having staff dedicated to walking through difficult decisions with patients and their families. Three areas of particular concern along these lines are those involving **beginning-of-life care, end-of-life care**, and **human subject research** within medical settings.

BEGINNING- AND END-OF-LIFE CARE

As medical science has advanced, the variety and complexity of decisions to be made has also expanded. Two places where this is particularly apparent are in beginning- and end-of-life care. When *Roe v. Wade* was decided in 1966, morning-after pills and various forms of non-surgical abortions weren't available. *In vitro* fertilization didn't exist, and medical science wasn't able to keep infants alive when they were born many months early. Provision and funding of contraception, provision and funding of abortion, and balancing parental, societal, and practitioner rights and responsibilities are all issues to be discussed in the context of an organization's mission, vision, and values.

Likewise, end-of-life care has become more complicated than in previous eras. Healthcare organizations now must pay close attention to obtaining advance directives and surrogate decision-makers, providing ethical care in the absence of clear directives, making crucial decisions about life-sustaining treatment, and balancing familial, societal, and practitioner rights and responsibilities.

Similarly, the *Cruzan* or *Quinlan* cases would have been much more complicated with today's increased array of end-of-life technologies. And we now face divergence between state and federal law about physician-assisted suicides. Of course, not every healthcare organization has the desire or the facilities to provide complicated care. In addition, the particular organization's mission and values will shape what it is willing to provide. Aside from the requirements of the Emergency Medical Treatment and Active Labor Act for those hospitals with emergency facilities and/or obstetrics departments, facilities are free to decide and publicize the types of care that their (often religious) standards will or will not allow them to provide.

RESEARCH IN HEALTHCARE SETTINGS

Privately sponsored medical research in smaller organizations has led to concern about appropriate human subjects oversight in those settings. **Institutional Review Boards (IRBs)**, committees to review human subject research proposals, are spreading beyond academic medical centers to provide protection for patients' rights in clinical research. Institutional Ethics Committees in most hospitals oversee a range of issues, and there are now Patient Advocate/Ombudsman Offices to speak for patients and families who may be unable to speak for themselves. In addition, each clinical profession has a code of ethics, as does the American College of Healthcare Executives Code of Ethics for administrators.

CONCLUSION

Health care is one of the most regulated industries in the nation. Laws have been put in place to protect patients based on ethical concerns and precedents. Every time an organization provides healthcare services, the potential for legal violations of patient's rights should loom large in the healthcare manager's consciousness. This chapter has provided you with the vocabulary and some context for addressing legal issues in healthcare organizations. Since these laws can change and the cases vary, it is incumbent upon the healthcare manager to stay abreast of developments in healthcare ethics and law.

DISCUSSION QUESTIONS

1. What distinguishes ethics from law? Are the ethics of all healthcare organizations the same? Why or why not?

2. Define and give an example of each of the following principles: respect for persons, beneficence, nonmaleficence, and justice.

3. What is the difference between civil law and criminal law? Do any cases ever constitute both? Give examples.

4. A physician went out of town for the weekend, leaving no one to cover for him while he was away. One of his hospitalized patients had a broken leg in a cast, and kept complaining that the cast was hurting him. The nurses attempted to reach the physician, to no avail. The odor in the patient's room became so overwhelming that nurses noted it on his chart and put air fresheners in his room. By the time the physician returned from his trip, the patient's leg was dead and had to be amputated. Who was liable in this case, the physician, the hospital, or both?

5. A woman arrives at a suburban emergency room in the early stages of labor. Both she and her husband speak little English, and the admitting clerk cannot obtain insurance information. The staff assume the mother (and child) are uninsured and unable to pay for healthcare services out-of-pocket. How soon can the hospital transfer the patient to another hospital?

6. An HMO appointment scheduler tells a 55 year-old, post-menopausal woman who has vaginal bleeding that the soonest she can be seen is in 6 months. The woman waits to see her physician at the HMO, and is told, after laboratory tests, that she has invasive endometrial cancer. The woman decides to sue the HMO for delay of care. Is the HMO liable?

REFERENCES

Beauchamp, T. L., & Childress, J. F. (2001). *Principles of biomedical ethics I* (5th ed.). New York: Oxford University Press.

Butler, P. (2003). Kentucky's 'Any Willing Provider' Law and ERISA: Implications of the Supreme Court's Decision for State Health Insurance Regulation. Washington, DC: National Academy for State Health Policy.

Callahan, D., & Jennings, B. (2002). Ethics and public health: Forging a strong relationship. *American Journal of Public Health, 92*(2), 169–176.

DHHS. (2003). Fact sheet: Protecting the privacy of patient's health information. Retrieved June 12, 2006 from http://www.hhs.gov/news/facts/privacy.html

Dresser, R. (2004). Schiavo: A hard case makes questionable law. *Hastings Center Report, 34*(2), 8–9.

Merriam-Webster's Dictionary of Law. (1996). Springfield, MA: Merriam-Webster, Inc.

Perry, F. (2002). *The tracks we leave: Ethics in healthcare management.* Chicago: Health Administration Press.

Stein, R. (2006, January 30). Health workers' choice debated: Proposals back right not to treat. *Washington Post*, A01.

Wickline v. California. (1986). 192 Cal App 3d 1630, 1636.

CHAPTER 14

Fraud and Abuse

Maron J. Boohaker

LEARNING OBJECTIVES

By the end of this chapter the student will be able to:

- Explain the difference between fraud and abuse;
- List examples of fraud and abuse and compare the extent of occurrences;
- Discuss the types of civil and criminal penalties incurred for violating rules and regulations;
- Describe the history of the False Claims Act and its application to health care;
- Discuss the managerial and organizational implications of the Emergency Medical Treatment and Active Labor Act (EMTALA);
- Explain the major objectives of the U.S. antitrust laws related to the healthcare industry;
- Describe the major provisions of the Stark I and Stark II laws and safe harbor regulations;
- List the major components of compliance, risk management, and internal control programs;
- Discuss *qui tam* and the whistle blower role; and,
- Explain the desirable role of a healthcare manager in fraud and abuse cases.

INTRODUCTION

Fraud and abuse have always been a concern to the federal government with regard to Medicare, Medicaid, and other federally-funded healthcare programs. Many remedies have been implemented through the years. In 1995, Operation Restore Trust (ORT) was put in motion by the United States Congress to give the Department of Health and Human Services (HHS) the investigative and enforcement authority necessary to deal with fraud and abuse violations. With ORT in motion, the delivery of healthcare in the United States has dramatically and definitively changed for the provider, the beneficiary and the payor of federally-funded healthcare benefits. Whether these measures were taken for political, fiscal, or quality of care reasons, the landscape has changed. The HHS Office of Inspector General (OIG) reported more than $20 billion in overpayments to healthcare providers in fiscal year 1997. This represents 11% of Medicare payments for that year (AMA OIG, 1998).

This chapter will focus on the beginnings of the fraud and abuse prevention programs that started with the decentralized home health agencies (HHA) and have broadened to include various types of compliance programs. The chapter will also look at the investigative processes used to uncover fraud and abuse, the enforcement role of governmental programs, and the responsibilities of employees of healthcare organizations.

For the federal government, ORT is a proven success. Billions of dollars have been restored to the program as a result of civil settlements, fines, or judgments related to healthcare fraud. Hundreds of defendants have been convicted of fraud, and thousands are now excluded parties from federal healthcare programs for those convictions.

WHAT IS FRAUD AND ABUSE?

Fraud is an intentional act of deception, while **abuse** consists of improper acts that are unintentional but inconsistent with standard practices. The more common forms of fraud and abuse are providers billing for services that were not provided or did not meet medical necessity criteria (false claims), for duplicate billing, for **upcoding** services to receive higher reimbursement, and for **kickbacks** for referrals.

HISTORY

The history of **compliance** as it relates to healthcare fraud and abuse dates back to the Civil War. The False Claims Act (FCA) was enacted in 1863 by the federal government as the primary civil remedy for fraudulent or improper health care claims. In 1986, the first major amendments were added to the FCA. These changes removed the clause requiring that there be specific intent to defraud the federal government and that the government need only show that the claim submitted is false and submitted knowingly. Violations of this act include fines of $5,500.00 to $11,000.00 per claim, plus up to 3 times the amount of the damages caused to the federal program (31 USC, 1986b). The Act's *qui tam* **provision** permits private individuals to file false claims actions on behalf of the federal government and receive 15% to 30% of any recovery (31 USC, 1986c). A *qui tam* (Latin for "who as well") is used to indicate that the plaintiff is bringing the action on behalf of the government "as well" as for himself. This individual is also known as a "**whistle blower**" or a "**relator.**"

While the number of civil healthcare fraud cases rose dramatically in the 1990s, the increase in the number of cases has stabilized since then, but the dollars recovered in suits and investigations has increased. In the fiscal year ending September 30, 2003, $1.7 billion was recovered through violations of the False Claims Act as it relates to healthcare fraud. This represents 81% of the total $2.1 billion recovered for the year as reported by the Department of Justice (DOJ) for fraud-related claims. Each U.S. Attorney now oversees healthcare fraud cases with a coordinator who works with the DOJ, the HHS OIG, the Federal Bureau of Investigation (FBI), state Medicaid fraud units, and other federal agencies.

OPERATION RESTORE TRUST

Operation Restore Trust (ORT) started in 1995 to counter charges about healthcare fraud and abuse. Initially, the program involved the five states with the heaviest volume of Medicare beneficiaries. The first services investigated were those provided outside of normal treatment facilities (e.g., hospices, home health agencies, etc.). These investigations led to recovery of $190 million from fraudulent healthcare activities. In 1997, the program was expanded to include 12 more states.

Operation Restore Trust now includes all 50 states and more healthcare delivery systems are covered. The program not only investigates and applies penalties for fraud, but also provides advisories to prevent violations. They use statistical data to select claims for audits and investigations. HHS has organized state and federal agencies to monitor activities under ORT. These activities include:

- Issuing of special fraud alerts to notify the healthcare community and the public about fraudulent activities by healthcare providers;
- Conducting studies and developing recommendations by the OIG and the Center for Medicare and Medicaid Services (CMS) for new programs and alterations to current programs to prevent fraud and reduce waste and abuse,
- Conducting surveys and inspections of long-term care facilities by CMS and state officials in search of fraudulent activities;
- Applying civil and administrative sanctions and recovery actions by the OIG and other law enforcement agencies;
- Conducting criminal investigations and making referrals by the OIG to the appropriate law enforcement agencies; and,
- Conducting financial audits by the OIG and CMS.

THE SOCIAL SECURITY ACT AND THE CRIMINAL-DISCLOSURE PROVISION

The Criminal-Disclosure Provision of the Social Security Act makes it a felony for a healthcare provider or beneficiary to possess "knowledge of the occurrence of any event affecting his initial or continued right to any such benefit or payment, or the initial or continued right to any such benefit or payment of any other individual in whose behalf he has applied for or is receiving such benefit or payment," to "conceal . . . or fail . . . to disclose such event with an intent fraudulently to secure such benefit or payment either in a greater amount or quantity than is due or when no such benefit or payment is authorized." Violation of this provision is a felony and may include punishment of up to 5 years in prison and/or fines of up to $25,000 (42 USC, 1987a).

This provision of the Social Security Act (SSA) also imposes a requirement to disclose overpayments to the government regardless of intent at the time the claim was submitted. By obligating this disclosure, the government may start collection efforts. If the provider acts in good faith to reimburse the program, it may limit its liability under the False Claims Act (FCA). It does not however, loosen any criminal liability under this provision.

Of particular importance to the OIG is the violation of the Criminal-Disclosure Provision involving the **Stark I and II Laws**. The Stark Laws were developed to prohibit physicians from referring their patients to providers in which they have a financial interest. Stark I was created to prevent physician referrals to laboratory services they benefit from monetarily. Stark II was adopted to limit physicians from referring patients to other ancillary providers in which they have a financial interest. The laws expressly state that a provider is not entitled to Medicare payments for services or items rendered in violation of Stark I and II restrictions on self-referral, regardless of intent. If a physician discovers after the fact that he has violated this law and knows he has received payment from Medicare, he has violated Stark laws and is subject to potential criminal liability if the error is not disclosed.

Examples of violations of the Stark Laws include paying a physician for a referral and a hospital offering rental space to a physician below fair market value. Physicians who receive benefits not given to other doctors or staff may be considered in violations of the rule, too.

At least two indictments are pending trial related to the Criminal-Disclosure Provision. These include several defendants who were charged with conspiracy to knowingly misstate certain interest expenses on providers' cost reports filed with the government. Documents show that the conspiracy involves the defendants knowingly failing to notify the government of the fiscal intermediary's audit error concerning interest expense. The defendants were convicted on the conspiracy count, but no separate finding was made on the failure-to-disclose allegation (42 USC, 1987b).

Another case involves three individuals in California who were charged with conspiracy to defraud the U.S. government in connection with a scheme to submit fraudulent medical necessity certification for certain medical equipment. These indictments are important to all directors and officers of for-profit healthcare providers because they show the government's intent to prosecute individuals under this dormant statute established for alleged non-disclosures made by a corporation. The combination of the Criminal-Disclosure Provision under the Social Security Act with the False Claims Act allows prosecutors to impose personal, criminal responsibility on officers and board members of for-profit providers who know, but fail to disclose to the government, that the provider is not entitled to those received Medicare payments.

THE EMERGENCY MEDICAL TREATMENT AND ACTIVE LABOR ACT

The Emergency Medical Treatment and Active Labor Act (EMTALA) was enacted in 1986 to prevent **patient dumping**. It is also known as the Anti-Dumping Act. It was used to prevent an emergency room from refusing treatment or transferring a patient to another facility because of inability to pay for treatment. The Act mandates that an appropriate **Medical Screening Exam (MSE)** be given to any patient who presents to any department that is established as a provider of emergent or urgent care. If a MSE is performed and shows an emergency condition exists, the patient must be 1) treated and discharged, or 2) admitted as an inpatient and transferred from the dedicated emergency department. The EMTALA obligations cease at this point. Also, in 2000, HHS enacted the "250 Yard Rule." This expanded the EMTALA rule to include any patient emergency that occurs within a 250-yard radius of a hospital that has an emergency room. In 2003, the Rule was adjusted to be less restrictive. Initially, this rule was applied to the radius around any healthcare provider site (hospital or clinic). In 2003, this rule was changed to apply only to healthcare providers that have an ER inside this 250-yard radius. This was to clarify that they were referring to true medical emergencies on thoroughfares around Emergency Rooms.

EMTALA also restricts the Emergency Room staff from discussing financial or insurance information until after the MSE has been performed and the emergent condition has been stabilized. As long as the treatment is not delayed, hospitals may continue the registration process.

The CMS has the authority to enforce EMTALA and can impose financial penalties on providers who do not comply. In addition, the OIG has separate authority to impose sanctions for EMTALA violations. Violators may incur monetary penalties of up to $50,000 per violation and have their Medicare program participation terminated. The final EMTALA rule became effective on November 10, 2003.

HOSPITAL COMPLIANCE WITH EMTALA

To avoid EMTALA violations, providers should:

- Require all clinical, administrative, and contact staff to review and understand the EMTALA requirements and to document this training;
- Ensure that all patients that have an emergent admission and either refuse or withdraw treatment, are offered a Medical Screening Exam and treatment before they leave the hospital. This refusal to accept treatment should be documented (informed consent);
- Ensure that the ER staff understands all statutory rules regarding transfer of patients to another facility; and,
- Enforce the requirement that prevents staff from asking for financial and accounting information before the Medical Screening Exam has been completed and the patient is stabilized.

THE BALANCED BUDGET ACT OF 1997

The Balanced Budget Act (BBA) added more enforcement tools for federal authorities. Through the following enforcement tools, the BBA:

- Mandates the permanent exclusion from federal healthcare programs of individuals convicted of three offenses constituting grounds for exclusion;
- Authorizes the Secretary of HHS to refuse to contract with a Medicare provider convicted of a single felony that the Secretary deems detrimental to the best interests of the Medicare program or its beneficiaries;
- Requires every explanation of benefits (EOB) form provided to Medicare beneficiaries to reflect a toll-free number for reporting of fraud, abuse, and waste in the Medicare program;
- Authorizes the exclusion of entities controlled by family members and members of the same household of sanctioned individuals;
- Creates new civil monetary penalties for contracting with individuals that the person knows or should know is excluded from participating in federal healthcare program;
- Requires **durable medical equipment** (DME) suppliers to disclose to HHS persons with an ownership or controlling interest in the supplier or in any subcontractor in which the supplier has a 5% or

greater interest, and to provide HHS with a surety bond of at least $50,000;

■ Requires diagnostic information when ordering diagnostic x-rays, DME, and certain prosthetic devices;

■ Replaces the reasonable charge method with fee schedules for items such as medical supplies, home dialysis supplies and equipment, and parenteral and enteral nutrients, equipment and supplies; and,

■ Requires a hospital's discharge plan to identify any referred provider to whom and in which the hospital has a financial interest or which has a financial interest in the hospital (Nahra, 1997).

ANTITRUST ISSUES

Antitrust laws were implemented to protect the citizenry from the negative effects of monopolies. Three Acts form the basis of antitrust law.

■ **The Sherman Antitrust Act**—Section 1 prohibits all conspiracies or agreements that restrain trade.

■ **The Clayton Act**—Section 7 of the Act prohibits mergers and acquisitions that may substantially lessen competition "in any line of commerce . . . in any section of the country." This was enacted in 1914.

■ **The Federal Trade Commission Act**—Section 5 of the Act prohibits various types of unfair competition.

The Department of Justice (DOJ) and the Federal Trade Commission (FTC) revised the Statements of Antitrust Enforcement Policy in Health Care in 1996. The revision was intended to ensure that policies did not interfere with activities that reduce health care costs.

FEDERAL ENFORCEMENT ACTIONS

In order to prevent violations of the Antitrust Act, Congress passed the Hart-Scott-Rodino Antitrust Improvements Act of 1976. This required hospitals, and all other parties who are entered into certain mergers, acquisitions, joint ventures, or tender offers to notify the DOJ and FTC before finalizing all agreements. This is a requirement for hospitals with assets greater than $100 million acquiring a hospital with more than $10 million in assets. The DOJ and FTC then decide if the transaction should be approved.

SAFE HARBOR/ANTI-KICKBACK REGULATIONS

There are two laws that have been enacted to prevent conflicts of interest in Medicare patient referrals. One is the **Stark II Law**, which prohibits physicians from referring patients to providers with which the physician has a financial relationship. This law is an extension of the **Stark I Law**, which only applies to physicians referring to laboratories in which they have a financial interest. These laws are also known as the Physician Self-Referral Law. The other law is the Anti-Kickback Act (42 USC, 1987a) that is designed to prevent the offer or payment of bribes or other remuneration as an inducement to refer Medicare patients for treatment or services. These rules, especially the Anti-Kickback statute, were so stringent that many providers were being wrongly accused of conduct that was not inherently illegal, leading Congress to ask CMS to develop and enforce safe harbor provisions.

Under Stark II, if a physician or immediate family member has a specified financial relationship with an entity, the physician may not refer Medicare or Medicaid patients to that entity to receive health services. Thus, the provision may be implicated when a referring physician has an ownership or investment interest, or when a physician or immediate family member receives compensation or other remuneration from the entity providing healthcare services.

Additionally, the recipient of the referral may not present a claim for any designated health services provided due to this referral. Any person who presents or causes presentation of a bill or claim for services "that the person knows or should know" is covered by the prohibition is subject to: (1) payment of a civil monetary penalty of up to $15,000 per service, (2) refunding of all monies improperly paid, (3) payment of treble (triple) damages, and (4) exclusion from participation in the Medicare and Medicaid programs.

ANTI-KICKBACK STATUTES

This is the law of choice for federal enforcement authorities. This Act imposes criminal liability for the knowing and willful payment, solicitation, or receipt of remuneration (remuneration is any kickback, bribe, or rebate, direct or indirect, overt or covert, in cash or in kind, and any ownership interest or compensation interest) in return for referring an individual to a person for, or in return for purchasing, leasing, ordering, arranging for, or recommending the purchase, lease, or order of items or services reimbursable by the federal healthcare program. This Act affects a vast array of healthcare industry business relationships.

Because this Act is so broad and vague in many instances, the HHS OIG, at the direction of Congress has issued narrow regulatory "safe harbors" that the OIG deems harmless and as such, "shall not be treated as criminal offense . . . and shall not be used as a basis for exclusion" from the federal healthcare programs (42 USC, 1987a). Activities outside of these safe harbors are not necessarily illegal, but it is often unclear at what point conduct crosses the line between a legitimate practice and a violation of the Anti-Kickback Act.

The Anti-Kickback Act, formerly known as the "Medicare and Medicaid Anti-Kickback Act," has broadened the original Act's reach to encompass all federal healthcare programs, excluding the Federal Employees Health Benefits Program, which is the healthcare program for federal employees. This was done in 1996 with the passage of the Health Insurance Portability and Accountability Act (HIPAA). In addition, the Balanced Budget Act of 1997 imposes civil monetary penalties of $50,000 for each violation of the Anti-Kickback Act and damages of up to 3 times the total amount of remuneration offered, paid, solicited, or received in violation of the Act (HR 2015, 1997).

Federal enforcement authorities continuously review application of the Act. They are currently reviewing doctors and drug samples, incentives for therapeutic switches, and provision of free goods or value-added services to nursing homes. OIG staffers have stressed that the most important aspect of the Anti-Kickback Act violation is the intent to induce referrals and that no safe harbor exists for conduct that may also benefit patients because enforcement authorities do not believe that such services are provided with only patients' interests in mind. At the American Society of Consultant Pharmacists Annual Convention in 1997, Assistant U.S. Attorney James Sheehan stated that, in the absence of a bright line test, federal prosecutors are applying a "smell" test to determine whether the provision of a free item or service rises to the level of the kickback (1997). In contrast to the Anti-Kickback Act, Stark I and II describe prohibited conduct explicitly. Unlike the Anti-Kickback Act, Stark I and II are strict liability statutes that do not require proof of intent, nor do they have regulatory safe harbors that give rise to gray areas.

SAFE HARBOR LAWS

Safe harbor regulations were put in place in 1987 by HHS after a Congressional mandate. Initially, 11 safe harbor provisions were implemented in 1991. These gave guidelines that, when complied with in full, would ensure compliance with this very vague statute. In 1993, the OIG proposed to include within the list of safe harbor provisions, payments made to surgeon-investors in **Ambulatory Surgery Centers (ASCs)**, provided that the facility was wholly owned by the referring surgeons and that these surgeons performed the surgery themselves on patients they had referred to the ASC. This safe harbor could be justified because the ASC facility was an extension of the referring surgeon's practice and of little risk for fraud and abuse.

On November 19, 1999, the HHS OIG published a final rule, which established 8 new safe harbors and clarified 6 of the original 11 that went into effect in 1991. With these additions and adjustments, there are now 23 safe harbors to immunize providers from criminal liability under the Anti-Kickback statute. The new ASC safe harbor contains four categories:

- Surgeon-owned ASCs,
- Single specialty ASCs,
- Multi-specialty ASCs,
- Hospital/physician-owned ASCs.

All of these new safe harbors have the following five requirements in common:

- The ASC must be certified under 42 CFR Pt. 416;
- Loans from the entity or other investors to physician investors are prohibited;
- Investment interests must be offered on terms not related to the volume or value of referrals;
- All ancillary services must be directly and integrally related to primary procedures performed at the ASC and none may be separately billed to Medicare or other federal healthcare programs; and,

■ Neither the ASC nor physicians practicing at the ASC can discriminate against federal healthcare program beneficiaries.

Both surgeon-owned and single-specialty ASC safe harbors, which differ only by types of physicians who may hold ownership interest in the ASC, impose an additional requirement that examines each investor's income from the ASC. Under this rule, one third of each physician-investor's medical practice income for the previous year must be derived from the physician's performance of surgical procedures at an ASC or hospital surgical setting. According to the OIG, this will ensure that a physician's investment in an ASC actually represents an extension of the physician's office.

The multi-specialty ASC safe harbor is identical to surgeon-owned and single specialty ASC safe harbors, but requires that at least one third of the physician's surgical procedures are performed at the ASC in which they are investing. Like the practice income test applicable to surgeon-owned and single specialty ASCs, this requirement is intended to prohibit passive investment among physicians in different specialties. This situation, according to the OIG, creates the greatest risk of prohibited payments or other remuneration for referrals.

The hospital/physician ASC is somewhat different from the above-described safe harbors. This safe harbor requires the same five criteria, but does not require the examination of practice income arising from the facility. Instead, the safe harbor imposes three stringent requirements on the hospital investor that may well keep all hospital/physician ASCs outside the scope of the safe harbor.

The most important feature of the new ASC safe harbor, may very well be the OIG's decision to do away with a requirement of 100% physician ownership. Under the final safe harbor, individuals who are neither an existing nor potential source of referrals are permitted to invest in the facility.

Also significant in the new safe harbors is the OIG's decision not to expand the scope of the safe harbor to include facilities that are not traditionally considered "surgical" facilities, such as lithotripsy centers, end-stage renal disease facilities, comprehensive outpatient rehabilitation facilities, radiation oncology facilities, cardiac catheterization centers, and optical dispensing facilities, despite support for inclusion.

STACKED PENALTIES

The government has successfully prosecuted cases under the FCA by contending that either the Stark laws or Anti-Kickback Statute violation constitutes making a false statement. These cases have primarily been ones in which a provider submits claims to the government certifying that, either implicitly or explicitly, all services or items were provided according to applicable laws.

MANAGEMENT RESPONSIBILITY FOR COMPLIANCE AND INTERNAL CONTROLS

According to the **American Institute of Certified Public Accountants** (AICPA), "**internal control** is a process effected by an entity's board of directors, management, and other personnel designed to provide reasonable assurance regarding the achievement of objectives in the following categories: reliability of financial reporting, effectiveness and efficiency of operations, and compliance with applicable laws and regulations."

Under the new structure of corporate compliance, it is important to note that the internal control of compliance programs is now the responsibility of the board, management, and other internal personnel. The responsibility clearly rests in the hands of management. The AICPA lists five interrelated components of internal control:

- **Control environment** sets the tone of an organization, influencing the control consciousness of its people. It is the foundation for all other components of internal control, providing discipline and structure.
- **Risk assessment** is the entity's identification and analysis of relevant risks to achievement of its objectives, forming a basis for determining how the risks should be managed.
- **Control activities** are the policies and procedures to help ensure that management directives are carried out.
- **Information and communication** are the identification, capture, and exchange of information in a form and timeframe that enable people to carry out their responsibilities.
- **Monitoring** is a process that assesses the quality of internal control performances over time.

CORPORATE COMPLIANCE PROGRAMS

The HHS OIG strongly recommends the adoption of a **corporate compliance plan** as it helps limit the risk of compliance errors and limits the liability of management and directors. An effective program can also limit liability under the Federal Sentencing Guidelines. Most importantly, an effective corporate compliance plan gives employees the guidelines necessary to follow the laws and allows management to know that the laws are being followed.

The OIG has published a list of "Seven Essential Elements of an Effective Compliance Program." They are part of the Federal Sentencing Guidelines. They include:

- *Establishing Compliance Standards of Conduct and Procedures.* The provider must organize its compliance materials, learn what laws and regulations govern its practices, and put into writing the steps necessary for a high-level compliance officer to be sure that laws are being obeyed.
- *Overall Compliance Program Oversight.* For the plan to be effective, a high level compliance officer must be appointed. This person will be at the highest level of management.
- *Due Care in Delegation of Authority.* There must be easy access to the compliance officer for the staff so problems may be reported and corrected. There must also be guarantees to the employees against retaliation for reporting compliance issues. In larger organizations, a 24-hour, 7 day-a-week compliance hotline is being utilized. This allows for confidential and anonymous reporting on potential issues.
- *Employee Training.* Education programs should be instituted for all employees and include periodic refresher courses.
- *Monitoring and Auditing Systems.* The monitoring program should include regular reports to the compliance officer and senior management. In larger corporations, the program will include compliance audits by internal and external auditors who are knowledgeable in federal billing regulations.
- *Consistent Enforcement and Discipline.* The OIG suggests that every plan contain disciplinary standards so that there are consequences for serious deviations from the organization's standards of conduct. Dis-

ciplinary action should apply to not only staff members, but to the supervisor who failed to detect the problem. The OIG also suggests that employers conduct background checks on new hires to ensure they are not excluded from Medicare or other federal government programs because of past involvement in health care fraud. The OIG has set up a national data bank that lists people who have been sanctioned for health care fraud.

- *Response and Corrective Action.* The OIG has established compliance guidelines and information on these may be found at the OIG website http://www.oig.hhs.gov/fraud/docs/complianceguidance/round table0700.pdf

For the compliance plan to be effective, all employees must be aware of the plan. The OIG will survey employees when auditing an institution to measure compliance knowledge and awareness. To develop an effective plan, the first step is to conduct a risk assessment facing the organization.

The greatest threat to healthcare compliance is erroneous or fraudulent billing. A snapshot of the corporation's billing practices should be created for a risk analysis under the supervision of organization attorneys, Once the risk areas are identified, a written compliance plan is developed. This written plan should be distributed to all personnel and training begins. Once the plan is in force and operational, it will only be effective if it includes management support, effective communication, continuous monitoring, and accountability.

CONCLUSION

This chapter has provided you with an overview of fraud and abuse and provided some examples of the same. Types of civil and criminal penalties incurred for violating rules and regulations have been discussed, the history of the False Claims Act and its application to healthcare has been reviewed, and managerial and organizational implications of a wide variety of antitrust, anti-kickback, and safe harbor laws and regulations have been reviewed. The terrain of health care can be rough, especially when it comes to compliance and prevention of fraud and abuse. It is now up to you to begin to apply what you've learned from this and other chapters.

DISCUSSION QUESTIONS

1. What is the difference between fraud and abuse? If a healthcare manager finds out that an employee is committing fraud, is the manager required to report it? What are the consequences of the manager's choices?

2. A physician and his colleague decide to set up a laboratory owned by a dummy corporation in their wives' names, and begin to refer patients to this laboratory. What (if any) laws have they violated?

3. A psychiatrist bills for ten hours of psychotherapy and medication checks for a deceased woman. Has he committed fraud or abuse? Can the deceased woman's estate press charges if the bills were sent to Medicare, and not to the family?

4. You are the new Compliance Manager for a healthcare organization. Describe the steps you will take to ensure that your compliance plan is legal and effective.

5. An attorney sees a plastic surgeon and is so happy with her face lift that she begins to refer all her friends and family. At her 6-month follow-up, she says, "So, Doc, I've sent you all these patients, where's my 30% cut of your fees?" What should the plastic surgeon do?

REFERENCES

American Institute of Certified Public Accountants (AICPA). Retrieved July 20, 2006 from http://www.coso.org/publications/executive_summary_integrated_framework.htm

American Medical Association, Office of General Counsel (AMA OIG). (1998). *Professional courtesy in the health care fraud and abuse context*. Retrieved June 12, 2006, from www.ama-assn.org/ama/pub/category/4615.html

Balanced Budget Act of 1997 (House Resolution 2015) (Public Law 105-33) Title IV, Subtitle D, Chapter 1, Section 4304 (b) (2).

Department of Health and Human Services, Office of Inspector General (HHS OIG). (1997). Semiannual Report, October 1, 1997–March 31, 1998. Retrieved June 12, 2006, from oig.hhs.gov/reading/semiannual/1998/98ssemi.pdf

Department of Justice (DOJ). (2003, November). Memorandum 613:11-10-03. Retrieved November 10, 2006, from http://www.usdoj.gov/opa/pr/2003/November/03_civ_613.htm

Kinkade, W. A. (2000). *Anti-kickback act safe harbor provisions finalized.* Retrieved June 12, 2006, from library.findlaw.com/2000/Dec/8/126843.html

Nahra, M. (1997). *New developments in federal fraud and abuse law: What every consultant needs to know.* Retrieved June 12, 2006, from www.ascp.com/public/pubs/tcp/1997/oct/newdev.html

Sheehan, J. (1997). American Society of Consultant Pharmacists Annual Convention, Scottsdale, AZ.

Title 31 United States Code (31 USC). 31 USC. The Federal False Claims Act. Money and Finance, Subtitle III. Financial Management, Chapter 37 Claims, Subchapter III. Claims Against the United States Government. (1986a).

Title 31 United States Code (31 USC). 31 USC §§ 3729 (7) et seq. (1986b).

Title 31 United States Code (31 USC). 31 USC §3730 (d1). (1986c).

Title 42 United States Code (42 USC). 42 USC 1320a-7b, 1903m Title 42 Consolidated Federal Registry (CFR) § 1001.952. (1987a).

Title 42 United States Code (42 USC). 42 USC CFR 489.24 and 42 CFR 413.65. (1987b).

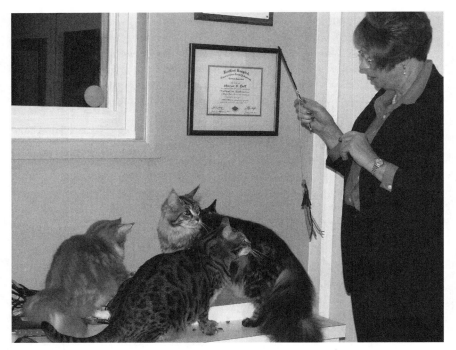

Managing health care is like herding cats. Courtesy of Dale Buchbinder.

CHAPTER 15

Healthcare Management Guidelines and Case Studies
Sharon B. Buchbinder
Donna M. Cox

INTRODUCTION

Case studies are widely used as learning devices in the education of managers and administrators. Case studies are taken from healthcare management situations and experiences in the real world and are written for students of healthcare management to analyze and resolve. They require the student to think, reason, develop critical thinking skills and analytic skills, identify underlying causes of problems, use creative abilities, make decisions, and deal with personality conflicts and change.

GUIDELINES

Based on a decade of experience using the case study method in the classroom and in faculty workshops, we recommend that students work in teams and use the following guidelines for case studies.

- Read (or watch) the case carefully several times. Become absorbed in the situation in such a way that you see yourself intimately involved with the personalities, problems, and conflicts.

- Decide what role you wish to play: the chief administrator in the case who must deal with the matter, or an outside management consultant who has been called in to advise top management on what to do.
- Determine what the major problem is—the real problem.
- Identify secondary and other problems.
- Analyze the factors behind the major and secondary problems. Apply reasoning to how and why the problems developed. Always answer the question WHY?
- Decide what actions you would take. Prepare a written report of the case using the following format.
  1. *Background statement.* What is going on in this case? What are the key points? Summarize the scenario in your own words without rewriting the case. Briefly describe the organization, setting, situation, who is involved, who decides what, etc.
  2. *Your role.* In a sentence or short paragraph, declare whether you are the chief administrator in the case or an outside consultant called in to advise. Regardless of your choice you MUST justify in writing WHY you chose that role. What are the advantages and disadvantages of each role? Be specific.
  3. *Identification of diversity issues and their impact in this case.* How do matters of race, color, ethnicity, gender, sexual orientation, age, national origin, religion, and/or disability appear in this case and what impact might they have? Be sure to include diversity issues in each section of the case study, identifying how they relate to the other sections, i.e., Major problems and secondary issues, Organizational strengths and weaknesses, Alternatives and resolutions, and Evaluation.
  4. *Major problems and secondary issues.* Specifically identify the major and secondary problems. What are the real issues? What are the differences? Can secondary issues become major problems? Analyze the causes and effects. What is *your* analysis of the case? While we only know what the case tells us, we need to think about underlying motivators while we read. Fully explain your reasoning.
  5. *Organizational strengths and weaknesses.* What are their strengths and weaknesses? How are they positioned in the marketplace? What strengths do they bring to the situation? What weaknesses do they need to address? This section can mirror, but should not be identical to the previous section.

6. *Alternatives and Resolution.* What alternatives do they have available to them? This is where you are being asked to "think outside of the box." Were there possibilities not suggested by the text? What feasible strategies would you recommend? What are the pros and cons? The best choice may not be affordable; as managers we have to "satisfice" i.e., make the best choice available at that time. State what should be done—why, how, and by whom. Be specific.

7. *Evaluation.* How will you know when you've gotten there? There must be measurable goals put in place with the recommendations. If you want to increase satisfaction, how will you measure it? Money is easiest to measure; what else can be measured? What evaluation plan would you have them put in place to enable them to assess if they are reaching their goals?

TEAM STRUCTURE AND PROCESS FOR COMPLETION

We recommend that teams select a team leader and a team recorder, although all should take notes. The team should decide how to divide up the tasks to be accomplished. In our classes, we expect to see written responses to the aforementioned questions, and the written, typed case studies to be a *minimum* of five pages long. Teams should indicate who had responsibility for different tasks/sections on the written materials that are handed in.

Team findings should be presented in no more than 10 minutes to the rest of the class. Individual grades are given for each of the student's designated sections and a group grade for the case study as a whole from peers on the presentation, plus, teammates are required to grade each other's efforts and teamwork within the group. The average of the three grades becomes each individual's case study grade. Copies of forms utilized for each (individual sections, group presentation, and teamwork) are provided in this chapter.

GUIDELINES FOR EFFECTIVE PARTICIPATION

1. Attend all team sessions. Eighty percent of life is showing up. It's important here too!

2. Prepare before coming to team sessions and take careful notes. Think about the project and be prepared for each session.
3. Help establish the purpose of the session and the direction to be followed by the group.
4. Have an open mind and be willing to modify your conclusions. Welcome the stimulation of having your ideas challenged.
5. Strike a balance between your speaking time and that of others.
6. Be respectful, considerate, and tactful of the feelings of others—*especially* when you disagree.
7. Present the substance of your thinking concisely and to the point.
8. Help the team reach some conclusions within the allotted time.
9. Really pull your weight on the team. Assist in accomplishing the work of the team by putting the needs of the group ahead of your own needs.
10. **HAVE FUN!**

I have indicated my evaluation of your paper for each of the following areas using a scale of 0 to 10, where 0 = Strongly Disagree and 10 = Strongly Agree. Therefore, the minimum number of points you could earn for each area is 0 and the maximum is 10. The points earned for each area are added up to give you the total score for your paper.

Name of Case Study

_____

Name of Section of Case Study (Circle One): Background statement and Identification of Role, Diversity Issues, Major Problems and Secondary Issues, Organizational Strengths and Weaknesses, Alternatives and Resolution, Evaluation.

The author(s) . . .

1. handed in the paper on time.   _____

2. utilized the format directed in the syllabus.   _____

3. used correct grammar, spelling and terminology.   _____

4. writing was clear and readable.   _____

5. accomplished the stated objectives.   _____

6. demonstrated an excellent understanding of
    relevant literature.   _____

7. demonstrated sound conceptual logic.   _____

8. demonstrated sound methodology and/or
    organization.   _____

9. discussion was appropriate and derived from
    available information.   _____

10. conclusions were logical and consistent with
    available information.   _____

TOTAL   _____

PROPORTION and GRADE   _____

FIGURE 15-1 Evaluation Criteria for Individually-Written Case Study Sections

Please indicate your evaluation of your peers' presentations for each of the following areas using a scale of 0 to 10, where 0 = Strongly Disagree and 10 = Strongly Agree. Therefore, the minimum number of points you could give for each area is 0 and the maximum is 10. The points earned for each area are added up to give the total score for the presentation.

The presenter(s) . . .

1. stated the purpose of the presentation clearly. _____

2. was well-organized. _____

3. was knowledgeable about the subject. _____

4. answered questions authoritatively. _____

5. spoke clearly and loudly enough to be heard. _____

6. maintained eye contact with the audience. _____

7. adhered to time constraints. _____

8. demonstrated sound methodology and/or organization. _____

9. covered the main points appropriate to the case study. _____

10. accomplished the stated objectives. _____

TOTAL _____

PROPORTION and GRADE _____

COMMENTS?

FIGURE 15-2 Peer Evaluation Criteria for Group Presentations

Your Name _____ **Project Name** _____

I have indicated my evaluation of my teammates' behavior for each of the following areas using a scale of 0 to 10, where 0 = Strongly Disagree and 10 = Strongly Agree. Therefore, the minimum number of points my teammates' could earn for each area is 0 and the maximum is 10. Points are added to give each teammate's score for team building behavior.

Names of teammates						
1. attended all team sessions.						
2. was well-prepared for each session.						
3. worked collaboratively to identify and meet session goals.						
4. was an active participant in group discussions.						
5. had an open mind, was willing to modify opinions or conclusions to keep project moving forward.						
6. presented ideas concisely.						
7. submitted assigned work on time.						
8. was considerate and tactful when interacting with teammates.						
9. submitted delegated work on time & fulfilled responsibilities as agreed.						
10. worked actively to achieve group consensus on issues/problems.						
Total Score Subdivisions						
I would be willing to work with this teammate again on another team. **(Answer ONLY YES or NO)**						

What Grade Do You Think The Team Should Earn for this Project?

FIGURE 15-3 Confidential Teammate Evaluation Form

Oops Is Not an Option

Maron J. Boohaker

Bill Salamander is a consultant working in the Medical Records Department of a medical center. As would any vendor doing business with this hospital, Bill's company has signed a Business Associate Agreement. This agreement confirms that the vendor will abide by the hospital's compliance and Health Insurance Portability and Accountability Act (HIPAA) policies.

Bill has friends all through town and they know how much access he has to patient information. One such friend is a personal injury attorney, Anna Anywaican. This attorney is full of ideas. One of her schemes includes a network of associates at hospitals around the state. She hadn't made inroads into this one facility, but now she had Bill.

It was a simple plan—Bill would provide Anna access to trauma patients and for every case he recruited, she would award him 10% of any monies she recovered.

In his first assignment, Bill was paid $25,000 after Anna's client accepted a settlement. However, Bill still had one problem. His access to the medical records was limited to post-discharge. Sometimes, a trauma patient's record would not arrive to the medical records department for months. Bill had to find help.

Bill decided to go to the Emergency Room and scout the third shift employees. Eventually, he comes to you, Micah Makaliving. On your break he asks you to provide him access to the patients that register in the ER as trauma patients. He offers you two choices: either pass out Anna Anywaican's cards or hand him a list of patient names and addresses. Bill will pay you 50% of what he makes. Micah, what will you do?

Building a Better MIS-Trap

Sharon B. Buchbinder

You are the CEO of a large health services organization in Florida. Your HSO has inpatient and outpatient facilities, home healthcare services, and every other service your patient population needs. You also have a world-renowned AIDS treatment center that has been considered by many to be a model for the rest of the United States. Your HSO has always enjoyed an excellent reputation and your quality of care is known to be excellent. You have been very happy in your work, knowing that your HSO provides good care to people who truly need it in a caring and cost-effective manner.

Your HSO has recently been featured in every media vehicle known to every man, woman, and child in the United States and beyond. The reason: someone downloaded the names of 4,000 HIV+ patients who had been seen in your world-renowned HIV clinic and sent the list to newspapers, magazines, and the Internet.

You and your Board of Trustees are completely blown away. The Board of Trustees is furious and wants to fire you. You have been able to convince them that they need to keep you on to fix the HSO's Management Information System (MIS). Their last words to you were "You had BETTER come back with plans for building a better MIS or you're fired!"

You hire a computer security consultant and she comes into your organization under disguise as a nurse manager to help you to determine where the security leak might be. She returns to you in 3 days with the following report.

"While I was under cover in your organization for a mere 3 days I observed the following breaches in computer security. These are the highlights (or low lights):

- Nurses log in with their passwords, walk away, and leave the system open and up and running;
- Dr. Jones leaves his password taped to the PC on a piece of paper;
- Fax machines and printers are often in areas of high traffic and in rooms without locks;
- With my one password, I was able to have remote access to every database in the hospital, including Human Resources, from my home;
- There are no programs reminding people to change their passwords on a regular basis;
- When I pretended to forget my password, other nurses gave me theirs; and,
- When I requested sensitive patient files on diskette, even after this incident, people rarely questioned me.

In short, you have a major problem with your MIS—and your staff!"
What should you do?

The Case of the Complacent Employee

Sharon B. Buchbinder

It was the end of an exhausting Wednesday for Bob Miller. He had spent all day with a 10-year-old girl who kept saying she was going home and taking all the pills she could find to kill herself. He had kept talking with her, trying to elicit what had triggered this response, as he'd simultaneously searched for her mother by phone. When the mother had arrived at his office, panic-stricken and crying, she had also been in need of support. It was four o'clock by the time the mother and daughter left. Now he had to document everything.

Bob looked up from the pile of papers on his desk as his office door opened. His boss stood there in her signature lime green suit, looking grim.

"Harriet! What brings you out today?"

She closed the door and looked around the cramped office.

"Do you have a chair, Bob? It would be good if I could sit down and chat with you."

"Um, sure, hold on a minute."

Bob stood up and grabbed a pile of papers off the threadbare visitor's chair. "There you go."

This couldn't be good. Not only were Harriet's visits rare, when she did appear at Louisa May Alcott Elementary School, they were always grab and grins, and then out she went. This was the first time she'd ever sat down in his broom closet of an office.

"So, Bob, how are you doing?" Her eyes bored into his head.

"Well, you know we're really busy here. Lots of kids with problems, families in crises, almost non-existent support systems, no money, no resources, the usual."

Harriet nodded, still staring at Bob.

Sweat trickled down his back. The office air-conditioner had broken 2 weeks before. He'd meant to write up a work order, but had been too busy. Today, for certain, after Harriet left, he was doing it.

"Bob, I feel really badly about this, and it's not as if we haven't given it a lot of thought. Administration has decided to cut your position."

"What?"

"There doesn't seem to be enough work here for a full-time child psychologist, Bob. This school will be covered part-time by a psychologist from Melville Middle School."

This can't be happening to me, Bob thought. I've fallen asleep at my desk and I'm having a nightmare. He pinched his leg under the desk. Nope. That hurt.

"I've been overworked here from day one," Bob said. "I never leave here before six o'clock. The principal told me the teachers and the kids love me! How did administration make this decision?"

"Remember those emails we sent out, asking you to complete those workload reports? You never answered them."

"Who has time to fill out workload reports when a suicidal child is sitting in your office, crying her heart out?"

"How about the monthly forms we asked you to complete, describing the population you serve and the kinds of problems you're seeing?"

"I have a hard enough time trying to keep up with the Medicaid paperwork so we can get some kind of reimbursement for the work I do here!"

"And, the newsletter, Bob? We never got any submissions from you."

"That piece of trash?"

Harriet flinched. "Some people think it's a very important form of communication for our school mental health professionals."

Bob had forgotten Harriet was the editor of "that piece of trash."

"Have you spoken to the principal? She loves me," he said. "The teachers love me. The kids love me! What are they going to do without me?"

"Principal Daniels did tell me she thought you were working hard, Bob. But, she also said she had no idea how many kids you were seeing, or how often. She said you pretty much kept to yourself."

"Kept to myself? Yeah, you could say that! I'm up to my eyeballs in work, I spend everyday with kids in crisis, the most emotionally draining work in the world, and I have an air conditioner that died 2 weeks ago!

When I eat lunch, it's at my desk, because I'm trying to keep up with the paperwork between crying, screaming kids, or being pulled into classrooms to help with a crisis, or to evaluate kids that teachers are worried about. Keep to myself? I can't even find myself!"

"I'm sorry, Bob. It's nothing personal."

Harriet stood to leave and Bob jumped to his feet.

"Why didn't you say something sooner? I've been doing my job! What could I have done differently?"

Managing Healthcare Professionals: Mini-Case Studies

Sharon B. Buchbinder
Dale Buchbinder

1. You are a new administrator at Jonestown Medical Center. You receive a telephone call from the nurse manager of the emergency room. Dr. Smith, an emergency room physician who is an employee of your hospital, has just reported for duty. The nurse manager suspects that Dr. Smith is intoxicated. What do you do?
2. You are the CEO of Sleepy Hollow Retirement Community and Nursing Center. A resident's family has come to you to complain that their loved one, who is on pain medication, is in intolerable pain. Her medications appear not to be working anymore. One of the family members states, "My 90-year-old mother saw the nurse put the pain medicine in her pocket." What do you do?
3. You are the practice manager of Docs R Us, Ltd., a large multi-specialty medical practice employing over 100 physicians. You are conducting a random review of billing for doctors in the practice and you discover that one of the internists in your group who treats mostly Medicare recipients has been checking off the wrong code for her procedures on the billing form. The procedures on the patient record do not match the billing form codes. You pull up her files for the past 3 months and find a pattern of upcoding. When you meet with her to review this miscoding, she becomes very defensive and angry. What do you do?
4. You are the assistant director of the hospital medical staff office at The Rural Outreach Community Hospital in a tiny town in Arkansas. It is your job to verify physician credentials for staff privileges. Your hospital receives an application from a physician for staff

privileges. On his application it states that he graduated from medical school in El Salvador. When you call to verify this, you are told that the medical school burned down 2 years ago and all the records were destroyed. What do you do?

5. You are a new administrator at a hospital, well known for pulmonary medicine. The physicians in the ICU, the ER, and the Department of Pulmonary Medicine have demanded to meet with you about the shortage of Respiratory Therapists. You stall them for 48 hours so you can gather data. What types of information will you need to collect to have an intelligent conversation with this powerful group of physicians?

6. Dr. White ordered an unusual dose of a medication. May Patterson, RN, sees the order and believes it to be the wrong dose. She calls Dr. White, who insists that she give the medication—as written. Nurse Patterson calls you, the administrator on call for the weekend, to resolve this crisis. What do you do?

Negotiation in Action

Daniel F. Fahey

The following Negotiation Case Study is designed to provide the student with a simulation of an actual negotiation scenario involving a medical group (or IPA) and an HMO. This case study will allow students to participate in a negotiation using real life issues so they may experience the actual negotiation process.

PROCESS

Approximately ten students are directly involved in the simulation. The IPA and HMO will each field a team of five to represent their respective interests as follows:

Majestic Health Plan (HMO)	EveryDoc IPA (Medical Group IPA)
Regional VP for Provider Relations (Chief Negotiator)	Director of Managed Care Contracting (Chief Negotiator)
Medical Director	Chief Executive Officer
Director of Utilization Management	Medical Director
Director of Pharmacy	Chief Operations Officer
Scribe or note taker	Chief Financial Officer

Other students may serve as observers and provide feedback regarding the process and outcomes of the negotiation.

Negotiations are expected to consume a minimum of six class sessions (one and a half hours each) including time for research and caucus. Students will be graded on participation and negotiating skills.

ASSOCIATED CASE DOCUMENTS

Associated with this case are the following three supporting documents:

- **Position Paper (Figure 15-4)**: A Position Paper has been provided to assist the medical group (IPA) with the negotiations. This Position Paper is *not* to be shared with the HMO.
- **Letter (Figure 15-5)**: A letter from the Majestic Health Plan HMO to EveryDoc IPA describes proposed changes that must be addressed during upcoming contract negotiations.
- **Attachment (Figure 15-6)**: The attachment to the letter above further details proposed changes to the agreement between the organizations.

EVERYDOC IPA

Capitation Rate: The current professional capitation rate is $40 per member per month (pmpm). Specialty costs have been increasing at over 15% per month, somewhat due to adverse selection as the result of a new large employer contract negotiated by Majestic HMO. The IPA has evidence that supports its position that a new capitation rate of $45 pmpm would allow the IPA to continue providing services.

OB Volume: The IPA has data that support the contention that its patient population has a substantially higher birth rate than other IPAs contracted with Majestic HMO. The IPA estimates that it should receive an additional $1 pmpm to offset the cost of providing obstetrical services to its members.

Stop-Loss Insurance: The current cost to the IPA for Stop-Loss Insurance, which is provided by the HMO, is $1.80 pmpm. The IPA has a bid from an outside insurance carrier in the amount of $0.60 pmpm. The IPA wants to be allowed to purchase the Stop-Loss at a lower amount and not have the HMO deduct the $1.80 pmpm from the IPA's capitation rate.

New Benefits/Procedures: The IPA wants language in the new agreement that prevents the HMO from offering new benefits or procedures which are not currently provided without consultation with the IPA and additional capitation for expensive procedures or services.

Retroactive Capitation Payment: The IPA wants the HMO to guarantee that capitation for new members added before the 15th of each month will be retroactive to the 1st of the month, instead of the current practice of increasing the capitation rate at the second month of enrollment.

Pharmacy Risk: The IPA is currently responsible for a portion of the pharmacy cost. The IPA wants the HMO to assume all risk for pharmacy cost with the new agreement.

Quality Improvement Incentive: The IPA currently receives an additional $1 pmpm if certain quality improvement measures are met, including better than average HEDIS and patient satisfaction scores. This effort consumes a great deal of resources and the IPA wants $2 pmpm.

Specialty Claims Processing: The IPA currently is required to reimburse specialists for services rendered within 45 days of submittal of a clean claim. This time period is too short and the IPA wants the period extended to 60 days.

FIGURE 15-4 Position Paper

MAJESTIC HEALTH PLAN OF THE INLAND EMPIRE, INC.

400 North Main Street
Any Town, USA 12345

December 10, 200X

Chief Executive Officer
EveryDoc IPA
100 Hospitality Way
Suite 500
Any Town, USA 12345

Dear CEO:

This letter is to inform you that Majestic Health Plan wishes to enter into negotiations for the contract year effective July 1, 200X. We apologize for the lateness of this letter but we have recently reorganized and this is the first opportunity we have had to enter into negotiation for the renewal of our agreement with your IPA affecting approximately 10,000 of our members assigned to your IPA.

We have enclosed our proposed changes from the current agreement. As you are well aware, this past year has not been kind to the managed care industry. A number of our competitors have either ceased business in the Inland Empire or have merged with other health plans. The business community continues to expect high quality care at relatively low premium levels. We have been informed recently by one of the major industry purchasing groups that they do not expect any increases in premiums for the coming year, which means that we are not in a position to enrich our agreement with you. Furthermore, the managed care industry continues to see escalating costs for medical services and must take specific measures to contain costs.

All this means that the coming year will be difficult for all concerned. We value our relationship with your IPA and hope we can reach agreement on a new contract before the termination date of the existing contract.

Sincerely,

John Jones

Vice President, Provider Relations

FIGURE 15-5 Negotiation Letter

The following are changes to the Agreement between Majestic Health Plan of the Inland Empire, Inc. (MHP) and EveryDoc Independent Physician Organization, Inc. (IPA), effective July 1, 200X.

1. The current capitation rate of $40 pmpm will remain in place for the duration of the agreement to take effect July 1, 200X and will continue thereafter unless modified by mutual written agreement.

2. The Division of Financial Responsibilities (DOFR) will be modified with the new agreement as set forth in the attached, which will become part of the new agreement. Among other issues in the DOFR, the revised DOFR will reflect that the cost of any prescription drugs not currently on the Formulary will be assigned to the IPA.

3. The new capitation rate will be paid based on an adjusted age-sex formula which will be prepared and presented before implementation of the new agreement.

4. We are requesting that the IPA expand its network of primary care physicians and specialists to the Palm Springs area. The details of this request will be discussed during the negotiations.

5. We will be making a change in the timing of capitation payments for newly enrolled members. Effective July 1, capitation for any new enrollee joining Majestic Health Plan will be paid beginning the second month of enrollment, except in the case of Medicare Seniors, which will be paid to the IPA within one month of receipt of funds from CMS.

6. Effective July 1, all specialist claims must be paid within 30 days of submittal. Any claim paid beyond 30 days will result in an automatic 10% penalty to the IPA and will be deducted from the next month's capitation payment.

7. Effective July 1, all referrals for liver transplant and bone marrow transplant will be to the Mayo Clinic as our Center of Excellence.

8. These negotiations depend on the successful completion of a new agreement with your PHO partner, St. Elsewhere Hospital.

9. We are asking that your IPA obtain and maintain Directors and Officers liability insurance for your Board in the amount of $5 million effective July 1, 200X.

10. Majestic Health Plan reserves the right to present additional negotiation issues by February 28, 200X.

FIGURE 15-6 Attachment

Similarities →

/

The Merger of Two Competing Hospitals: A Case Study

Mary Anne Franklin, Dale Mapes,
Audrey McDow, and Karin Mithamo

This case highlights the process of merging two fully accredited hospitals, both of which have a full complement of state-of-the-art diagnostic technology, including MRI and CAT scanners, 24-hour physician-staffed emergency care centers, and specialized women's centers. Both of these facilities are located in a community of 60,000 in the southeastern part of Idaho.

The success of the merger hinges on the timely resolution of several issues that the executive staff implemented; mutually, enhancing solutions in the areas of: 1) Leadership; 2) Culture Adaptation; 3) Human Resource Management; 4) Staffing; and 5) Benefit Issues.

OVERVIEW

Hospital A: Porter Regional Medical Center (PRMC)

Located on the east side of town, Porter Regional Medical Center (PRMC) was a for-profit hospital, consisting of 110 hospital beds, 8 of which were reserved for transitional care. PRMC was a privately-owned facility. Mountain Health Care (MHC), a large healthcare organization in the Rocky Mountain region, owned the facility. Built in 1990, the facility was designed to efficiently handle patient flow from the emergency room to the pharmacy and to be a point of referral for more complicated patient conditions. PRMC services consisted of general and same-day surgery and full-service rehabilitation and radiology departments. Other services included a kidney dialysis center, on-site retail pharmacy, a regional Red

Cross blood bank, 24-hour laboratory, home health, Ominous/Home IV, and a women's center, including obstetrics, and numerous other amenities.

Other assets owned by PRMC were the adjacent medical office buildings, a day care center, the land on which an assisted living center was located adjacent to the hospital, and the sports medicine complex adjacent to the state university's arena. These assets represented 188,000 square feet of facility space housed on 63 acres. The hospital employed 450 personnel.

For 2001, the hospital's operating budget was $34 million. However, in the same year, the hospital experienced a $1 million loss and a projected $500 thousand loss for 2002. After 3 years of red ink, PRMC decided to liquidate.

Hospital B: Banner Regional Medical Center and Turner Geriatric Center (BRMC)

Built in 1951, Banner Regional Medical Center (BRMC), a county-owned hospital, was over 50 years old. Located on the west side of town, the hospital structure included 154 inpatient beds and a geriatric healthcare center that consisted of 100–106 beds, 13 transitional care beds, and 7 rehabilitation beds. Completed in 1998, a medical office building with a parking structure was located adjacent to the hospital. The campus consisted of 561,366 square feet of building space, housed on 6 acres. The hospital's operating budget for 2001 was $79 million. BRMC had a reserve fund of $20 million earmarked for major renovations to the existing facility's emergency room and intensive care unit. BRMC's services included the Herman Cancer Center, Family Centered Care (Ob/Gyn), a newborn intensive care unit, a women's center, Life Flight (mobile intensive care), a regional pediatric unit, a geriatric center, and a sports/industrial medicine clinic. The hospital had a staff of 914 employees.

While the majority of the services were housed at BRMC, the home health administrative offices and the physical therapy departments were housed at different locations within the same town. For strategic planning purposes, management knew that the hospital's viability depended on the necessary action to expand and renovate the facility to meet the needs of its current market.

The stage was set for the consolidation of the two competing hospitals: PRMC, crippled with 3 years of losses and BRMC, struggling with aging facilities. The process would take the next 3 years (2002–2005) to complete the merger and create a new facility. BRMC's board of directors offered the facility to the county, so as not to let an outside organization compete for its resources and patients. The county would pay $25 million, to be paid in increments of $15 million at the time of purchase and $10 million over the next 2 to 3 years, interest free. The CEOs of PRMC and BRMC, Pat Herman, MHA, FACHE, and Scott Johns, MBA, had applied for the single, hospital management slot. A consulting firm from Seattle was hired to review resumes, experiences, and job performances of both men. In the end, the commissioners voted to hire Herman, who had over 20 years as an administrator for a Catholic institution and had been the chief communication officer for a military academy.

CONSOLIDATION

In fall of 2001, the chairs of each hospital's board met to discuss options for cutting healthcare costs, addressing the shortage of healthcare personnel and improving the delivery of health care in the community. In spring of 2002, a letter of intent to consolidate was sent from BRMC to MHC. In the summer of 2002, an agreement was solidified with the following requirements: 1) the consolidated hospital would have a new name; and, 2) a transitional team, including the previous CEO of PRMC, would be assembled to deal with management changes and employee benefit packages.

Other requirements included a new mission statement; a policy that no workers would be laid off as a result of the merger; and a newly elected 15 member-hospital board, comprised of 10 BMRC board members and 5 PMRC members. Public meetings were held by board members and hospital administrators to answer questions and explain the merger process. During the meetings, the public voiced concerns that consolidation would destroy competition in the area, leading to an increase in healthcare costs and a decrease in services and quality. In preliminary employee meetings, the staff expressed concerns over seniority, job placement, compensation, and benefit packages.

LEADERSHIP

Leadership style at BMRC could be characterized as participative, autonomous, and self-governing. As CEO of BRMC, Pat Herman's initial job was to rebuild the executive team that had been depleted by the retirement of the outgoing CEO, the serious illness of the Director of Nursing Services, and the departure of the Vice President of Human Resources.

PRMC operated as a subsidiary of MHC, whose corporate office made all policy and strategic management decisions. Lower-level managers were not highly involved in the decision-making processes at MHC. Management therefore, was highly-structured and centralized. Consequently, the management team at PRMC relied on the corporate office for the day-to-day operations of the hospital.

To embrace the new entity, the community decided to name the consolidated hospital Portsmith Regional Medical Center. At the time of the merger, there was a combined staff of over 1400 employees. The staff at both PRMC and BRMC in duplicate management positions had to compete for their jobs. Approximately 90 employees decided to retire. By the conclusion of streamlining positions, 1200 employees were part of the new organization.

Herman conducted 30 to 40 meetings with the staff and met weekly with the managers to answer their questions and concerns. The employees were encouraged to express their feelings. Employees were given access to the EAP program, social workers, and one employee relations person to help cope with their fears and apprehensions.

CULTURE ADAPTATION

Cultures in organizations are manifested in language, physical settings, values, symbols, and formal procedures. As a single entity, BRMC had developed an autonomous, independent, self-directed culture. PRMC's culture was much less independent and relied heavily on the corporate office for its decision making, policy development, and for its operating procedures. These factors greatly influenced the culture of each organization and the final impact on the consolidation of the new entity.

PRMC and BRMC referred to each other in competitive language. There were many references to "them" versus "us" within the organizations. The language was indicative of the entrenched processes, cultures, loyalty, and systems that had to be addressed in the consolidation.

Both organizations had symbols that represented their cultures. Each organization had a logo that symbolized who they were and what they represented. PRMC had a vision and mission statement developed and de-fined by the corporate office, while BRMC, on the other hand, did not have a clearly-defined mission and vision statement. Although BRMC's board and Pat Herman had determined their vision and mission state-ments for the future, these statements were not clearly-defined and were not communicated to the staff.

HUMAN RESOURCE MANAGEMENT

In 2003, a new Vice President of Human Resources, Dale Miller, was re-cruited from a Catholic healthcare system in Kentucky to handle the newly-merged hospital. Miller had extensive experience in mergers and ac-quisitions. Soon, he realized that the merger included more than the con-solidation of duplicated services. The merger also brought together two different hospital boards, two separate groups of physicians and staff, and two different benefit packages.

STAFFING

There were several major staffing concerns for the consolidated hospital. Six months prior to consolidation (spring of 2002), PRMC and BRMC had to develop a joint medical structure that included: leadership, creden-tialing, bylaws, rules and regulations, and peer review. Both hospitals had three medical staff leadership positions: Chief of Staff, Vice-Chief and Secretary, for a total of six physicians. A process was developed to consol-idate these six positions to four. Four of the existing physicians' names were recommended to the medical staff, and subsequently, the staff voted to retain all four to lead the new, consolidated medical staff. BRMC's Dr. Gene Roberts became the new chief of staff of Portsmith Regional Med-ical Center.

The next step required evaluating the different bylaws, rules, and regu-lations for each medical staff at PRMC and BRMC. Through a ballot, the two medical staffs decided to adopt bylaws, rules, and regulations that re-flected their joint decision-making efforts. Credentialing the two medical staffs required interventions by a legal team. Since every physician must be credentialed every 2 years, both hospitals had to develop a timeline that would meet JCAHO's standards that would keep physician's credentials current as the time of consolidation. For example, if a physician's time for credentialing would put him/her out of compliance, then the credentialing timeline had to move to the shortest time in order to maintain his/her current license. Since each hospital had different peer review/quality standards, the newly elected medical executive team and staff voted to modify and adopt PRMC's more stringent, well-documented standards. By the time of consolidation (October 1, 2003), 160 physicians at PRMC and 180 medical staff at BRMC had completed a smooth transition with only 5 physicians choosing to leave.

Another staffing issue was with the nursing department. An analysis of the combined workforce revealed that in nursing services, the ratio of RNs to LPNs was disproportionate (70% LPN to 30% RN). This ratio was opposite what was needed for the planned high-tech services to be offered by the merged organization, which included cardio-vascular, open-heart, heart cauterization labs, cancer centers, and four call centers of excellence. These centers of excellence required a higher level of specialty nursing than was needed previously. The nursing staff ratio needed to be changed to a 60:40% RN to LPN ratio as rapidly as possible.

In addition, the staff analysis revealed that the skill levels of other existing staff needed to be developed rapidly in order to perform in a more technically-advanced environment that included: picture archiving computerization systems, electronic medical records, and new patient systems technology.

BENEFITS

Each hospital offered its employees benefits that included: sick leave, paid time-off, health insurance, life insurance, and retirement plans. Paid time-off and sick leave were accrued at different rates at each hospital. BRMC was self-insured, while PRMC offered its employees a fully-insured healthcare plan. In addition, healthcare coverage, deductibles, premiums, and out-of-pocket costs varied between the hospitals. PRMC employees feared that they would lose benefits if they moved to the BRMC retirement system. In the end, 90 BRMC employees opted to leave the organization for fear of losing their benefits. Another group opted to stay in order to obtain a better benefits package.

Two months later, the newly formed board and executives, including Herman and Miller, met at a planning retreat in Jackson, Wyoming to decide how to best resolve leadership, culture adaptation, human resource management, staffing, and benefits issues.

QUESTIONS

1. What specific steps should the board take to create an executive team to manage the newly created organization?
2. Given the diversity of cultures embedded in the merged organization, what should the management team do to facilitate a working culture in the new organization?
3. How should management deal with the physical structures at the time of the consolidation?
4. How should the duplication of services and departments be handled?
5. What are the risk management issues and legal issues associated with the merger?
6. How can the board and administrators calm the fears of the staff before, during, and after the consolidation?
7. How do the physicians work with administration to share power and resources within the new consolidated hospital?

The Orchestra:
A Narrative in a Minor Key

Leonard H. Friedman
Spence Meighan

OVERTURE

In the contemporary literature of health care management, metaphors are a common vehicle used to help the reader arrive at a common understanding of a word, phrase, or event. They may even help to explain something totally unrelated. In the modern literature on leadership, managers are urged to move away from simply doing the work of administration and instead think of themselves as teachers, coaches, and even ringmasters. In each of these cases, a particular metaphor may evoke a different way of thinking and practice.

Hospitals, physician practices, managed care organizations, academic health centers, skilled nursing facilities, and others across the healthcare continuum have always represented an important challenge to management. Today, the challenges are even greater. One example is the feeling of powerlessness that many physicians are experiencing, particularly in relation to constraints on caring for their patients, severely constricted reimbursement, and the effects of increasingly large damage awards in negligence cases. All of these factors combine to compromise effective and lasting relationships between physicians and their patients.

In our combined experience, both in the scholarly study of healthcare organizations and the actual practice of medicine and administration, the tensions that exist between the clinical, administrative, and governance aspects of healthcare delivery appear to be more difficult today than at any time in the past. What can be done to help physicians, administrators, and governing board members work together in a more collegial and productive manner? Before telling you our ideas, it might be useful to share with you a tale that uses the metaphor of a symphony orchestra to illustrate the relationships and organizational dynamics that exist in many healthcare organizations.

THEME AND VARIATION

Not very long ago, in a community not very far from here, there existed a very special orchestra. The Philharmonic Healthcare Orchestra (or PHO as it came to be known) was composed almost exclusively of physicians, with a small handful of nurse practitioners, physician assistants, and an even smaller number of non-specialty nurses playing minor parts. The lead role in each instrumental section of the orchestra was assumed by a physician (who was as it just so happened, board certified in his/her non-primary care area of specialization). This was only proper given the many extra years of study that these specialists needed in order to be expert in their chosen field. These section leaders had devoted many years to their study of music and to perfecting the art of playing their instrument. Each of the sections (violin, percussion, trumpet, etc.) were made up of physician players who, while expert and quite talented in their own right, had not quite achieved the virtuoso status of the section leader. Non-physician members of the orchestra were assigned the responsibility of setting the stage, turning the music sheets on cue, helping bring the instruments to perfect tune for each performance, and doing other ancillary duties as might be required by the real musicians.

Every good orchestra requires a conductor who can bring out the best in each performer. Beyond simply dressing up in an expensive tuxedo and waving the baton to the beat of the music, the conductor is expected to know and be able to draw out the capabilities of each musician, and then blend the sounds to create a final product that is both pleasing to the ear and that honors the musical intent of the composer. The conductor of PHO was Alexandra Stewart, who was hired 3 months ago and given the task of bringing the orchestra to new heights of performance and renown. Ms. Stewart earned a master's degree from the nationally accredited program at the University of Musicology. Given her training, Stewart believed that she was well-prepared in the art and science of conducting. Coupled with many years of experience conducting lesser-known physician orchestras, Stewart was thought by the board of directors to be the ideal replacement for the previous conductor, Michael Highland, who had been terminated after having served less than a year as the conductor of PHO. As the Executive Director of the PHO board explained it to Ms. Stewart, the previous conductor had his contract revoked because the members of the orchestra (and by extension, the board) had lost confidence in Mr. Highland's ability to lead PHO and elevate it to its proper stature. Too often, he ran afoul of the orchestra members and made many of them angry by asking them to play the music according to his wishes and by expecting them to play off the same musical score. He should have known that angering the musicians was absolutely unacceptable, and so the board had no alternative but to question his leadership skills. While everyone agreed that Highland was a good and capable conductor, he just didn't have the "right stuff" to lead this orchestra, which inevitably led to his short tenure.

Endorsing the hire of Ms. Stewart was the board of directors of PHO and their chairman, Mr. Howard Gold. The board consisted of a large number of persons from the community who were well known and highly regarded in the areas of philanthropy, marketing, finance, the law, and politics. The board members had no detailed knowledge about musical matters (aside from their role as members of the audience) but in spite of these apparent deficiencies felt entirely competent to evaluate governance and leadership. The board also included a representative from the members of the orchestra, in this case, Dr. Mark McLung, a cardiothoracic surgeon who was also the first violin in the orchestra.

The search for a new conductor had been both lengthy and tedious. PHO advertised in all the major conductors journals, sought out candidates at the major conductors' professional meetings, and in fact, hired a conductor search firm to help identify possible new leaders. Out of a list of over two dozen applicants, the top three candidates were brought out to meet the interview team. As is the case in most interviews, the positive aspects of the organization and the key stakeholders were emphasized and problematic persons or situations were either hidden away or ignored entirely. The two other candidates brought out for an interview had major shortcomings. One was clearly an authoritarian leader and the players were unanimous in downgrading this candidate. The other person had considerable experience in group dynamics and while he was affable enough, several of the players were suspicious of his overly warm and caring personality, which immediately ruled him out as a serious contender.

Unfortunately for Stewart, she did not ask the types of questions during the interview that might have made clear the real reason why Highland's contract had been abruptly terminated.

The board came to believe that Ms. Stewart had the leadership qualities and experience to not only bring out the best in the members, but would also help PHO attain financial stability and meet the musical needs of the community. Her arrival was marked by great hope and expectation by the orchestra, board, and community.

MOLTO AGITATO

Despite the relative joy and high expectations that Stewart's arrival engendered among many people in the community, trouble was already beginning to brew among some of the musicians of PHO. A certain amount of history had been omitted during Ms. Stewart's interview with the board. The members of PHO had an unfortunate tendency to practice together only when they felt it was absolutely necessary. During several practices (and in a particularly embarrassing moment during an important concert), the musicians would often not play from the same page of music because they could not agree upon the particular tune that they would play together. In fact, the incident that precipitated the termination of the previous conductor (Highland) was a particularly egregious example of this unwillingness to play as one. One night, before a standing room only audience at the concert hall, while the majority of PHO had started the *William Tell Overture*, a group of trumpet and trombone players broke away and began playing John Phillip Sousa's *Stars and Stripes Forever*. It was only until the board intervened after the concert that the renegade brass players reluctantly agreed that there would be no further disruptions.

Another very touchy subject was starting to surface surrounding the role of nurses in the orchestra. While in the "old days" nurses were willing to do the supportive (some would call menial) tasks required to make the orchestra play together, now more and more of the nurses (particularly the nurse practitioners) were demanding the right to actually play the instruments during a live performance. In fact, in her role as a conductor at a previous physician orchestra, Stewart had tremendous success with nurse musicians and was able to convince the physicians to allow them to play in the background (although never in a section leader or soloist role). This information had filtered to the musicians of PHO and rumors had already begun that Stewart had been hired with the intent of replacing them with lower paid performers of far lesser skill and stature. It was bad enough that primary care musicians who could play several different instruments as the need dictated had infiltrated their ranks several years ago. These multi-instrument players were grudgingly accepted but only on the condition that they would never lead a section and all musical decisions would need to take place after consultation with their single instrument colleagues.

Alexandra Stewart soon learned about the discontent among the musicians and was rightfully concerned that these rumblings and unsubstantiated rumors might soon build into something far worse. Her first inclination was to call a general meeting of the orchestra members, but that was soon abandoned as no time could be agreed upon when most members could attend. As an alternative, Stewart called a meeting of the various section heads with the objective of gaining their support and understanding of the charge that she had been given by Mr. Gold and the board. The results of the meeting were particularly unsatisfactory, and in fact, probably made matters worse than before as this highly edited transcript of the meeting illustrates:

> McLung: "I appreciate the fact that PHO might have had difficulties in the past but that was due exclusively to a lack of leadership on the part of the previous conductors and the board, coupled with an unwillingness to allow the orchestra members to perform the music in a way they see fit. The players must be given the freedom to perform in a manner commensurate with their training and skill. There should be no interference by non-players."

> Stewart: "Unfortunately, that is the essence of the problem here. We must perform as an integrated whole without fracturing into dozens of individuals who insist on doing their own thing. Can't you see that?"

> 1st Clarinet: "Who are you to lecture us on playing together? When was the last time you picked up an instrument, much less played it in front of thousands of adoring fans?"

> Stewart: "Just for your information, I studied piano for 10 years before I decided to become a conductor."

> 1st Cello: "It's obvious that you have no talent for making music, otherwise you would have continued your study and risen to our level. Besides, even if you wanted to play with us you would be prohibited given the rules of the musicians' union."

Several of the players learned that Ms. Stewart's father had been a gifted violinist. This discovery emphasized to the orchestra members that she would have been a player if she had possessed the talent and that her career as a conductor was a second choice based upon her limited abilities.

CRESCENDO

Immediately after the meeting with Stewart, McLung called all the section leaders and other influential musicians together in a closed-door session to decide what to do about the problematic conductor coupled with the perceived lack of board support. The meeting took place in the basement of McLung's home and was quite a scene. The tone of the meeting started in a hostile fashion and became increasingly intense as the members aired both their real and imagined grievances. Dr. McLung made it clear that he and his fellow cardiac surgeons and violinists had a limited interest in PHO given that they had formed their own quartet, which they affectionately named the Heartstrings. Since he received greater applause and admiration as the star of the quartet, he expressed his thought that playing in the orchestra was a relative waste of his time and talent. The gastroenterologist members who had formed a wind ensemble echoed this same sentiment. All agreed that they made far more money playing as either soloists or in small ensembles than as part of the symphony orchestra.

Some of the more generalist members of PHO had a different perspective from those who claimed that membership in the orchestra meant virtually nothing to them. The general surgeons took a position that they needed the orchestra in order to play the entire symphonic repertoire. It became clear that carving out specialty players would greatly diminish the quality of the music and would severely limit the scope of what pieces the orchestra could perform.

It seemed as though the only thing the group could decide on was that Stewart was just the latest iteration of a conductor who did not respect the training and position of the orchestra members. If she would only allow the orchestra to decide for themselves what the audience wanted to hear, and then trust them to play the right melodies, then all these problems would vanish.

At the same time the musicians of PHO were meeting to discuss the abysmal state of affairs between themselves and their conductor, Alexandra Stewart was ensconced at the annual meeting of the professional conductors' association. This group was composed of both full and assistant conductors from across the country and was the largest such association anywhere. They had active student chapters that allowed young apprentices the opportunity to network with older and more seasoned conductors. The association meeting was full of educational sessions, social

activities, and numerous opportunities that allowed the members to recognize and celebrate one another's accomplishments, and give each other
awards and tributes. Stewart had risen to a significant leadership position
within the association and, in fact, represented the conductors in her region of the country. That day, Stewart chaired the plenary session which
featured as its keynote speaker, Dr. Pat Patterson, one of the country's
foremost physician musicians who, that morning, spoke on the necessity
of building and sustaining relationships between the orchestra members,
conductors, and board of directors. After a careful and systematic study of
physician orchestras across the country, Patterson concluded that those
who were truly great, and produced the finest music year after year, had at
their core a culture of trust, communication, and a shared vision between
and among all three groups. Talent, virtuosity, size, geographic location,
plus any number of other variables had little or nothing to do with long-
term success. In fact, many of the most successful orchestras had no individual stars either as musicians or as conductors. Rather, all the parties
agreed that success was built upon shared decisions, building a common
culture, and trusting one another to do what was in the best interests of the
orchestra and their respective communities.

Needless to say, Patterson's remarks set off quite a commotion in the
hall. Conductor after conductor challenged Dr. Patterson, with the overall sentiment being that the musicians (and particularly the section directors) had historically viewed the rest of the orchestra as their personal
entourage to do with as they wished. Conductors complained of musicians
making unreasonable demands for the newest and finest instruments, concert halls, and expensive recording contracts, despite declining attendance
and ticket prices set by a small group of the largest brokers. How could the
poor conductors hold together the integrity of the orchestra when it
seemed as though none of the members had any interest in listening to
what they had to say and often resisted any and all changes proposed?
Without even trying to respond to individual complaints and allowing
each person the opportunity to tell their story, Dr. Patterson calmly looked
around the room and asked when was the last time any of the conductors
sought their musicians' input on decisions of substance to their orchestra.
A hush fell over the room as the conductors looked at one another and
simply shrugged or looked down at the floor. Finally Stewart spoke up and
acknowledged that, while the members of the orchestra were not always
brought into the decision process, there was good reason for this omission.

Both conductors and orchestra members were very busy people and conductors were hired to make the many decisions that affected the orchestra. Musicians were there to make beautiful music—they were not trained to conduct. After all, if the musicians simply allowed the conductors to do their jobs, they in turn would allow the musicians to do theirs.

FINALE

On the flight back home from the conference, Stewart had the opportunity to think carefully about Dr. Patterson's comments and to make her own assessment of the organizational environment in which she functioned. Stewart could not help but reminisce how quickly the musical world had changed since she first began conducting professionally. At the start of her career, there had been literally thousands of orchestras, both in big towns and small, with audiences that truly seemed to appreciate the efforts of everyone associated with the orchestra. Some of these orchestras had international reputations, while others were just well known in their local communities, but regardless of their size or standing, everyone seemed happy. There were plenty of resources to operate the orchestra, the musicians generally seemed contented (although squabbles did sometimes break out), and the communities appreciated whatever it was the orchestra decided to play even if it was not exactly what they wanted to hear.

Being the conductor had its rewards—enhancing both financial status as well as standing in the community. Association with the musicians was generally limited to a few brief rehearsals and then the performance. Whatever the conductor and musicians wanted, the board typically approved. Musicians played for the joy of making music and therefore, the conductor's job was relatively simple. Everyone was a member of one big happy family.

However, recent changes had dramatically changed the ways in which the orchestra operated. Federal and state agencies had developed strict standards for all members of the orchestra. The funding for community orchestras became more and more restrictive, forcing many orchestras to merge or to close outright. This was most pronounced in the smaller, more rural orchestras, but even the larger, more urban orchestras were not immune from this shrinkage. The result was that the remaining orchestras were forced to compete with one another for both audience and talented musicians.

The audience itself had become much more demanding and even fickle. No longer were they willing to listen quietly to whatever the orchestra served up that evening. Many started complaining about rising ticket prices and began comparison shopping to find the best orchestra at the best price. Outside groups sprang up to give the communities a measure of the quality of the orchestra. Conductors and boards could search a database to assess the quality of the musicians as measured by the number of times they had played off-key or (worse yet) had been asked to leave an orchestra for some reason or another. Rather than see the musicians as valued professionals, many conductors (Stewart included, as she admitted to herself), now viewed musicians as nothing more than any other employee of the orchestra who demanded high salaries, complete professional autonomy, and came with inflated assessments of their own abilities. Why was it so difficult for the musicians to admit that the world had changed? thought Stewart. Why would they not accept the new way orchestras had to operate and just be grateful they had a place to play their instruments? How could it be that the musicians expected the world to continue as it had in the past, with no recognition of the demands of today?

Unbeknownst to Stewart, while she had been away at the conductors' conference, the section leaders of PHO had scheduled a lunch meeting with Chairman Gold and a handful of other board members. After doing away with the pleasantries and chitchat about one another's upcoming overseas trips or golfing safaris, Dr. McLung presented a proposal to Mr. Gold on behalf of a large number of section leaders and other PHO musicians. Briefly stated, the musicians were not at all happy with the way in which they were being treated by Stewart since she arrived. They acknowledged that there had been some problems in the past with members launching off into their own preferred music, and not taking the time and effort to learn how to play together. Their concern was that Stewart should have recognized this problem and dealt with it early in her tenure. She simply did not provide the kind of leadership that was necessary to bring PHO the prominence they so richly deserved. If only Stewart had listened to the concerns of the musicians and particularly the section heads and then acted on them, we would not be having this conversation today. Dr. McLung said, "While she is a very nice person and a seemingly capable conductor, the other members of the orchestra simply believe that Stewart is simply not the right person at this time for PHO. What would be particularly helpful is if the orchestra could have significant input on the selection of the next conductor."

When she walked into her office the next morning, Stewart found an urgent message asking that she contact Mr. Gold immediately. She called Gold on his private phone line and was asked to find time to meet with him later that afternoon with the agenda being a discussion of the future direction for the orchestra. At the appointed hour, Stewart entered Mr. Gold's beautifully decorated office. The walls were covered with fine art and photographs of Mr. Gold shaking hands with local and national dignitaries, along with proclamations from civic and community leaders speaking to the importance and influence of his work enhancing the excellence of PHO. Choosing his words carefully, Gold sought to provide Stewart with the background necessary to help her understand the necessity to bring the orchestra to prominence and the concern about the perception of the musicians about her shortcomings as a leader. Just as Gold was getting warmed up, Stewart interrupted him with some information of her own. On the flight home from the conference, she had been weighing an offer that had been made to her by a brand new start-up orchestra to be their very first conductor. While the salary was not quite what she was earning at PHO, Stewart was intrigued by the opportunity to start from scratch in a new community, with musicians who were just learning to play with one another and were enthusiastic about the potential of making wonderful music together. The more she thought about her situation at PHO, the more attractive the offer seemed. So attractive, that Alexandra Stewart handed her resignation letter to Gold then and there.

Gold stared at Stewart blankly. He was fully intending to terminate her, but on his terms. Gold mumbled out something about what are we going to do without a conductor? Stewart consoled Mr. Gold by saying, "My presence will not be missed." She continued, "Unless the players want to play well together and are committed to doing that, then it does not really matter who conducts the orchestra, now does it?" She concluded, "You will be able to find somebody to lead your orchestra and I will do all I can to make the transition as smooth as possible." Mr. Gold appeared to be quite happy with this particular outcome.

CODA

In times long ago, fables were among the most popular forms of literature. Not only were they widely consumed by many readers, the objective was to teach a lesson about one or more of life's many virtues. What we have attempted to accomplish with *The Orchestra* is to provide the opportunity for the reader—whether physician, administrator, governing board member, or student of health care management—to think carefully and reflect on the absolute necessity of these groups to work in harmony with one another. Healthcare delivery at the start of the 21st century is in a very fragile state. Buffeted by the demands of payers and commercial insurance companies, physicians and hospitals are forced to demonstrate increasing levels of value for the services they provide. Patients are becoming ever more savvy and sophisticated in their healthcare purchasing decisions, as evidenced by the direct advertisement of prescription drugs and exponential growth in the use of the Internet to access health Web sites. Competition between and among healthcare providers has poisoned relationships among professionals without the intended effect of lowering prices. Physician Hospital Organizations, which started with much fanfare as a way to align the financial incentives of both groups, have proved to be a failure overall, as evidenced by their rapid disintegration.

In our work as students of the U.S. healthcare delivery system, we suggest that given these realities, it is more important now than ever before, that physicians, administrators, and governing boards learn to work together in ways that are meaningful to all parties. Returning to a system where power is concentrated in one group or another is antithetical to the goal of shared governance. Simply getting along with one another is not adequate. Decisions must be made in an atmosphere of trust, honesty, and goodwill. We leave the specifics on how to accomplish this to each of you and your organizations. However, as was so aptly stated during the flight of Apollo 13 in 1970, "Failure is not an option." The imperative is for all parties to put historical hurt feelings, pride, and animus aside for the goal of everyone, creating beautiful music that ultimately benefits the person who needs it most: the patient.

Labor and Delivery Dilemma

Brenda Freshman
Louis Rubino

Ms. Garcia, the Nurse Manager of Labor and Delivery, calls Dr. Kim to ask for orders on Mrs. Ford, a full-term woman who presents herself unexpectedly for delivery at Lakeview Memorial Hospital. Ms. Garcia is concerned, since she did not receive advanced notice or the required prenatal record on Mrs. Ford.

Dr. Kim gets very upset with the phone call, saying that he just completed a delivery and was trying to get a couple hours of sleep. He swears and says he will be there shortly and to start prepping for a C-section. Ms. Garcia is agitated at Dr. Kim's response and she feels her shoulders and neck tense up. Ms. Garcia could tell that Mrs. Ford was not expecting a C-section based on her comments when taking a history.

Dr. Kim enters the unit as Alice, the L&D nurse, is putting the baby monitor on Mrs. Ford. He condescendingly snaps, "Who taught you how to do it that way?" and takes over. Ms. Garcia is nearby and asks Dr. Kim why he intends to do a C-section. Dr. Kim ignores her inquiry since he has a full schedule ahead of him and does not want to take the time to wait through labor for a vaginal birth. He instead barks an order to the nurse to release Mrs. Ford to the surgery nurse.

Dr. Kim leaves to scrub for surgery. Ms. Garcia hears Alice crying and goes over to her. She puts her arm around Alice and says, "Don't let him get to you, sweetie. Dr. Kim is a real jerk."

Sexual Harassment at the Diabetes Clinic

Kenneth L. Johnson
Barry G. Gomberg

PART A

The diabetes clinic is one of four academic hospital-based clinics Tim Jorgenson has been managing for the past 3 months. Tim earned an MBA and has worked in hospital administration for about 5 years. This is his first experience as a medical group manager. While the clinic staff members are impressed with Tim's management background, he has no clinical experience, so some of the nurses and a few of the physicians are questioning Tim's ability to understand their needs.

All four of the clinics Tim has been hired to manage are connected by a rear hallway and are home to physicians from the internal medicine department. The diabetes clinic is located at the western end of the area, next comes the general internal medicine clinic, then the oncology clinic, and finally the infectious disease clinic. Physicians using the diabetes clinic are specialists in endocrinology, however, they do not keep the clinic busy every day of the week. When the endocrinologists are not using the rooms, they are used by gastroenterology, pulmonary, and cardiology specialists. The other connected clinics represent general internal medicine and rheumatology, infectious diseases, oncology, and the heart and lung transplant programs. Some of the physicians bring their own nurses to the clinics when they work there, but in the diabetes clinic alone, Tim manages four clerks, two medical assistants, two licensed practical nurses (LPNs) and four registered nurses (RNs), who serve whatever group of doctors happens to be using the clinic. Among the four clinics, the different specialties practice on different days. Monday is very busy with endocrinology

GI patients, general internal medicine, infectious diseases, oncology, and some pulmonary. Tuesday is heavy cardiology, pulmonary, oncology, and internal medicine. Wednesday is heart transplant, pulmonary, and so on. Tim never seems to have enough rooms or enough staff to meet the demands. That includes the overwhelming number of phone calls and check-ins handled by the clerks at the front. He is always concerned about turnover and works hard to keep the staff he has.

While the other three clinics seem to be functioning well, the diabetes clinic never seems to run smoothly. In particular, Tim is concerned about the lack of comradery and teamwork among the staff. The nurses seem to be more concerned about each other's work habits than they are of their own. One of the medical assistants, just out of high school, doesn't respond to the nurses' requests and has come to Tim arguing that she shouldn't report to the nurses. One of the LPNs has worked for the clinic for 12 years and doesn't like the newer RNs taking over. Some of the RNs think their first priority is the physicians, even if it means putting coworkers and clinic patients on the back burner. Other RNs think the patients in the clinic should come first.

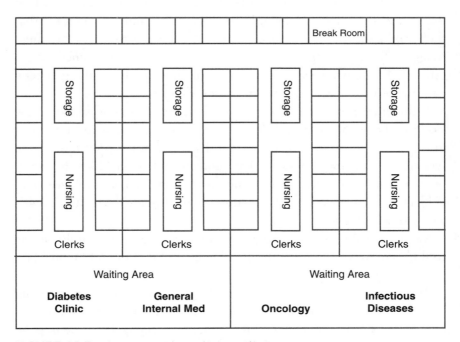

FIGURE 15-7 The Internal Medicine Clinics

Tim has decided to hold regular staff meetings with all four clinics combined in order to discuss some of the issues he has noticed. No minutes of previous staff meetings or training sessions exist in the clinic. He's not sure what has happened in the past.

While the clinical staff struggles a bit, Tim is pleased that he has a group of clerks who seem to be comfortable with their jobs, are well-trained, and seem to be able to handle the overwhelming challenges they are faced with each day in the clinic. It is one of the clerks, however, a young woman named Maggie Connelly, who has made it to the top of Tim's list of worries.

Maggie has been a clerk at the diabetes clinic for nearly 3 years. She works most specifically with the endocrinologists who have expressed their appreciation for her work. She's one of the few clerks working for Tim who can take the sometimes heated demands of the endocrinologists in stride. In fact, she shows no fear and has earned their respect. Tim's concern centers around a few comments made by one of Maggie's coworkers, who indicated that Maggie speaks and jokes openly with other clerks—all women—about sex, sometimes talking about her dates the night before. While no official complaints have come to Tim's attention, he has sensed from a couple of her coworkers that Maggie may be creating a situation that is uncomfortable for them. In the back of his mind, Tim knows that the entire endocrinology team will soon be moving to a new building. Maggie will be moving with them and will most likely be joined by another clerk who will be a new hire. She will no longer be working directly with the other clerks who have shown some concern.

William Peterson is the only male clerk in the four-clinic area and now works in the oncology area. William is a 22-year-old man who has worked in the oncology clinic for about 8 months. William has proven to be the type of individual who always solves problems. He is well liked by everyone he works with and Tim wishes that more of his employees had William's initiative. William is also the type of individual who likes to visit and joke with his coworkers.

While focusing on the diabetes clinic, prioritizing the problems he could begin to work on, Tim heard a knock on his door and found Maggie standing there.

"William's bugging me," she said. Maggie came in and began telling Tim she was feeling very uncomfortable with William. "He's always stopping by my station and making jokes about sex," she said. "Sometimes he touches me on the arm or shoulder and it really makes me feel uncomfortable. He does the same thing any time we both end up together in the break room or some other area of the clinics when no one is around."

"Wow, I haven't seen that in William when I'm around," said Tim. "Have you asked him to stop?"

"Well, no, not really," Maggie said.

"Tell me more about it. How long has this gone on?"

"Maybe for 2 or 3 weeks," Maggie answered.

"Have other people been around you when this has happened," Tim questioned?

"I don't think so."

"What would you like me to do?" Tim asked sincerely. He knew not to just ignore her, even though the irony of the situation struck him immediately.

"Well, I can't work here with him around," she answered.

What would you do in Tim's situation?

PART B

Tim has decided on a couple of alternative solutions to the problems presented by Maggie and William. First, Tim discussed with Maggie what she wanted him to do. She indicated that she just wanted William to leave her alone. She isn't asking that he be fired. As a result, Tim has spoken with William and indicated Maggie's concerns. William indicated that he was surprised to learn that Maggie was so bothered by what he considered friendly chats. In fact, he felt they had a good relationship. Tim suggested to William that he be courteous and respectful with Maggie, but avoid being alone with her. This not only protects Maggie, Tim thinks, but it will protect William from any allegations that aren't true since witnesses will be nearby.

Tim has also decided to pursue training for his entire staff. This training will include specifics about harassment, i.e. what it is, what it's not, policies surrounding the issues, the rights of those involved, how to document and report it, and other important concerns. A second type of training will focus on communication skills. Tim suspects that part of the problem in his clinic is due to the fact that some people might not be able to communicate that they are offended, and some, perhaps as in the case of William, may not know that what they say and do may be offensive to others.

As he is preparing his training outline and deciding how to approach his staff on this issue, Maggie again comes to his office. Now, she alleges, William has gone too far. She reports, "He grabbed my butt." Again, she has no witnesses.

Does this change what Tim should do? If so, what does he do now?

Seaside Convalescent Care Center

H. Wayne Nelson

Mindy Alternot has been the administrator of Seaside Convalescent Care Center (SCCC) for 7 months. This was her first job after earning her Nursing Home Administrator's license, and despite her initial enthusiasm, she began having second thoughts about her career choice. Things weren't going well at SCCC. Actually, things hadn't gone well there for several years. Mindy had hoped to turn things around, but the facility's last survey was terrible. The inspectors had found several deficiencies indicating a pattern of "potential for more than minimal harm" to the residents. There were other significant problems relating to resident care, resident rights, and quality of life. Consequently, SCCC was denied payment for new admissions and was being fined $3,000 a day for non-compliance.

Mindy blamed her nurse's aides (NAs). After all, they provided over 90% of the hands-on patient care. She found it nearly impossible to find good ones, and even when she did, she couldn't keep them. Their turnover rate was well over 100% a year (not rare in troubled facilities). Even those who seemed to enjoy working with the elderly would inevitably leave during the summer when it was easy to find more lucrative tourist-trade work.

Mindy had tried to motivate her aides by improving their training and by making their job more meaningful. She tried to encourage their input in matters related to patient care—and wanted to work with the licensed nurses to make the aides part of the total primary care team (which didn't sit well with the nurses). She wanted the aides to assume more responsibility for solving everyday resident problems. Moreover, she tried to build good relationships with them. She wanted to lead by being visible, available, engaged, and in tune with what was going on in the interactive caregiving environment. After 2 months of "beating her brains out" trying to build relationships, Mindy finally conceded to her Director of Nursing Services, Ann, that the task was hopeless. This was a bitter pill for Mindy who had been warned by Ann that "touchy feely schoolbook approaches," just wouldn't work with this crowd.

Ann was a top-notch nurse and a veteran nursing manager. She found the nurse's aides to be a sullen lot, generally, and very hard to manage. Her experience showed them to be young, immature, poorly educated, untrustworthy, undependable, and condescending (to residents), with very poor work habits and almost no motivation. "Besides," she complained "most of them barely speak English, and even those that can, don't really like working here—they do it only because they can't get work elsewhere."

Mindy didn't buy this at first, but quickly became frustrated by the aides' lack of commitment. Soon, she resigned herself to the fact that she couldn't develop the aides' competence, especially when they left even before they really got to know their jobs or the patients' individual needs. Moreover, because she had to maintain the minimum required staff-to-patient ratios, she couldn't be too choosey, and was compelled to hire warm bodies just to avoid fines.

Stressed, exhausted, and feeling defeated, Mindy began to resent her ignorant and "uncaring" nursing assistants, and began to avoid them. By her third month at SCCC she had delegated their direct oversight to Ann. Mindy felt that this was feasible because Ann had worked in nursing homes for years and had a clear vision and the strength of character to whip a poorly motivated work force into shape. Ann was a strict disciplinarian who understood how to deal with workers who only wanted a paycheck.

"You set clear rules and guidelines, you punish infractions, and you ride them all the time," she explained. "It sounds tough, but unskilled and reluctant workers need clear direction and they only respect strong, determined leadership. You know, there is such a thing as being too supportive—and this type of work force sees that type of boss as a sucker."

Ann set about to "clean the place up." But due to the high turnover and staff shortages, Ann required a good deal of overtime. Double-shifting was not uncommon. Ann knew that this would take a toll on the aides' resilience, but she reasoned that it's "better to use 'em while you got 'em, as they'll quit for better bait during the tourist season anyway."

This delegation of responsibility to Ann allowed Mindy to focus on managing the budget—where Mindy had excellent skills. In fact, she was highly adept at all the technical aspects of managing a nursing home. Do you think that this change in management responsibility will bode well for Seaside Convalescent?

Staffing at River Oaks Community Hospital: Measure Twice, Cut Once

Dawn M. Oetjen, Woody D. Richardson,
and Donna J. Slovensky

The CEO began the meeting. "The census for all units and all programs has decreased dramatically from 75% inpatient occupancy to just 50%. The Community Residential Center occupancy, formerly at 90%, has fallen to 40%; and we've dropped from 40 outpatients/partial hospitalizations a week to 15! With these decreased census numbers, we must make staff reductions." Now Debbie Davis, Director of Operations, and the other directors knew the reason for the emergency executive committee meeting. The CEO not only expressed concern, but also mandated that each of the directors make staff reductions in their departments. "Have your recommendations ready for tomorrow's regularly scheduled meeting, and remember no department shall remain untouched . . . period."

RIVER OAKS COMMUNITY HOSPITAL (ROCH)

River Oaks Community Hospital (ROCH) was a 70-bed, private, for-profit healthcare facility established to treat alcohol/drug abuse and mental illness. Built on vacant farmland, the facility, which had been in existence for 10 years, sat well hidden in a growing urban area surrounded by shopping malls and neighborhoods. Competing facilities and their proximity to ROCH are shown in Table 15-1.

ROCH had adult, youth, and residential inpatient units and outpatient and partial hospitalization programs. The adult unit, outpatient, and partial programs treated individuals 18 years of age and older. The youth unit, outpatient, and partial programs treated children from 3- to 17-years

TABLE 15-1   Market Area Facilities

Type of Facility/Programs	Miles Away
New private for-profit general hospital/inpatient and outpatient psychiatry units	2
Private for-profit alcohol and drug rehabilitation center	2
State-owned hospital/inpatient and outpatient psychiatric units	7
State-owned alcohol and drug treatment facility	10
Established private for-profit general hospital/inpatient and outpatient psychiatry units	10
Several private psychiatric practices offering outpatient programs	2–15
Private for-profit community residential program	50

of age. Some exceptions were made with 17- and 18-year-olds, depending on their maturity level (e.g., an immature 18-year-old might be placed on the youth unit and an independent, mature 17-year-old might be treated on the adult unit). The community residential center (CRC) was fairly unique in the clientele it treated. It treated very violent youths, ages 12 to 17, who needed long-term (4 months or longer) psychiatric and/or addiction treatment in a structured environment. The partial hospitalization program provided treatment for both adults and youths.

Outpatients reported to their respective units between the morning hours of 7:00 and 8:00 a.m. and were free to leave after the last session, usually around 5:00 p.m. The outpatient program provided adults and youths several group and individual sessions to choose from every week.

STAFFING

ROCH maintained around 100 employees working on 3 shifts (24-hour coverage), 7 days a week, and 365 days a year. The executive management team consisted of the Chief Executive Officer and Directors of Operations, Nursing/Clinical Staff, Finance, Marketing/Advancement, and Outpatient/CRC Services.

With a new master's degree in health administration and 8 years of experience in healthcare management, Debbie had been in her position as the Director of Operations for only a few weeks. Her responsibilities included the following departments: Medical Records (two full-time employee), Utilization Review (one full-time and one part-time employee), Quality Management, Risk Management, Housekeeping (two full-time employees), Maintenance (two full-time employees), Dietary Services (five full-time employees), Education/School (two full-time employees), and an administrative assistant (one full-time employee). Two of the departments, Quality Management and Risk Management, were not staffed, and Debbie was performing those duties.

ROCH, in addition to clinical treatment, also provided educational services with one full-time teacher for the youth unit and one for the CRC, and one full-time and one part-time dual-diagnosis educator for adults who acted as "counselors" for other adult patients. Two full-time activity therapists were also on staff to provide recreational and creative activities and programs throughout the day to all patients. The youth educators reported to Debbie while the dual-diagnosis educators reported to the Director of Nursing.

Despite the diverse clinical and special programs offered at ROCH, admissions were declining. This was partly due to the increasing competition from both inpatient and outpatient facilities (new and established) and private practice physicians (solo and group practices) in the area. A second cause was attributable to recent reimbursement changes due to an increased number of managed care-type insurers. These changes encouraged shorter lengths of inpatient stay with more intense treatments and more outpatient visits and partial hospitalizations. Whereas an inpatient may have been allowed 21 to 28 days of treatment in the past, current reimbursement allowed for 14 days.

THE REACTION

After the CEO left the conference room, Debbie looked around for reactions from the other directors. They looked dumbfounded, but only for a few seconds. Heated and emotional statements filled the air for the next 10 minutes. A sampling from the other directors included the following:

> I am already functioning with a skeleton crew. I cannot, no, make that *will* not, allow my staff to be cut anymore, it's just not safe! Sure, this might help meet today's budget, but what about a few months down the line? Fire today, re-hire tomorrow, then fire 'em again—that's a great way to build a quality staff.

Debbie chimed in with "I'm already doing two of my employees' jobs in addition to my own . . . if we keep these cutbacks up, I'm going to be admitted here myself."

DEBBIE'S DILEMMA

Debbie left the conference room, went to her office, and closed the door. Was it too late to return her diploma and sign up for a residency instead? Her mind (and eyes) wandered out to the courtyard where she saw a few of her employees eating lunch. These same employees had, just 2 days ago, shared with her their concerns of downsizing and their feelings of being overwhelmed with their workloads. They had asked Debbie to consider hiring some temporary staff to help them get caught up, and she agreed to look into it. At the time, it did not seem unreasonable, even with low census numbers, due to a scheduled site visit from the Joint Commission for Accreditation of Healthcare Organizations (JCAHO) less than a year away. She had planned on requesting temporary help for the Quality Management, Medical Record, and Maintenance Departments. Quality Management and Medical Record requirements for the JCAHO were some of the most important, detailed, and time-consuming parts of the entire survey. She knew extra attention and time should be given to each area for 1 to 2 years prior to the survey and with less than a year until the visit, ROCH was already behind. Maintenance also needed extra staff to ensure that the facility was in compliance in terms of safety, cleanliness, and appearance.

With this new mandate, not only were these moot points, but Debbie now needed to consider how to "get blood from a stone." She had one day to create a new staffing plan for her departments that reflected the required staff reductions. She pulled out the "cheat sheet" that she had created to help her identify each of her employees (Table 15-2) and the staffing sheet (Table 15-3) she was given at the meeting only an hour ago. It was going to be a long night.

TABLE 15-2 Staff Profiles for Debbie's Direct Reports at ROCH

Name	Department/Position	Full or Part Time	Years with ROCH	Years in Field	Sex	Age	Performance Appraisal Score (4 being best)
S. Buford, RRA	Medical Records/Supervisor	Full	8	17	F	49	3.25
D. Fitzgerald	Medical Records/Clerk	Full	3	13	F	52	3.5
S. Carpenter	Medical Records/Transcriptionist	Part	2	5	F	27	3
M. Burke	Housekeeping/Housekeeper	Full	10.0	35	F	58	4
T. Snyder	Housekeeping/Housekeeper	Full	7	10	F	32	2.75
D. Bogues	Maintenance/Interior Specialist	Full	10	20	M	41	4
T. Dimatteo	Maintenance/Exterior Specialist	Full	1.5	22	M	40	3.25
A. Pensa	Dietary—Cafeteria/Cook	Full	10	37	M	55	2.75
J. Jones	Dietary—Cafeteria/Cook	Full	3	6	M	28	3.75
P. Tucker	Dietary—Cafeteria/Server, Preparer	Full	10	20	F	37	4
C. Black	Dietary—Cafeteria	Full	1	3	F	24	3
T. Burns	Dietary—Cafeteria/Server, Preparer	Full	2.5	8	M	32	3
M. Carter, RD	Dietary—Cafeteria/Dietician	Full	1	7	F	29	3.75
Y. Fredericks, RN	Utilization Review/Case Reviewer	Full	10	20	F	42	4
B. Stephens, LPN	Utilization Review/Case Reviewer	Part	6	12	F	36	3.75
P. Johnson	School—Education/Teacher (youth unit)	Full	10	12	F	34	4
B. Patterson	School—Education/Teacher (CRC unit)	Full	3	22	F	45	3.75
P. Stanton	Administrative/Assistant	Full	7	25	F	47	3

TABLE 15-3 ROCH Staffing Report

Department Positions	Shifts		
	7:00 a.m.–3:00 p.m.	3:00 p.m.–11:00 p.m.	11:00 p.m.–7:00 a.m.
Nursing			
R.N. (nurse)	**6** (2/2/2)	**6** (2/2/2)	**3** (1/1/1)
R.N. Supervisors	2	2	1
P.C.A. (patient care assistant)	3 (1/1/1)	3 (1/1/1)	3 (1/1/1)
A.T. (activity therapist)	2	—	—
S.W. (social work)	3 (1/1/1)	—	—
S.W. Supervisor	1	—	—
Intake (admission screeners)	2	1	1 (on call)
Intake Supervisor	1	—	—
D.D. (dual diagnosis educators)	1.5	—	—
Nursing Director	1	(on call)	(on call)
Operations			
M.R. (medical records)	1.5	—	—
M.R. Supervisor	1	—	—
Maintenance	2	(on call)	(on call)
Housekeeping	2	—	—
Dietary—Cafeteria	3	2	—
Dietician	1	—	—
Q.M. (quality management)	(vacant)		
R.M. (risk management)	(vacant)		
U.R. (utilization review)	1.5	—	—
Teachers—School	2	—	—
Administrative Assistant	1	—	—
Operations Director	1	(on call)	(on call)
Marketing			
Marketing Associates	2	—	—
Administrative Assistant	1	—	—
Marketing Director	1	—	—
Finance			
Business Office Staff	7	1	—
Operator	1	1	—
Business Office Supervisor	1	—	—
Administrative Assistant	1	1	—
Finance Director	1	—	—
Outpatient/CRC			
Staff	2	1	1
CRC Supervisor	1	(on call)	(on call)
Outpatient Supervisor	1	—	—
Administrative Assistant	1	—	—
Director	1	(on call)	(on call)
Administrative			
CEO	1	—	—
Administrative Assistant	1	—	—

Heritage Valley Medical Center: Are Your Managers Culturally Competent?

Velma Roberts

Heritage Valley Medical Center was very proud of its reputation for providing quality services for all citizens in the community. Over the last 20 years, the Medical Center had flourished, and both staff and health professionals in the organization were committed to its shared values and its respect for all patients and their families. Services were provided to a community whose residents were 80% Caucasian, 15% African American, and 5% Hispanic. However, in the last 5 years, the population had gradually changed to 50% Caucasian, 40% African American, and 10% Hispanic and Asian American. The Center's occupancy rates were down to 40%, given that many of their traditional, more affluent, private-pay patients had moved out into the suburbs to escape the urban sprawl that comes with development.

The Medical Center administrator first noticed a change when the patient mix became more diverse. After the State Health Indigent Care Fund was established, Medicaid reimbursement increased, making it comparable to those of managed care organizations. It was strategically imperative to capture this new market and these potential revenues, particularly since most of the indigent and Medicaid recipients were minorities. Heritage Valley started a major marketing campaign and developed alliances with physicians, community clinics, and public health agencies to increase their referrals of Medicaid and indigent patients to capitalize on this new source of revenue.

By year 3 of this strategic initiative, the increase in minority patients had jumped from approximately 10% to 40% (primarily African American and Hispanics). Many of the Hispanics were immigrants with work permits for the construction boom in the affluent areas of the county and surrounding suburbs. Even though there was an increase in minority patients, the ethnicity of the service providers remained at their previous levels. Eighty-five percent of the clinical staff members, including physicians, nurses, laboratory technologists, pharmacists, and therapists were Caucasian. There were two African-American managers and one Hispanic manager. The executive management team was 100% Caucasian, with one female. The majority of the support and administrative staff (secretaries, human resource technicians, nurse's aides) were African American. In some of the support areas (e.g., dietary or environmental services), the staff was 100% African American. There was little turnover, and the clinical and support staff were like family, since the majority of them had worked at Heritage for over 15 years, and shared similar values and principles about valuing every patient and treating each patient with respect.

At a management meeting with administrative directors and the Vice President of Community Relations, Ms. Harper, shared the results of a recent patient satisfaction survey which indicated that while 80% of the Caucasian patients were very satisfied with their care, only 30% of African Americans, 10% of Hispanics, and 20% of Asians were satisfied. She was very concerned about the reasons for dissatisfaction. At the top of the list for all three ethnic groups was the reason "I don't feel welcomed here." The second was "people talk down to me," and the third was "the nurses don't seem to understand me." When asked for feedback and how to improve these results, the nursing director immediately defended her staff. She made it clear that she had one of the most caring, attentive, and qualified nursing staffs in the county. She could not understand how these minority patients could be so ungrateful.

"These people will never be satisfied unless they can get something for nothing. Half of them can't even speak English and the others mess up the King's English so badly you don't know what they want. We can't help it if these people are uneducated, can't speak the language, and don't know how to communicate with professional people. My nurses and nurse aides are doing the best they can to work with these people, even when they are too limited to understand basic information."

Following this feedback, several other managers also voiced their support for the nursing staff because their employees had complained about these same issues. They wanted to let the vice president know their opinions, of which the following comments were representative:

- Most of these patients won't even look us in the eye. We can hardly get any information out of them.
- It takes twice as long to deal with Hispanics and Asians because they can barely speak English. They should learn to speak English and get with the program. It's not the employees' fault that these people can't speak the language.
- There is absolutely no excuse for those Black patients. They were born here and still cannot speak English. We have done everything for them—given them a free ride for education, jobs, and housing. If anything, they are driving away our few remaining paying patients with their loud conversations and by bringing family members and children with them who are always acting ghetto and foolish.
- These patients are not satisfied? Has anybody considered what *we* have to put up with? These people are just ungrateful complainers!

The two African-American managers were asked what they thought about the patients' feedback. Both of them agreed with their colleagues, saying:

Those Hispanics and Asians need to learn how to speak English. This is America—what do they expect? We can only do so much. As for those Asians, they should speak up and stop being so passive. You can't get them to talk; they bring every family member with them and they speak Chinese or Vietnamese while you're trying to help them. Sometimes I think they are talking about us right in front of our faces. Plus, they think they are better than other minorities; they are cliquish and they don't want to be a part of anything. How can we ever understand them when they won't talk to us?

The male Hispanic manager was very upset about the African Americans and Caucasians feedback about Hispanics. He felt that Hispanic patients were being unnecessarily targeted because they were the most vulnerable. He knew that they were hard-working people just trying to make a living doing work no one else would. To blame them for the way they felt about their treatment at the Medical Center was wrong. He went on to say the following:

How dare the African-American managers say anything? They are only here because of affirmative action and diversity initiatives. The only reason they are agreeing with the White managers is because they want to keep their jobs. The Blacks are ashamed of their culture and are afraid to be associated with the low income Black patients, even though they probably came from the same ghetto neighborhood.

Ms. Harper was completely shocked and dismayed at the responses of these managers. As she left the meeting, she was at a loss as to how to explain these attitudes to the Medical Center's executive team. And more importantly, what could be done to change these managers' beliefs and attitudes about minority patients? Or was it too late?

Humor Strategies in Healthcare Management Education

Rosalind Trieber

Educators and managers have a critical role in creating a learning environment that initiates emotion, attracts attention, creates meaning, and subsequently, builds lasting memories. When we learn in such a rich environment, it then becomes possible to apply what we've learned to a real life situation. Research demonstrates that there is a significant correlation between humor and leadership effectiveness (Priest & Swain, 2002). Organizational culture supports the use of humor by leaders in appropriate ways. In addition, the humor employed by managers and leaders achieves three specific ends: 1) it reduces stress in the workplace, 2) it helps employees understand management concerns by enhancing communication patterns, and 3) it motivates followers (Davis & Kleiner, 1989). A majority of good leaders are shown to have quick wit, see the point of jokes, maintain group morale through extraverted humor vs. mean-spirited humor, have infectious laughs, and tell humorous satires in dialect (Priest & Swain).

The greatest challenge in the college classroom is to prevent death by lecture with material that is thought to be boring, difficult, and stress-producing. According to Mehrabian's Communication Model, what determines a speaker's impact on an audience is based on the following: (a) *what* you say accounts for 7%; (b) *how* you say it accounts for 38%; and (c) how you *look* accounts for 55%. The rate of retention of material also varies, depending upon the instruction mode used, as follows: (a) lecture and reading—15% retention rate; (b) audio-visual—20%; (c) demonstration—30%;

(d) discussion group—50%; (e) practice by doing—75%; and (f) teaching others—90% (NTL Institute for Applied Behavioral Science, n.d.).

Humor and collaborative strategies have a significant role in teaching. The goal of collaborative learning is to develop autonomous, articulate, thinking people (Sawyer, 2004).

The use of humor in the classroom has the ability to grab students' attention, increase interest in the topic, make topic learning fun, and facilitate understanding of the topic (Berk, 2003).

How can educators use effective humor strategies to help students learn to develop the capacity to relate effectively to others, cooperate and achieve agreed outcomes, as well as develop an understanding of themselves and of the groups (teams) to which they belong? Studies suggest that people learn in direct proportion to how much fun they are having (Pike, 1989). The following case study of a health care management team combines both fun and learning by using exaggeration in a dramatization, combined with exaggerated non-verbal behavior, spontaneous responses, and class participation.

CASE: TO DISCHARGE OR NOT TO DISCHARGE (KOPPET, 2001)

Overview

All participants, other than the interpreter, are instructed to speak in a nonsense language, as if they are from a foreign country or cannot speak the same language. Gibberish can be anything, such as blah, blah, unah, hoah, etc. Everyone practices a minute of gibberish to get the idea.

Topic Identification

In this case the patient did not want to be discharged from the hospital. The daughter was not sure about the options her mother had in terms of recovery. The surgeon and occupational health therapist felt the patient was ready to go home, with an occupational therapist making home visits.

The Task

The task is to provide explanations to both the patient and her daughter as to why the patient would have a successful recovery having the occupational therapist make home visits.

Players

Five volunteers and the remaining students in the class assume the roles below:

- A 65-year-old hospitalized female recovering from hip replacement surgery who does not speak English.
- A 30-year-old female daughter of the patient who had a hip replacement and does not speak English.
- An occupational health therapist assigned to the case who does not speak the same language as the patient or her daughter.
- The surgeon who only speaks English.
- An interpreter who speaks the foreign language of the patient and her daughter as well as English.
- The remaining students in the class.

Procedure

The case role play should proceed as follows:

- The *patient*, in very animated body language and with multiple inflections using gibberish, explains her concerns.
- The *interpreter* explains the patient's concerns in English to everyone.
- The *daughter* responds with her concerns with animated body language and gibberish.
- The *interpreter* explains the daughter's concerns, in English, to everyone.
- The *occupational* therapist explains how she can be helpful to both the patient and the daughter, in gibberish.
- The *surgeon* explains to everyone his prognosis and how accessible he would be if necessary, in gibberish.

Tips and Added Guidelines:

While conducting the dramatization, keep in mind the following:

- The only person who speaks English is the interpreter.
- The class also has the opportunity to ask questions that can be interpreted into gibberish by the interpreter.
- This process can last from 5–10 minutes.

- Whatever is said in gibberish or English is correct.
- The idea is to accept the information (that which is being said), acknowledge it, add more information, and lead to new discoveries.
- The interpretations should be based on the information taught in class.

Questions

The following questions are intended to facilitate learning.

- These questions are to be asked of the volunteers and the class:
  - What communication cues do we have other than words?
  - Did the translation match the interpretations you made in your heads?
  - What did you learn about the group in general?
  - How did people contribute to the success?
  - How did you feel about what you communicated to the group?
  - How or what helped you learn?
  - What did you learn?
- These questions are asked specifically of the volunteers who played the specific roles:
  - How did it feel to communicate without words?
  - How do you feel about what you created as a group?

Outcomes

Below is a list of desired outcomes of this case study:

- Everyone is involved.
- Team building occurs because everyone is helping each other be successful.
- Everyone is actively listening to one another.
- There is a conscious review of the material needed taught by the instructor.
- Participants learn to think spontaneously and recover from mistakes.
- Everyone has fun and rarely forgets the substantive learning points.

REFERENCES

Berk, R.A. (2003). *Professors are from Mars® and students are from Snickers®*. Sterling, VA: Stylus Publishing.

Davis, A., & Kleiner, B. H. (1989).The value of humor in effective leadership. *Leadership and Organizational Development Journal, 10*(1), 1–3.

Koppet, K. (2001). *Training to imagine*. Sterling, VA: Stylus Publishing.

NTL Institute for Applied Behavioral Science (NTL). (n.d.). http://www.ntl.org/

Pike, B. (1989). *Creative training techniques: Tips, tactics, and how-to's for delivering effective training*. Minneapolis, MN: Lakewood.

Priest, R., & Swain, J. E. (2002). Humor and leadership effectiveness. *HUMOR: International Journal of Humor Research, 15*(2), 169–189.

Sawyer, R. K. (2004). Creative teaching: Collaborative discussion as disciplined improvisation. *Educational Researcher, 33*(2), 12–20.

Electronic Medical Records in a Rural Family Practice Residency Program

Carla Wiggins
Emilie Cellucci

Family Practice Medicine (FPM) is a family practice residency program associated with a state university located in the U.S. intermountain west and with a neighboring hospital, Rural Medical Center (RMC). Physician residencies are post-doctoral training programs and a physician doing post-doctoral training in the specialty of Family Practice completes a 3-year residency program. FPM describes itself as "committed to clinical excellence, academic productivity, fiscal responsibility, and service to our supporting institutions and the community."

In the late 1990s, physicians at FPM were evaluating strategies to assist them in clinical medical research. Determining that the primary impediment was their paper medical records system, they began to seek grant funding to establish an Electronic Medical Record (EMR). After receiving the grant, the director of FPM, Dr. Joe Clark, brought together a committee composed of local practitioners, the university, and the hospital to assess system needs. This committee evaluated a number of systems, narrowing them to three viable, wireless-enabled, EMR systems. Eventually, Centricity from General Electric was selected.

Recognizing the difficulty in obtaining qualified professional IT staff in a rural environment with wage constraints, FPM hired a graduating senior from the university, Anne Wright, to provide the principle IT support throughout the initial implementation and subsequent rolling out of additional features. Wright created specifications for the necessary system infrastructure, and priced the system. A wireless network configuration using Dell computers as a backbone was acquired, as well as tablet PC's and other necessary software to further enable a wireless EMR.

To help facilitate system implementation, Clark contacted professional colleagues and a family medical practice in the northern area of the state to provide guidance for her staff. Eventually, this became an ad hoc steering committee for system implementation, and all potential configuration conflicts were deferred to this group.

In addition to being responsible for the acquisition and performance of the hardware and software, Wright was also the project manager for EMR implementation, coordinating the entering of patient information and system integrations. Additional functions of Wright's position included network administration and support, as well as training for the system. She also implemented interfaces between the hospital's system and Centricity, and a medical voice recognition system.

The project was initiated by sending one of the third-year residents, Jack Hopkins, to the northern part of the state to observe the use of the Centricity system. Upon his return, a project task of entering data for each patient's last three visits was initiated, starting with the letter A. Because FPM cut back on appointments in this phase, some headway was made in entering patient information. However, it was winter, and the cold and flu season was upon the state. The strategy was altered and a full appointment schedule reinstated, to provide necessary patient healthcare. Prior to patients' arrivals, their information and the data from their last three appointments were recorded into the system. After this "stop-gap" data entry, the entering of the patient records from A-Z was continued. This forced the physicians to utilize the system early on, weaning them from the paper system. An additional facet of the EMR was to have remote system access for the physicians. Simultaneously, Wright and Hopkins assisted the faculty and residents in system training and home computer access, creating a consistent operating environment at remote computing sites.

Wright began to create a series of system interfaces between Centricity and the various hospital systems. For example, laboratory results from the hospital were immediately input into the system, being instantly available for analysis. With each feature added by Wright, with each milestone of data entry accomplished, the physicians and residents began to rely completely upon the new system. Wright then supervised the remodeling of the file room and directed the removal of all paper records.

As the project moved forward, discussions began regarding the extension of the EMR to additional clinics and the initial goal of enhancing research capabilities began to broaden. By creating remote accessibility, Wright had demonstrated the feasibility of extending the EMR to other intermountain west clinics in the region and state. This ability to extend the EMR to remote sites set the stage for the greater goal of leading EMR implementation for rural healthcare providers in the state.

There were a number of drivers for the emergence of the larger goal. First, the goal of improved quality and availability of the data had been satisfied. Second, FPM was beginning to realize improved healthcare delivery with the data now easily available to them, both while meeting with patients, and then later when analyzing patient data. Third, it was obvious to FPM that healthcare services might be enhanced throughout the state by the implementation of EMR in local and regional clinics. Most local clinics could not afford the upfront costs of IT investment. If FPM could help rural providers overcome the barrier of the initial financial investment, FPM could have a strong positive impact on the health of the citizens of the state.

Looking forward, it is Wright's belief that by implementing an EMR at the residency program and by creating an adequate infrastructure, the EMR at FPM can be expanded to handle a practice management system for the entire rural clinic network. She envisions a resource that can be shared with little capital investment on the part of the other clinics.

DISCUSSION POINTS

1. Three overarching competencies skilled health IT professionals need to possess are:
   a) Environmental Knowledge
   b) Understanding of Healthcare Data, Structure, and Content
   c) Administration and Leadership Abilities in Information Management

   Are these competencies demonstrated in this case study, and if so, by whom?

2. In addition to the hospital and the university, who are FPM's stakeholders? Create a stakeholder map and describe the attributes of each relationship.

3. Create a job description for Anne Wright. She is a critical point for success or failure. What does that mean? Provide examples.

4. How would you measure the success of the residency's EMR thus far? What would you measure and how would you measure it?
5. Discuss FPM's original goal, and how and why it expanded. Create a new and improved goal statement for the expanded goal.

Evaluate the process by which Anne Wright implemented the changes she made. Can you suggest any improvements? The physicians and the residents began to rely upon the new system quickly. Why do you think the outcome was one of support for Anne as opposed to resistance to the changes?

Medication Errors Reporting at Community Memorial Hospital

Eric Williams
Grant Savage

Francis Ballentine, RN, MSN, VP for Nursing Services, has a problem. A recent Joint Commission inspection found several deficiencies at her hospital, including incomplete reporting of medication errors. The CEO gave her 6 months to fix this situation. Francis, who had been on the job for less than a year, already knew that the reporting of medication errors was problematic. She often found it difficult to complete her own monthly report on the number and causes of medication errors. She did not receive timely incident reports from every department, and many times these reports were incomplete. She also suspected that some incidents were going unreported.

In her investigation, Francis learned that although there was a clearly defined process (Figure 15-8) in the procedure manuals that each floor used, the process seemed to be inconsistently applied when a medication error occurred. She also knew that there were some other issues, but could not pin them down without some additional investigation. From her observations, she estimated that 20–30% of medication error incident reports were not completed correctly, not completed on a timely basis, or not completed at all.

The next step of her investigation was to discuss the situation with the Director of Quality Improvement, Ally Ray. Together they agreed it would be worth creating a QI team to study the current work process of "reporting medication errors." The discussion ended with Ally asking Frances to put together the necessary information to present to the hospital's quality council for approval of the QI project. In the next quality council meeting, the Medication Errors Quality Improvement (MEQI) project was approved.

The initial meeting of the MEQI project team consisted of representatives from the pharmacy and the six hospital units (north, south, east,

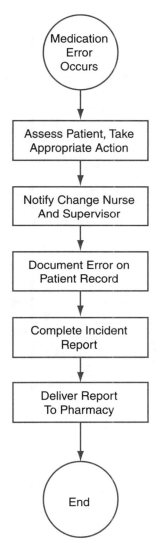

FIGURE 15-8 Medication Error Reporting Flowchart

west, northeast, southeast) who were knowledgeable about the reporting of medication errors. The meeting was devoted to training on basic TQM/CQI principles and tools. The group decided to use the FOCUS-PDCA framework as their guide for completing the MEQI project. The group had clearly completed the first two steps: *F* (Find a process to improve) and *O* (Organize a team that knows the process).

The second meeting focused on the *C* part of the framework—to clarify current knowledge of the process. Several MEQI members were surprised when Francis pulled out the current medication error reporting process (Figure 15-8). In preparation for the third meeting, each team member was asked to develop a cause and effect chart (Fishbone or Ishikawa diagram; Figure 15-11) based on their discussions with other unit members. This began work on the *U* part of the framework—to understand the sources of variation. Additionally, the six hospital units were asked to create a daily checklist of medication errors for the month of July (Figure 15-10). Pharmacy would keep a corresponding checklist of medical error incident reports received (Figure 15-9). Comparing the two checklists would allow for the identification of the number of missing reports and reveal other patterns.

The third meeting turned out to be a fruitful one. To open the meeting, Francis presented a chart (Figure 15-9) showing the incident reports received from each unit for each day in July, 2003. She also showed the corresponding checklist of medication errors from each unit (Figure 15-10). A comparison of these two charts revealed three things: 1) only 66% of er-

Unit	T 1	W 2	T 3	F 4	S 5	S 6	M 7	T 8	W 9	T 10	F 11	S 12	S 13	M 14	T 15	W 16	T 17	F 18	S 19	S 20	M 21	T 22	W 23	T 24	F 25	S 26	S 27	M 28	T 29	W 30	T 31
N	1		1		1	1	1			1		1	1	1	1			2		1				2				1		1	
S				1	1		1	2		1		1	1	1		1			1			1			2		1				
E		2		1			1	1			1						1							1							
W							1						1	1			1		1				1		1				1		
NE	1		1			2		1		1	1		1	1			1	1	1						1			2			
SE					1				2							1						1									1

FIGURE 15-9 Report Received by Pharmacy for July

Unit	T 1	W 2	T 3	F 4	S 5	S 6	M 7	T 8	W 9	T 10	F 11	S 12	S 13	M 14	T 15	W 16	T 17	F 18	S 19	S 20	M 21	T 22	W 23	T 24	F 25	S 26	S 27	M 28	T 29	W 30	T 31
N	1		1	1	1	1	1			1		1	1	1	1			2	1	1				2	2	1	1	1		1	
S	1		1	1	1	1	1	2		1		1	1	1	1	1			1	1		1	1				2				
E		2		1		1	1	1			1	2					1			1				1		1				1	
W	1			1	1	1	1				1		1	1		1	1	1	1				1		1		1	1	1	1	
NE	1	2	1	1	1	2		1		1	1	1	1	2	1		1	1	1						2		1	2	1		
SE					1				2					1	1	1	1	1	1			1									2

FIGURE 15-10 Combined Unit Checklists for July

rors identified on the unit checksheet were also reported on the pharmacy checksheet; 2) the east, west, and southeast units had the poorest reporting record; and 3) the number of errors reported declined during the weekends.

After a break, each team member reported on their cause and effect diagram and the team, after several hours of discussion, created a composite cause and effect diagram (Figure 15-11). As a further refinement to the diagram, each of the ten team members was asked to vote for the two most important causes of problems in the medication errors reporting process (these are indicated by the stars that appear next to a number of the process problems identified in the cause and effect diagram; more stars reflect more votes that the problem is serious). The composite cause and effect diagram (Figure 15-11) shows three principle causes: 1) vague policy (5 votes), 2) vague forms (4 votes), and 3) nurses unsure of reporting procedure (4 votes).

The *S* part (*Select a solution*) began with Francis asking the team to individually create a list of potential solutions. A composite list of solutions was then created and discussed. From this discussion a two-prong solution emerged. The committee decided to 1) revise the policy and forms and 2) retrain all staff on the policy and forms with special attention to the three problem floors and weekend staff.

Once the solution was determined, the team moved to the *P* part (*Plan the solution*) of the PDCA cycle. In the fifth team meeting, Francis tasked two subgroups to make specific plans about how to carry out the plan. The first subgroup recommended that the QI team implement the policy and form revision and a second group, made up of human resources staff, would design and implement a Web-based training program. Over the next three meetings, the QI team focused on revising the policy and forms. Once this was done, the human resources staff prepared the Web-based training program.

The *D* or "*Do*" part of the process began with a general announcement to the hospital staff and a series of meetings between the QI team and the nurse manager of each wing to discuss the implementation of the new policy, forms, and training program. Over the next month (September), each floor was familiarized with the policy and forms, reinforced with the on-line training program. The committee set a goal of 95% of medication errors being reported on time. To see if this goal would be met, checksheets,

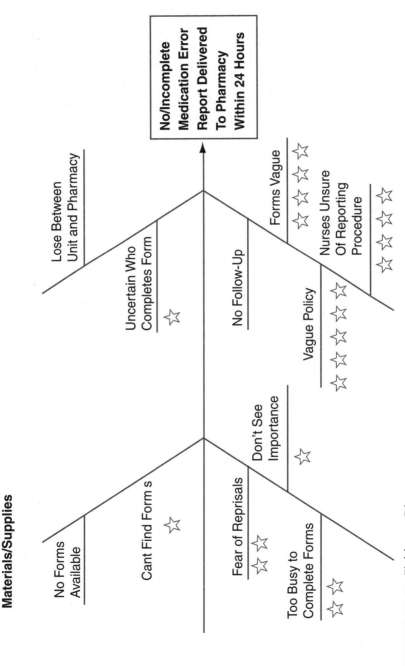

FIGURE 15-11 Fishbone Diagram

like those prepared for July, were also prepared for September through December.

The *C* or "*Check*" part of the cycle began with an initial examination of the September data, which revealed a modest improvement, with 72% of medication error reports received (up from 66% in July),but showing the same problems with certain units and the weekend shift. The QI team was somewhat dismayed by the results and felt that the online training was not being taken seriously. The team then asked the CEO to meet with the wing nurse managers to reinforce the importance of medication error reporting. The October data revealed that 87% of medication error reports were received and that the three problem units improved considerably. The weekend reporting problem remained. The data showed improvement through November and December, with 93% and 96% of medication errors being properly reported. The three problem units still had lower reporting rates, but the gap had narrowed considerably. The weekend reporting remained somewhat lower than the weekday report.

The *A* or "*Act*" part (Acting to hold gains) began in mid-January with a meeting between the CEO and the QI team. The CEO praised the team's hard work and success. One member of the QI team asked about the weekend problem. Both the CEO and QI team recognized this as an issue, but decided to continue to monitor the reporting process via the two checksheets. They did ask the human resource department to continue to use the online training program in their orientation sessions. At the end of this meeting, the QI team disbanded. Francis continued to monitor the reporting process while Ally moved on to helping other QI teams within the hospital.

INDEX

A

AACN (American Association of Colleges of Nursing), 247–248

AAMC (American Association of Medical Colleges), 232

AAN (American Academy of Nursing), 19t

ABC Inventory method, 223

ABMS (American Board of Medical Specialists), 235

Abuse
  antitrust issues, 364
  in billing for services, 358
  Criminal-Disclosure Provision of Social Security Act and, 360–362
  definition of, 358
  EMTALA and, 362–363
  Operation Restore Trust and, 358, 359–360

Accept/reject decision, 228

Access to care restrictions, for health insurance, 163

ACCME (Accreditation Council for Continuing Medical Education), 233

Accounting
  financial, 198
  managerial, 198

Accounts receivable management, 219–221, 220t

Accreditation Council for Continuing Medical Education (ACCME), 233

Accreditation Council for Graduate Medical Education (ACGME), 233

Accreditation of hospitals, 88–89, 140

Accrediting agencies, 200

Accrediting agency, initiatives for system improvement, 113–114

ACGME (Accreditation Council for Graduate Medical Education), 233

ACHCA (American College of Health Care Administrators), 19t

ACHE. *See* American College of Healthcare Executives

ACHE (American College of Healthcare Executives), 17–18, 18t, 19t

Achievement, need for, 27

ACPE (American College of Physician Executives), 19t

Acquired Needs Theory of McClelland, 27

Act, in FOCUS-PDCA framework, 101

Action Inquiry, 52

Active errors, 109

Activities of daily living (ADLs), 251

Activity-based costing, 213

Adam's Equity Theory, 28

Adjourning, of teams, 312

ADLs (activities of daily living), 251

Administrative skills, for information technology professionals, 149–150

Advanced practice nurses (APNs), 253–255

Advertising methods, for, recruitment, 279–280

Advocating, in Tobert's Action Inquiry, 52

Affiliation, need for, 27

Age/aging
  cultural views on, 333
  health/medial care needs and, 269
  uninsured population and, 189, 190t

Age Discrimination in Employment Act, 274t

Agency for Healthcare Research and Quality (AHRQ), 112, 116

Agent Orange, 186

AHRQ (Agency for Healthcare Research and Quality), 112, 116

AICPA (American Institute of Certified Public Accountants), 369

Airlines industry team building model, 316

Alderfer's ERG Theory, 26

Allied health professionals, 232, 234, 255–257

AMA (American Medical Association), 159, 176, 306

Ambiguity, 47

Ambulatory Surgery Centers (ASCs), safe harbor regulations, 367–368

"Amenities of care," 83–84

American Academy of Nursing (AAN), 19*t*
American Association of Colleges of Nursing
        (AACN), 247–248
American Association of Medical Colleges
        (AAMC), 232
American Board of Medical Specialists (ABMS),
        235
American College of Health Care Administrators
        (ACHCA), 19*t*
American College of Healthcare Executives
        (ACHE), 17–18, 18*t*, 19*t*
American College of Physician Executives
        (ACPE), 19*t*
American College of Surgeons' Hospital
        Standardization Program, 88
American Dental Association, 88
American Health Information Community,
        establishing, 123
American Institute of Certified Public
        Accountants (AICPA), 369
American Medical Association (AMA), 159, 176,
        306
American Nurses Association (ANA), 248
American Nurses' Credentialing Center Magnet
        Recognition Program, 248
Americans with Disabilities Act (ADA), 274*t*
ANA (American Nurses Association), 248
Analyze, in DMAIC, 102
Analyzing processes, for data collection,
        107–108
ANCC Commission on Accreditation, 249
Ancillary staff, 234
Antibiotics, overuse of, 85
Anti-Dumping Act. *See* Emergency Medical
        Treatment and Active Labor Act
Anti-Kickback statutes, 365–367, 369
Antitrust issues, 364
Any Willing Provider laws (AWP), 352
APNs (advanced practice nurses), 253–255
Artifacts, in organizational culture, 327
ASCs (Ambulatory Surgery Centers), safe harbor
        regulations, 367–368
Asian cultures, 333
Assault, 348
Assessments, flawed, 43
Association for University Programs in Health
        Administration (AUPHA), 19*t*
Assumptions, sharing, 48–49
Attention processes, perceptions and, 42–43
Attribution error, 45–46

Attribution theory, 45–46
AUPHA (Association for University Programs in
        Health Administration), 19*t*
Automated patient billing, 138
Autonomy, 345
Avoidance learning, 27
AWP laws (Any Willing Provider laws), 352

B
Bad debt, 210
Balanced Budget Act of 1997 (BBA)
        enforcement tools, 363–364
        key provisions, 171–172
        Medicaid and, 177, 181
        Medicare and, 176, 209
Baldrige, Malcolm, 96
Bar coding, 144
Bargaining, in teams, 319
Barriers, to strategy execution, 75
Basic health insurance policies, 162
Batched information requests, 139
Battery, 348
BBA. *See* Balanced Budget Act of 1997
Beginning-of-life care, 353–354
Beliefs
        perceptual expectations, 44–45
        sharing with others, 49–50
Belonging needs, 26
Benchmarking, 89, 221, 284
Beneficence, 345–346
"Best practices," 83, 89
Beta blockers, underuse of, 84
Bias, 49
Billing for services, fraud and abuse in, 358
Bioethics, 17
BLS (Bureau of Labor Statistics), 231–232
Board certified physicians, 235
Board eligible physicians, 235–236
Board of directors, 14, 202–204
BPQA (State Boards of Physician Quality
        Assurance), 234
Breach of duty, 348
Break-even point, 213–214
Bridge to Excellence (BTE), 114–116, 124
Budget calendar, 225
Budgeting
        definition of, 224
        importance of, 224–225
Budget management, 224–228
Budget period, 224

Budgets
definition of, 224
types of, 225–226
Bundle payments, for hospital and physician
services, 206
Bureau of Labor Statistics (BLS), 231–232
Business Associate Agreement, 383
Business process reengineering, 102–103

C
Canadian Medical Association, 88
Capital assets, long-term investments in, 200
Capital budgeting, 226–228
Capital budgets, 226–227
Capital rationing, 228
Capitated financing systems, 124
Capitated rate, 164
Capitation, 206, 209
Care indicators, 89–90
Care Management for High Cost Beneficiaries,
127
Care processes
effective, 118–119
non-routine, 119–120
routine types, 119
Case flow, 218
Case mix, 208
Case studies, 383–447
effective participation, guidelines for, 377–378
evaluation criteria, 379f
group presentations, peer evaluation criteria
for, 380f
guidelines for, 375–377
on Management Information System,
384–385
on managing healthcare professionals,
389–390
merger of two competing hospitals, 397–403
purpose of, 375
teammate evaluation forms, 381f
team structure and process for completion, 377
Cash advances, 219
Cash budgets, 225–226
Cash conversion cycle, 218
Cash inflows, 226
Cash outflows, 226
Catastrophic coverage health insurance policies,
162
Causation, in tort, 348
CBCs (criminal background checks), 235, 244

Center for Quality Improvement and Patient
Safety, 116
Centers for Medicare and Medicaid Services
(CMS)
accreditation and, 141
enforcement of EMTALA, 362
healthcare payments and, 65, 125
healthcare system improvement and, 90, 116
Medicaid cost control measures, 180–181
Medicare financing and, 174
national healthcare expenditures, 156–157,
156t
Premier Hospital Quality Incentive
Demonstration, 125
reimbursements for hospital services, 207–208
CEO (Chief Executive Officer), 152, 203
Certified Nurse Midwives (CNMs), 254–255
Certified nurses' aides (CNAs), 251–253
Certified Registered Nurse Anesthetists
(CRNAs), 254
CEUs (continuing education units), 249
CFO (Chief Financial Officer), 138, 140, 152,
203–204
CGFNS (Commission on Graduates of Foreign
Nursing Schools), 250
CHAMPVA program, 184, 186
Charges
allowable or approved, 216
determinants of, 215–216
fee-for-service, 205
goals/objectives for, 215
minus a discount or percentage, 205
setting, 214–215
vs. prices, 214–215
Charity care, 210
Chart abstractions, 106
Chart audits, 106
Check sheets, 106
CHI (Consolidated Health Informatics
Initiative), 123
Chief Executive Officer (CEO), 152, 203
Chief Financial Officer (CFO), 138, 140, 152,
203–204
Chief Information Officer (CIO), 140, 152, 204
Chief Operating Officer (COO), 203
Children of Women Vietnam Veterans
Healthcare Program, 186
Choice, as intrinsic reward, 31
Chronic Care Improvement Program, 126
CIO (Chief Information Officer), 140, 152, 204

Civil laws, 347
Civil Rights Act, 274*t*
Clarify, in FOCUS-PDCA framework, 100
Clayton Act, 364
Clinical Nurse Specialists (CNSs), 254
Closed-panel health maintenance organizations (HMOs), 164
CME (continuing medical education), 236
CMS. *See* Centers for Medicare and Medicaid Services
CNAs (Certified nurses' aides), 251–253
CNMs (Certified Nurse Midwives), 254–255
Coaching, 10, 11*t*
COBRA (Consolidated Omnibus Budget Reconciliation Act), 274*t*
Code of Ethics, 17–18, 18*t*
Codex Hammurabi, 86
Codman, Ernest, 87
Coercive style of leadership, 10, 11*t*
Cognition, 41
Cognitive biases, 43–45
Co-insurance, 161
Collaboration. *See* Teamwork
Collection period, for accounts receivable, 219, 220
Collective bargaining, 294
Collective organizational action, 52
Commission on Graduates of Foreign Nursing Schools (CGFNS), 250
Committees, 305
"Common cause" variations, 94, 105
Common law, 347
Common schemas, 46
Communication
    barriers, 50
    cross-cultural, 331, 332–333
    definition of, 50
    e-mail, 145
    failure, 50
    successful, 50
    team, patient-centered, 315–316
    in teams, 317
Compensation, employee, 32, 283–286
Competence, as intrinsic reward, 31
Competition
    human resources management and, 269
    setting charges and prices and, 216
Competitive Rivalry, 63, 65–66

Compliance
    with EMTALA, 363
    history of, 359
    program oversight, 370
    standards, establishment of, 370
Comprehensive health insurance policies, 162
Comptroller, 203
Computerized Physician Order Entry (CPOE), 143–144, 149, 151
Confidentiality, 148, 345
Consolidated Health Informatics Initiative (CHI), 123
Consolidated Omnibus Budget Reconciliation Act (COBRA), 274*t*
Consumer-driven health plans, 166, 168–169
Consumerism, Mission, Vision, and Values, 67
Consumers, power of, 63, 64
Contingency Theory of Leadership, 5
Continuing education units (CEUs), 249
Continuing medical education (CME), 236
Continuous Quality Improvement (CQI)
    customer focus of, 97
    data-driven decision making, 98
    definition of, 97
    detection of latent errors, 109–110
    dimensions of, 97–98
    employee empowerment and, 98
    executive leadership in, 98–99
    FOCUS-PDCA framework, 99–101
    goals, 292
    in health care, 96–99
    history of, 6, 94–96
    medical uncertainty and, 118–121
    PDCA cycle model, 95, 95*t*
    statistical process control and, 97
    in strategic planning, 98–99
Contraception, 354
Contracts, legal, elements of, 347
Contractual allowance, 208
Control
    in DMAIC, 102
    of strategic plan, 73, 74*f*
Control activities, for internal control, 369
Control environment, for internal control, 369
Controller, 203
Control limits, 105
COO (Chief Operating Officer), 203

Copayments, 161
Corporate compliance plan, 370–371
Corporate culture, diversity in, 327–329
Cost accounting, 211–214
Cost allocation, 212–213
Cost drivers, 213
Cost information, recording/analyzing, 200
Costs
    allocation of, 212–213
    allowable, 216
    associated with accounts receivable, 219
    classification of, 211–212, 212t
    control of, 211, 221
    estimates, 216
    healthcare, 40, 60
    of inventory, 222
    of nursing turnover, 309
    plus percentage for growth, 205
    product, determination of, 213
    projected, 205
    of teamwork, 310–312
Cost sharing, 161
Costs/revenues, 198–229
Coupling, 110–111
CPOE (Computerized Physician Order Entry),
    143–144, 149, 151
CPT-4 (*The Physician's Current Procedural
    Terminology*, fourth edition), 209
CQI. *See* Continuous Quality Improvement
Credentialing, of physicians, 235–239
Credit, willingness to extend, 219
Crew resource management, 316
Criminal background checks (CBCs), 235,
    244
Criminal-Disclosure Provision, of Social
    Security Act, 360–362
Criminal laws, 347
CRNAs (Certified Registered Nurse Anesthetists),
    254
Crossing the Quality Chasm (Institute of
    Medicine), 82, 84, 108, 115
Cultural competency, 323–337
    case study, 429–432
    diversity staff training and, 329–330
    in workplace, 331–337
Cultural frameworks, in healthcare management,
    326–329
Current liabilities, 217

Customer focus, of Continuous Quality
    Improvement, 97

D
Dartmouth Atlas of Health Care, 85–86
Data, for Continuous Quality Improvement, 98
Data collection methods, 69, 70t
Data collection tools, 106–107
Davis, Michael M., 306
Decision rules, 228
Declaration of Helsinki, 345
Deductibles, 161
Defamation of character, 348
Defensive practice of medicine, 117
Deficit Reduction Acts, 92, 181
Define, in DMAIC, 102
Definition, rigorous, 104
Delegation of authority, 370
Deming, W. Edwards, 94–95
Deming cycle, 95, 95t
Department managers, capital budget requests,
    227
Department of Defense (DOD)
    financing, 187, 187t
    TRICARE plan, 181–183, 182t
Department of Health and Human Services (HHS)
    Office of the National Coordinator for Health
        Information Technology, 122–123
    Operation Restore Trust, 358, 359–360
Department of Justice (DOJ), 364
Diagnosis-related groups (DRGs), 92–93, 171,
    208
Direct contracting health insurance plans, 166
Disease Management Demonstration for
    Chronically Ill Dual-Eligible
    Beneficiaries, 126–127
Disease Management Demonstration for Severely
    Chronically Ill Medicare Beneficiaries, 126
Disease management programs, 287
Disease-specific health insurance policies, 162
Disincentives, from medical malpractice
    litigation, 117
Distributors, 222
Diversity. *See also* Cultural competency
    definition of, 324–325
    leadership, 8–9
    management of, 326–329
    training, 335–336

DMAIC, 102
DME (durable medical equipment), 363–364
Doctoral degrees, in nursing, 243
DOD. *See* Department of Defense
DOJ (Department of Justice), 364
Donabedian, Avedis, 83
DRGs (diagnosis-related groups), 92–93, 171, 208
Drug-drug interactions, 85
Durable medical equipment (DME), 363–364
Duty, toward harmed party, 348

E
EAPs (Employee Assistance Programs), 289–290
ECFMG (Educational Commission for Foreign Medical Graduates), 241
E-commerce, 222
Economic incentives, for national health information technology infrastructure, 123–127
Economic market conditions, in setting charges and prices, 215–216
Economic order quantity (EOQ), 222
Education
    of nurses, 243–247
    of physicians, 232–233
Educational Commission for Foreign Medical Graduates (ECFMG), 241
Effective care (evidence-based medicine), 118–119
E-Health (Telehealth), 144–145
EHRs (electronic health records), 122
EI (emotional intelligence), 7–8, 8*t*, 330
Eisenhower administration, 169
Elasticity of demand, 215–216
Electronic health records (EHRs), 122
Electronic medical records (EMRs)
    adoption of, 143
    advantages over paper records, 142–143
    reimbursements for, 151
    in rural family practice residency program case study, 438–441
    systems for, 142
E-mail communication, 145
EMCRO (Experimental Medical Care Review Organizations), 91
Emergency Medical Treatment and Active Labor Act (EMTALA), 65, 349–350, 362–363
Emotional intelligence (EI), 7–8, 8*t*, 330

Empathy
    emotional intelligence and, 7, 8*t*
    "tough," 8
Employee Assistance Programs (EAPs), 289–290
Employee empowerment, Continuous Quality Improvement and, 98
Employee Retirement and Income Security Act of 1974 (ERISA), 274*t*, 352
Employees
    with attitude problems, 45
    benefits for, 286–288
    compensation for, 283–286
    complacent, case study on, 386–388
    counterproductive behaviors, 24
    discipline/enforcement, 370–371
    as drivers of organizational performance, 271–272
    hard-to-motivate, 32
    hiring process, 280–281
    "inner game" of, 42
    interaction with manager, 39
    interviewing/selection process, 280–281
    job analysis, 275
    job descriptions, 277
    learning methods, focus on, 34
    manpower planning, 275–277
    motivation
        failures, 25
        individual, 24–25
        from managers, 24–25
    negotiations, 280–281
    orientation, 281–282
    performance appraisals, 290, 291*f*, 292–294
    recruitment, 277, 279–280, 279*t*
    responsibility for their own motivation, 34
    retention of (*See* Retention, employee)
    revitalization of, 34
    staffing needs (*See* Staffing needs)
    strengths, 34
    termination of, 293–294
    training/development of, 282–283, 370
Employee satisfaction
    egocentric *vs.* other-centered, 33
    motivation and, 31–33
Employee Staff Manual, 281
Employee suggestion programs (ESPs), 296–297
Employer-sponsored initiatives, for system improvement, 113
EMRs. *See* Electronic medical records

EMTALA (Emergency Medical Treatment and Active Labor Act), 65, 349–350, 362–363
Ending cash, 226
End-of-life care, 353–354
End Result System, 87, 89
Enterprise Resource Planning System (ERP), 146–147
Enthusiasm, of leader, 13
Environmental knowledge, of IT professionals, 147–148
EOG (explanation of benefits), 363
EOQ (economic order quantity), 222
EPOs (Exclusive Provider Organizations), 165
Equal Pay Act, 274t
Equipment acquisition, consignment method of, 222
Equity Theory of Adam, 28
Equivocal information, 47
ERG Theory, 26
ERISA (Employee Retirement and Income Security Act of 1974), 274t, 352
ERP (Enterprise Resource Planning System), 146–147
Error-reporting systems, mandatory, 116
Espoused beliefs and values, in organizational culture, 327
ESPs (employee suggestion programs), 296–297
ESRD Disease Management Demonstration, 126
Esteem needs, 26
Ethical principles, 84
Ethics
    ACHE Code of, 17–18, 18t
    biomedical concerns, 353–354
    concepts of, 344–346
    of countries relying on IMGs, 240–241
    law and, 343–344, 344t
    managed care organizations and, 351–352
Ethnicity, as diversity, 324–325
Event schemas, 46
Evidence-based medicine (effective care), 118–119
Exclusive Provider Organizations (EPOs), 165
Execution, of strategic plan, 75–76
Executive orders, 347
Existence, in Alderfer's ERG Theory, 26
Expectancy Theory, 28, 45
Expectations
    for employees, 33
    perceptual, 44–45

Expenditures, healthcare, 156–157, 156t
    funding sources, 157, 158f
    national, 156–157
Expense budget, 225
Experimental Medical Care Review Organizations (EMCRO), 91
External auditors, 200
External dimensions, in managing diversity, 326–327
Extinction, 28
Extrinsic factor theories of motivation, 27–28
Extrinsic incentive bias, 32
Extrinsic rewards, 24, 30, 32
Eye contact, 332, 333

F

Factoring receivables, 219
Fair Labor Standards Act, 274t
False Claims Act (FCA), 359, 361, 369
False imprisonment, 348
Family Medical and Leave Act (FMLA), 274t
FCA (False Claims Act), 359, 361, 369
Federal government, goals for HIT infrastructure, 121–122
Federal government initiatives, for system improvement, 112–113
Federal Sentencing Guidelines, 370–371
Federal Trade Commission (FTC), 364
Federal Trade Commission Act, 364
Fee-for-service model
    for financing systems, 124
    for health insurance coverage, 160–161
    indemnity insurance and, 163
    TRICARE plan option, 181–182
Fee schedule, by CPT code, 206
Fidelity, 345
Fiduciary duty, 350
Field tests, of indicators, 89
FIFO (first-in, first-out), 223
Finance departments
    accounting functions, 198
    finance functions, 199
Finance staff, 227
Financial accounting, 198
Financial Committee, annual review, 222
Financial forecasts, 68
Financial management
    accounts receivable management, 219–221
    budget management, 224–228

Financial management (*cont.*)
  charges, setting, 214–215
  cost accounting, 211–214
    allocation of costs, 212–213
    break-even analysis, 212–213
    classifying costs, 211–212, 212*t*
  definition of, 198
  functions of, 198–199
  materials and inventory management, 221–223
  objectives for, 199–200
  objectives of, 199–200
  purposes/function of, 198–199
  responsibility for, 202–204
  working capital management, 217–218
Financial reports, 200
Financial risk, of healthcare organizations, 200
Find, in FOCUS-PDCA framework, 99
First-in, first-out (FIFO), 223
Fishbone diagram, 107
Five Forces Model, 63
Fixed assets, 226
Flexible health benefits, 287
Flexible or variable pricing, 216
Flexible spending accounts, 168, 288
Flexner, Abraham, 306
Flexner Report, 87–88, 306
Flowcharting, 100, 107
FMLA (Family Medical and Leave Act), 274*t*
Focused, Unpredictable, and Novel (FUN)
  approach to motivation, 33
FOCUS-PDCA framework, 99–101
Followership, 3–4
Foreign educated nurses, 249–250
Foreign Medical Graduates (International
  Medical Graduates), 239–241
Forming, of teams, 312
For-profit healthcare organizations
  financial goals of, 201
  tax status, 201–202, 202*t*
  vs. not-for-profit, 200–202, 202*t*
"Four Layers of Diversity," 326–329
Framing, in Tobert's Action Inquiry, 52
Fraud
  adoption of corporate compliance plan and,
    370–371
  antitrust issues, 364
  in billing for services, 358
  civil remedies, 359
  Criminal-Disclosure Provision of Social
    Security Act and, 360–362
  definition of, 358
  EMTALA and, 362–363
  enforcement tools, Balanced Budget Act and,
    363–364
  federal enforcement actions, 364
  Operation Restore Trust and, 358, 359–360
  patient referral kickbacks (*See* Referrals,
    patient)
  response and corrective action, 371
  safe harbor regulations, 367–368
  stacked penalties, 369
Free-rider syndrome, 317
Frequency chart, 107–108
Frustration-regression principle, 26
FTC (Federal Trade Commission), 364
FUN (Focused, Unpredictable, and Novel)
  approach to motivation, 33
Fundamental attribution error, 45
Future service volumes, 276–277

G
GAAP (Generally Accepted Accounting
  Principles), 203–204
Gainsharing, 285
Generally Accepted Accounting Principles
  (GAAP), 203–204
Geographic mapping, 106
Geographic pricing, 216
Gerontophobia, 333
GME (Graduate Medical Education), 233
Goal Setting Theory, 28
Goal-sharing programs, 285
Governance, 14–15, 15*t*
Governing body approval, of capital budget, 228
Government, healthcare coverage and, 159–160
Government regulators, 200
Graduate Medical Education (GME), 233
The Great Man Theory, 4
Green Belts, 102
Group model health maintenance organizations,
  164
Growth, in Alderfer's ERG Theory, 26
Guidelines for Teamwork, 317, 318*f*

H
Hall, Edward T., 331
*Hallmarks of the Professional Nursing Practice
  Environment*, 247–248
Hart-Scott-Rodino Antitrust Improvements Act
  of 1976, 364

HCFA (Health Care Financing Administration), 90, 93. *See also* Centers for Medicare and Medicaid Services
HCPCS (Healthcare Common Procedure Coding System), 208–209
Health care, aims of, 108
Healthcare, culturally-sensitive, 334–337
Healthcare financial management. *See* Financial management
Healthcare Financial Management Association (HFMA), 19*t*
Health Care Financing Administration (HCFA), 90, 93. *See also* Centers for Medicare and Medicaid Services
Healthcare industry, as high hazard industry, 111
Healthcare management, cultural frameworks in, 326–329
Healthcare managers. *See* Managers
Healthcare market, consumer influences on, 64
Healthcare occupations employment, projected growth in, 269, 270*t*
Healthcare organizations
    financial risk, control of, 200
    for-profit
        financial goals of, 201
        tax status, 201–202, 202*t*
        vs. not-for-profit, 200–202, 202*t*
    governing bodies, 202–204
    not-for-profit (*See* Not-for-profit healthcare organizations)
    organizational behavior issues in, 40–41
    performance, employees as drivers of, 271–272
    sensemaking in, 47–48
    tax status, 200–202, 202*t*
Healthcare professionals, 231–257
    allied health professionals, 255–257
    categories of, 231–232
    home health aides, 251–253
    managing, mini-case studies on, 389–390
    midlevel practitioners, 253–255
    nurses (*See* Nurses)
    nurse's aides, 251–253
    physicians (*See* Physicians)
    teams of (*See* Teams)
Healthcare provider, legal responsibilities of, 349–350
Healthcare Service Organizations (HSOs), 271
Healthcare settings, research in, 354

Healthcare spending, national, 156–157, 156*t*
Healthcare system improvement
    assessing, 115–116
    challenges, 116–121
Healthcare workforce, power of, 63
Health data, content/structure of, 148–149
Health information. *See* Information
Health information technology (HIT). *See* Information technology
Health insurance, 156–193
    access to care restrictions, 163
    benefits, types of, 162
    for catastrophic expenditures, 158–159
    consumer-driven health plans, 166, 168–169
    costs, statistics on, 188, 189*t*
    cost sharing, 161
    coverage, 159, 187–188, 188*t*
    demand for, 159
    as employee benefit, 287
    expansion of public sector coverage, 160
    forms of payment, 160–161
    group policies, 159
    history of, 159–160
    intent of, 158
    key concepts, 158
    moral hazard, 162
    plan characteristics, comparison of, 167*t*
    policy limitations, 161–162
    private, 157, 160, 163–166
    Provider Choice, 163
    reimbursements, 159, 204–210
    social evolution of, 169–173
Health Insurance Portability and Accountability Act (HIPAA)
    case study, 383
    challenges of, 150
    confidentiality of patient information and, 350–351
    enactment of, 65, 274*t*
    penalties, 148–149
    respect for persons and, 345
    security standards of, 148
    training/employee orientation and, 282
Health maintenance organizations (HMOs)
    accreditation, 114
    characteristics of, 167*t*
    closed-panel, 164
    enrollment, 166*t*
    forms of, 164
    group model, 164

Health maintenance organizations (HMOs)
(*cont.*)
independent Practice Association, 165
negotiation case study, 391–396
open-panel, 164
routine healthcare and, 119
staff model, 164
TRICARE plan option, 181–182, 182*t*
Health Plan Data and Information Set (HEDIS),
114, 184*t*–185*t*
Health Reimbursement Arrangements (HRAs),
168
Health relationships, as intrinsic reward, 31
Health Savings Accounts (HSAs), 168–169
HEDIS (Health Plan Data and Information Set),
114, 184*t*–185*t*
Herzberg's Two Factor Theory, 26–27
Heuristics, 43
HFMA (Healthcare Financial Management
Association), 19*t*
HHAs (home health agencies), 171, 358
HHS. *See* Department of Health and Human
Services
Hierarchy of need, 25–26
Hill-Burton legislation, 150
HIPAA. *See* Health Insurance Portability and
Accountability Act
Hippocratic Oath, 86
Histogram, 108
HIT (health information technology). *See*
Information technology
Holding costs, 223
Holidays, 287
Home health agencies (HHAs), 171, 358
Home health aides, 251–253
Home Health Resource Groups, 171
Hospital Compare, 125
Hospital Outpatient Prospective Payment System
(OPPS), 171
Hospital Quality Alliance (HQA), 115
Hospital Quality Initiative, 124–125
Hospital Rewards Program, Leapfrog Group, 124
Hospitals
accreditation of, 88–89, 140
alignment with physicians, 307
compliance with EMTALA, 363
departments, involved in accounts receivable
management, 220–221, 220*t*
Medicaid/Medicare reimbursements, 207–208
outpatient department services, 171

Hospital-surgical health insurance policies, 162
Hourly rated positions, 284
HQA (Hospital Quality Alliance), 115
HRAs (Health Reimbursement Arrangements),
168
HSAs (Health Savings Accounts), 168–169
HSOs (Healthcare Service Organizations), 271
Human resources management, 266–297. *See
also* Employees
administrative view of, 266
environmental forces and, 268–269, 268*t*,
270*t*, 271
examples of, 267
legislation and, 273, 274*t*
recruitment
advertising methods for, 279–280
responsibilities for, 277, 279*t*
retention of employees (*See* Retention,
employee)
strategic perspective of, 266
Humor strategies case study, 433–436
Hygienes, in Herzberg's Two Factor Theory, 26

I

ICD-9 (International Classification of Disease),
208
ICU (Intensive care unit), nurse residency
programs, 245
IHI (Institute for Healthcare Improvement),
114, 116
Illness beliefs, cultural aspects of, 332
Illustrating, in Tobert's Action Inquiry, 52
IMGs (International Medical Graduates),
239–241
Immigration Reform and Control Act, 274*t*
Implementation, of strategic plan, 72–73, 73*f*
Improve, in DMAIC, 102
IMSystem (Indicator Measurement System),
113–114
Incentive compensation plans, 285–286
Income, 199, 217
Indemnity insurance, 163, 164
Indemnity plans, characteristics of, 167*t*
Independent auditor, 204
Independent Practice Association (IPA)
description of, 165
negotiation case study, 391–396
Indicator Measurement System (IMSystem),
113–114
Individual proficiency, drive for, 49

Information
  ambiguous and equivocal, 47
  batched requests, 139
  collection methods, 69, 70*t*
  and communication, for internal control, 369
  external, 141
  internal, 140
  processing, heuristics and, 43
  providing to users, 141–142
  users of, 141
Information technology (IT), 137–152
  accelerated adoption of, 123
  adoption of, 150–151
  applications, 142–147
  challenges, 150–152
  financial investment in, 151
  health manager role in, 147–150
  historical overview, 138–140
  interoperability and, 151–152
  national infrastructure development, 121–127
    aligning economic incentives for, 123–127
    barriers to, 122
    goals for, 121–122
    projects, 122–123
  standards, intra-organizational, 151
Information technology professionals
  administrative/leadership skills, 149–150
  environmental knowledge of, 147–148
  health data knowledge of, 148–149
Injury or damages, in tort, 348
Innovations in Technology, 63, 64–65
Inquiring, in Tobert's Action Inquiry, 52
In-service training programs, 222
Inspirational leadership, 8
Institute for Healthcare Improvement (IHI),
    114, 116
Institute of Medicine (IOM), 81–82
  Crossing the Quality Chasm, 82, 84, 108, 115
  definition of healthcare quality, 82–83
  Medicare quality assurance, 93
  recommendations for improving system
    quality, 115–116
Institutional Review Boards (IRBs), 354
Integrated delivery systems, 166
Intensive care unit (ICU), nurse residency
    programs, 245
Intentional torts, 348
Interactiveness, 110
Interdisciplinary health teams. *See* Teams
Internal Assessment, 61, 67–69

Internal auditor, 203–204
Internal control, 369
Internal dimensions, in managing diversity, 326
International Classification of Disease (ICD-9),
    208
International Medical Graduates (IMGs),
    239–241
International Organization for Standardization
    (ISO 9000 certification), 103
Interoperability, as information technology
    challenge, 151–152
Intrinsic factor theories of motivation, 28
Intrinsic rewards, 24, 30–32
Invasion of privacy, 348–349
Inventory, performance, evaluation of, 222
Inventory management, 221–223
Investing, in long-term capital assets, 200
IOM. *See* Institute of Medicine
IPA. *See* Independent Practice Association
IRBs (Institutional Review Boards), 354
Ishikawa diagram, 107
ISO 9000 certification (International
    Organization for Standardization), 103
IT. *See* Information technology

J
JCAH (Joint Commission on Accreditation of
    Hospitals), 88–89
JCAHO. *See* Joint Commission on Accreditation
    of Healthcare Organizations
JIT (Just-in-time inventory method), 223
Job analysis, 275
Job burnout, of physicians, 242–243
Job descriptions, 277, 278*f*
Job pricing, 284–285
Job satisfaction
  organizational climate and, 247–248
  physicians and, 242–243
Johnson, President Lyndon B., 169
Joint Commission on Accreditation of
    Healthcare Organizations (JCAHO)
  health information and, 140, 141
  leadership standards, 17
  quality improvement initiatives, 113–114,
    116
  quality of care indicators, 89
  retention of nursing staff and, 245
Joint Commission on Accreditation of Hospitals
    (JCAH), 88–89
Judgment, systematic errors of, 43–44

Juran, Joseph M., 95–96
"Juran Trilogy," 96
Justice, 346
Just-in-time inventory method (JIT), 223
J-Visa, 241

K
Kennedy, President John F., 169
Kennedy-Kassebaum Bill (Public Law 104-191), 148
Kerr-Mills Act, 169
Key financial indicators, 68–69
Kickbacks, for referrals, 358

L
Labor and Delivery dilemma case study, 415
"Laborists," 63
Labor relations, 294–296
LANs (Local Area Networks), 139
Last-in, first-out (LIFO), 223
"Late adopter" stance, 64
Latent errors, 109
Law
    biomedical concerns, 353–354
    concepts, torts, 347–349
    ethics and, 343–344, 344t
    as leadership barrier, 15–16
    legal concepts, 346–347
    managed care organizations and, 351–352
    patient rights and, 350–351
    provider responsibilities and, 349–350
Leader-Member Exchange Theory, 5–6
Leaders
    challenging to think in strategic context, 69
    charismatic, 6
    competencies of, 3, 3t
    focus of, 2, 2f
    professional associations for, 19, 19t
    of teams, 314
    transformational, 6
Leadership
    barriers/challenges of, 15–17, 16t
    competencies, 11–12, 12t
    contemporary models, 6–10, 7t, 8t, 10t
    Contingency Theory of, 5
    in Continuous Quality Improvement, 98–99
    diversity, 8–9
    domains, 12, 12t
    emotional intelligence and, 7–8, 8t
    ethical responsibility of, 17–18, 18t

followership and, 3–4
future concerns and, 18–20
governance and, 14–15, 15t
history, in United States, 4–6
input, for Internal Assessment, 69
inspirational, 8
Path-Goal Theory of, 5
protocols, 12–14, 13t
servant, 9
situational approach, 5
skills, for information technology
    professionals, 149–150
spirituality, 9, 10t
strategy execution and, 76
style approach, 5
styles, 10–11, 11t
vs. management, 1–3, 2f, 3t
Leadership theories, in United States, 7, 7t
Leapfrog Group, 113, 116, 124
Learning, managing and, 48–49
Learning organizations, practices or disciplines
    in, 49
Legislation. *See also specific legislation*
    human resource management and, 273, 274t
    major healthcare-related, 170–173
    regulatory environment, 63, 65
    regulatory issues, in setting charges and prices,
        215
Licensed Practical Nurses (LPNs), 250–251
Licensed Vocational Nurses (LVNs), 250–251
Licensure, of physicians, 234–235
Life insurance benefits, 287
LifeMasters, 127
Lifetime limit, on health insurance benefits, 162
LIFO (last-in, first-out), 223
Liquidity, 218
Listening, in Tobert's Action Inquiry, 52
Local Area Networks (LANs), 139
Locke's Goal Setting Theory, 28
Long-term capital assets, budgeting for, 226–228
Loss leaders, 211
LPNs (Licensed Practical Nurses), 250–251
LVNs (Licensed Vocational Nurses), 250–251

M
Major medical health insurance policies, 162
Malcolm Baldrige National Quality Award, 96
Malpractice, 349
Managed behavioral healthcare organizations
    (MBHOs), 114

Managed care health plans, 163–166, 166*t*

Managed care organizations (MCOs)
  contracts, 219
  legal/ethical concerns, 351–352
  prospective reimbursements, 205–207

Management, healthcare
  history of, 306–307
  learning and, 48–49
  methods, for teams, 316–319
  mini-case studies, 389–390
  motivation case study, 421–422
  motivation of workforce, 23–24
  organizational behavior contributions to, 39
  organizational behavior field (*See*
    Organizational behavior)
  vs. leadership, 1–3, 2*f*, 3*t*

Management education, healthcare, humor
  strategies case study, 433–436

Management Information System (MIS) case
  study, 384–385

Management theories of motivation, 28–29

Managerial accounting, 198

Managerial ethics, 17

Managers
  budgeting importance for, 224–225
  cognitive principles in human interaction,
    41–42
  competencies of, 3, 3*t*
  financial, 204
  in financial analysis/decision making, 199
  focus of, 2–3, 2*f*
  in information technology, 147–150
  judgments on employee motivation,
    31–32
  management philosophy of, 44
  role of, 147–150
  in strategic planning, 76–77
  in strategy execution, 76–77
  teamwork and, 307

Mangers
  staff member questions for, 313

Manipulation, *vs.* motivation, 32

Mapping processes, for data collection, 107

Market Assessment, in Situational Assessment,
  61, 63–66

Market Volume Forecast, 66

Maslow's hierarchy of need, 25–26

Master Black Belts, 102

Master's of Science in Nursing (MSN), 243

Materials management, 221–223

MBHOs (managed behavioral healthcare
  organizations), 114

MBTI (Myers-Briggs Type Indicator), 314–315

MCAT (Medical College Admission Test), 232

McClelland's Acquired Needs Theory, 27

McGregor's Theory X and Theory Y, 29, 44

MCOs. *See* Managed care organizations

Meaningful work, as intrinsic reward, 31

Measure, in DMAIC, 102

Measurement, in quality improvement, 104–105

Measure reliability, 104

Medicaid
  administrative services, 178
  Balanced Budget Act of 1997 and, 171–172
  benefits, 177
  cost control measures, 180–181
  creation of, 160
  eligibility requirements, 177–178
  establishment of, 88, 91, 170
  expenditures, 178–180, 179*f*, 180*f*
  federal financing and, 178
  introduction of, 138
  patient referrals Anti-Kickback Act and,
    365–367
  provider services, 178
  reimbursements, 207–209
  requirements for HSOs, 271
  services, mandatory, 177
  vs. VA programs, 184*t*–185*t*

Medical College Admission Test (MCAT), 232

Medical education system
  quality in, 87–88
  reorganization of, 306

Medical equipment, submission of fraudulent
  medical necessity certification for,
  361–362

Medical errors, 81–82, 85
  prevention of, 143–144
  reporting, 117

Medical Group Management Association
  (MGMA), 19*t*

Medical malpractice litigation, 117–118

Medical records access, case study, 383

Medical Savings Accounts (MSAs), 168

Medical Screening Exam (MSE), 362

Medical uncertainty, accounting for, 118–121

Medicare
  Advantage Plans, 172
  Balanced Budget Act of 1997 and, 171–172
  creation of, 160

Medicare (*cont.*)
enrollees, growth in, 174
establishment of, 88, 91, 170
expenditures, 174–176, 176*f*
historical development of, 169–170
introduction of, 138
Part A, 173
Part B, 173
Part C or Medicare+Choice, 172, 173–174
Part D, 172–173, 174
patient referrals Anti-Kickback Act and, 365–367
PFP initiatives, 124
quality assurance program, 113
reimbursements, 207–209
requirements for HSOs, 271
revenue sources, distribution of, 174, 175*f*
solvency of, 176–177
vs. VA programs, 184*t*–185*t*
Medicare Care Management Performance Demonstration, 125
Medicare Health Care Quality Demonstration, 125–126
Medicare managed care, 172
Medicare Modernization Act, 122, 125–126
Medicare Payment Advisory Commission (MedPac), 127
Medicare Prescription Drug Improvement and Modernization Act, 168, 172–173
Medication errors
Computerized Physician Order Entry and, 143–144
reporting, case study on, 442–447
MediGap policies, 162
MedPac (Medicare Payment Advisory Commission), 127
Mental distress, 348
Mental models
definition of, 47
discussing and revising, 48–49
examination and testing of, 49–50
surfacing and challenging, 49
Mergers, hospital
case study, 397–403
patient-focused care model for, 310–312
Metaphors, 404
MGMA (Medical Group Management Association), 19*t*
Midlevel practitioners, 234, 253–255
Midwives, nurse, 254–255

Military personnel health insurance. *See* Veterans Health Administration
Minicomputers, introduction of, 138
Minimum standards, establishment of, 87
Minority ethnic populations, in United States, 323–324
MIS (Management Information System) case study, 384–385
Mislabeling, 111
Mission, Vision, and Values (MVV), 61, 66–67
Mission statement, definition of, 67
Misuse of resources, 84, 85–86
Money, as motivation, 32
Monitoring
for internal control, 369
of strategic plan, 73, 74*f*
Moral hazard, 162
Motivate, definition of, 24
Motivation
case studies, 386–388, 421–422
combination of factors in, 32
definition of, 24
emotional intelligence and, 7, 8*t*
of employees
individual, 24–25
by managers, 24–25
employee satisfaction and, 31–33
rewards for, 24, 30–34
strategies for, 33–34
vs. manipulation, 32
of workforce, as managerial task, 23–24
Motivation theories
extrinsic factor, 27–28
intrinsic factor, 28
management, 28–29
needs-based, 25–27
Motivators
effective, 33
in Herzberg's Two Factor Theory, 26–27
MSAs (Medical Savings Accounts), 168
MSE (Medical Screening Exam), 362
MSN (Master's of Science in Nursing), 243
Multicultural organization, 330
MVV (Mission, Vision, and Values), 66–67
Myers-Briggs Type Indicator (MBTI), 314–315

N
National Business Coalition on Health (NBCH), 113

National Committee for Quality Assurance (NCQA), 113, 114, 116
National Council Licensure Examination (NCLEX), 244
National Council Licensure Examination-Practical Nurse (NCLEX-PN), 251
National health spending, 156–157
National Labor Relations Act, 274t, 295
National Labor Relations Board (NLRB), 295
National Practitioner Data Bank (NPDB), 117–118, 238–239
National Quality Forum (NQF), 112
National Residency Matching Program (NRMP), 233
National security, 151–152
Nationwide Health Information Network architecture, 123
NBCH (National Business Coalition on Health), 113
NCLEX (National Council Licensure Examination), 244
NCLEX-PN (National Council Licensure Examination-Practical Nurse), 251
NCQA (National Committee for Quality Assurance), 113, 114, 116
Need, Maslow's hierarchy of, 25–26
Need for achievement, 27
Need for affiliation, 27
Need for power, 27
Needs-based motivation theories, 25–27
Negative reinforcement, 27–28
Negligence, 348, 349
Negotiations case study, 391–396
Net income, 217
Net working capital, 217
Network model HMO, 165
Nightingale, Florence, 86–87, 306
NLRB (National Labor Relations Board), 295
Non-compliance, 120
Non-criteria-based capital budgeting, 228
Nonmaleficence, 346
Norming, of teams, 312
Not covered or uncompensated care, 210
Not-for-profit healthcare organizations
    business-oriented, tax status, 201, 202t
    charity care, 210
    financial goals of, 202
    government-owned, tax status, 201, 202t
    tax status, 201, 202, 202t
    vs. for-profit organizations, 200–202, 202t

NPDB (National Practitioner Data Bank), 117–118, 238–239
NPs (nurse practitioners), 254
NQF (National Quality Forum), 112
NRMP (National Residency Matching Program), 233
NRPs (nurse residency programs), 245
Nurse practitioners (NPs), 254
Nurse residency programs (NRPs), 245
Nurses
    advanced practice or APNs, 253–255
    foreign educated, 249–250
    Licensed Practical or LPNs, 250–251
    Licensed Vocational or LVNs, 250–251
    registered (See Registered nurses)
Nurses' aides
    motivation case study, 421–422
    training, 251–253
Nursing education, outside the U.S., 249–250
Nursing profession, development of, 305–306
Nursing school curriculum, 243–244
Nursing shortages, 63
Nursing specialties, 248–249
Nursing staff
    patient-to-nurse ratios, 246
    retention, strategies for, 245–246
    turnover, 244–245, 309

O
OBRA (Omnibus Reconciliation Act), 171
Obstetricians
    problem behavior case study, 415
    supply and demand of, 63
Occupational safety and health, 288
Occupational Safety and Health Act, 274t
Office of the National Coordinator for Health Information Technology, 122–123
OIG, 367, 368, 370–371
Omnibus Reconciliation Act (OBRA), 171
Open-panel health maintenance organizations, 164
Operating budget, 225
Operation Restore Trust (ORT), 358, 359–360
Opportunity costs, 310
OPPS (Hospital Outpatient Prospective Payment System), 171
Organizational behavior, 38–55
    contribution to management, 39
    definition of, 38–39
    influence of thinking on, 41–42

Organizational behavior (*cont.*)
  as interdisciplinary field, 38–39
  issues in health organizations, 40–41
  key topics in, 39
Organizational buy-in, for strategy execution, 76
Organizational culture, diversity in, 327–329
Organizational dashboard or scorecard, 73, 74*f*
Organizational research, Action Inquiry
      approach, 52
Organizational theory, 39
Organizational Volume Forecast, 68
Organize, in FOCUS-PDCA framework, 99
Orientation, employee, 281–282
ORT (Operation Restore Trust), 358, 359–360
ORYX® initiative, 114
Ouchi's Theory Z, 29
Out-of-pocket expenditures, for healthcare, 157,
      158, 161
Outpatient care, demand for, 40
Outpatient Prospective Payment System (OPPS),
      171
Overestimations, 43
Overuse
  of resources, 84, 85–86
  of services, 124
  of unnecessary medical services, 117

P
Pacesetting style of leadership, 10–11, 11*t*
PACs (Picture Archive Communication
      Systems), 64–65
Paid-time-off (PTO), 286
Pareto chart, 107–108
Participants, in strategic planning, 76
Participative style of leadership, 10, 11*t*
PAs (physician assistants), 232, 255
Path-Goal Theory of Leadership, 5
Patient accounts. *See* Accounts receivable
Patient care delivery, appropriate, 221
Patient-centered care model, team
      communication and, 315–316
Patient dumping, 362
Patient-focused care model, teams in, 310–312
Patient information, 140
Patient mix, 208
Patient-provider communication, 145
Patient rights, legal aspects of, 350–351
Patient Safety Task Force, 112–113
Patient-to-nurse ratios, 246
Payers, power of, 63, 64

Pay-for-performance initiatives, 114–115
Pay-for-performance (PFP) programs, 124–127,
      285
Payroll, 200
PCPs. *See* Primary care physicians
PCs (personal computers), 139
PDCA (Plan-Do-Check-Act) cycle model, 95,
      95*t*, 99
Peer Review Improvement Act of 1982, 92
Peer review organization (PRO), 92–93
Perception
  attention processes and, 42–43
  definition of, 42
  sensemaking and, 47–48
  sharing, 48–49
  systematic errors of, 43–44
Per diagnosis payments, 206
Per diem payments, 205
Performance
  high, promotion of, 34
  improvement, 81–129 (*See also* Continuous
        Quality Improvement)
  history of, 86
  standards, 116
Performance appraisal systems, 290, 291*f*,
      292–294
Performing, of teams, 312
Personal computers (PCs), 139
Personality, in managing diversity, 326
Personal schemas, 46
Personal space, cultural aspects of, 331, 332
PFP programs (pay-for-performance programs),
      124–127, 285
PHOs (physician-Hospital Organizations), 166
Physician assistants (PAs), 232, 255
Physician Group Practice Demonstration, 125
Physician-Hospital Organizations (PHOs),
      166
Physicians
  alignment with hospitals, 307
  board certified, 235
  board eligible, 235–236
  cognitive biases of, 43–44
  credentialing of, 235–239
  criminal background checks, 235
  educational requirements, 232–233
  failure to embrace teamwork, 307
  gap between educational and employment
        placements, 237–238
  incompetent, 238–239

International Medical Graduates (IMGs), 239–241
as leadership challenge, 16
licensure requirements, 234–235
number of, 232
obstetricians, supply and demand of, 63
as patient advocates, 352
premedical programs for, 232
primary care, 240–242
problem behavior case study, 415
problem behaviors, 307
referrals, Stark laws I and II, 361
reimbursements to, 208–209
relationship with nurses, 246–247
residency training programs for, 233–234
resistance to acknowledge nurses as professionals, 247
review of credentials, 238–239
The Physician's Current Procedural Terminology, fourth edition (CPT-4), 209
Physician Self-Referral Law, 365
Physiological needs, 25
Picture Archive Communication Systems (PACs), 64–65
Placement within the organization, diversity and, 327
Plan-Do-Check-Act (PDCA) cycle model, 95, 95*t*, 99
Planning, in FOCUS-PDCA framework, 100–101
Pledging receivables as collateral, 219
Point-of-service plans (POSs), 157, 165, 166*t*, 167*t*
Politics, social insurance development and, 169–170
Position descriptions, 277, 278*f*
Positive reinforcement, 27
POSs (point-of-service plans), 157, 165, 166*t*, 167*t*
Poverty status, 178
Power, need for, 27
Power of Consumers and Payers, 63, 64
Power of the Healthcare Workforce, 63
PPOs. *See* Preferred Provider Organizations
PPS (prospective payment system), 60, 92, 171
Preconceptions, 43
Preference-sensitive care, 118, 119, 120
Preference-sensitive services, 124
Preferred Provider Organizations (PPOs)
characteristics of, 164–165, 167*t*

enrollment, 166*t*
NCQA and, 114
TRICARE Extra, 181–182, 182*t*
Pregnancy Discrimination Act, 274*t*
Prejudices, 334
Premier Hospital Quality Incentive Demonstration, 125
Prepayment, of health insurance coverage, 160, 161
Prices
determinants of, 215–216
goals/objectives for, 215
published, 214
setting, 199
vs. charges, 214–215
Pricing tactics, 216
Primary care physicians (PCPs)
employment of, 240–241
IMGs, 240
turnover of, 241–242
PRIME, 181–182, 182*t*
Privacy, of healthcare data, 148
PRO (peer review organization), 92–93
Probationary period, 292
Problems
in healthcare management, tame *vs.* wicked, 313
identification, 51, 99
oversimplification of, 43
Problem solutions, 43, 51
Problem solving
phases of, 51
in teams, 319
thinking and sensemaking in, 50–51
Process variation, 105
Products, inelastic *vs.* elastic, 215
Professional associations, 19, 19*t*
Professional charges, 216
Professional healthcare workers, autonomy of, 40
Professionalism, 13
Professional Standards Review Organizations (PSROs), 91–92
Profitability, improvement of, 221
Profitability index, 228
Progress, as intrinsic reward, 31
Proposal evaluators, for capital budget, 227–228
Proposal reviewers, for capital budget, 227
Prospective payment, 124
Prospective payment system (PPS), 60, 92, 171
Prospective reimbursements, 205–207

Protocols, leadership, 12–14, 13*t*
Provider Choice health insurance, 163
Proximic theory, 331
PSROs (Professional Standards Review
    Organizations), 91–92
Psychiatric health aides, 251–253
PTO (paid-time-off), 286
Public Law 104-191 (Kennedy-Kassebaum Bill),
    148
Punishment, 28

Q

QA. *See* Quality assurance
QIOs (Quality Improvement Organizations), 91,
    93, 113, 116, 125
Quality, healthcare, 81–82
    components of, 83
    CQI (*See* Continuous quality improvement)
    definition of, 82–84
    fundamental questions, 84
    history of, 86
    importance of, 84–86
    Joint Commission on Accreditation of
        Hospitals and, 88–89
    multiple stakeholder perspectives and, 83–84
    problems
        misuse, 84, 85–86
        overuse, 84, 85–86
        underuse, 84, 85–86
    problems, for healthcare processes, 120
    systems perspective, 83
Quality assurance (QA)
    actions, 90
    history of, 86–87
    personal accountability and, 90
    quality problems and, 120–121
    standards, 89
    tracking and trending, 89–90
Quality improvement
    key concepts, 103–105
        measurement, 104–105
        process variation, 105
        statistical process control, 105
    models
        business process reengineering, 102–103
        CQI (*See* Continuous quality
            improvement)
        ISO 9000, 103
        medication errors reporting case study,
            442–447

Six Sigma, 101–102
system thinking and, 108–111
teams, 304–305
tools, 106–108
Quality Improvement Organizations (QIOs), 91,
    93, 113, 116, 125
Qui tam provision, 359

R

Racial groups
    uninsured population and, 189, 190*t*
    in U.S. population, 323–324
Radiology personnel shortages, 63
RBRVS (Resource-Based Relative Value System),
    171, 208
Recognition programs, differences in, 32
Recruitment, 268–269
    advertising methods for, 279–280
    responsibilities for, 277, 279*t*
Reengineering, 102–103
Referrals, patient
    Anti-Kickback statutes, 365–367
    safe harbor regulations, 367–368
    Stark Laws I and II, 361, 365
Registered nurses (RNs), 243–250
    burnout, 246
    continuing education for, 249
    criminal background checks, 244
    educational requirements for, 243–244
    foreign educated, 249–250
    job dissatisfaction, 246
    job satisfaction, organizational climate and,
        247–248
    new, concerns of, 244–246
    number of, 232
    relationship with physicians, 246–247
    specialties for, 248–249
    staff turnover, 244–245
Regulations, 347
Regulatory Environment, 63, 65
Rehabilitation Act, 274*t*
Reimbursements, 40, 204
    modified on basis of performance, 205
    to physicians, 208–209
    prospective, 205–207
    for providers, Medicare and Medicaid,
        207–209
    retrospective, 205
    by uninsured individuals, 209–210
Reinforcement Theory, 27–28

Relatedness, in Alderfer's ERG Theory, 26
Relator (whistle blower), 359
Reliability, 104
Reorder point (RP), 222
Research
    ethical principles of, 345–346
    in healthcare settings, 354
    in teams, 319
Residency training programs, for physicians,
    233–234
Resource-Based Relative Value System (RBRVS),
    171, 208
Resources
    allocation of, strategic planning and, 60
    misuse of, 84, 85
    overuse of, 84, 85
    underuse of, 84, 85
Respect
    for leader, 13
    for persons, 345
Respiratory therapists (RTs), 256
Respondeat superior, 348
Retention, employee
    benefits and, 286–288
    compensation for, 283–286
    Employee Assistance Programs and, 289–290
    employee suggestion programs and, 296–297
    labor relations management and, 294–296
Retirement benefits, 287–288
Retrospective reimbursements, 205
Revenue budget, 225
Rewards
    definition of, 24
    for desired behavior, 33
    extrinsic, 24, 30, 32
    intrinsic, 24, 30–32
    performance-enhancing, 33
    tailored, 33–34
    tailoring to individual, 32
Risk assessment, for internal control, 369
Robert Wood Johnson Foundation (RWJF), 114,
    245
Roe v. Wade, 353–354
Role schemas, 46
Rollout, of strategic plan, 72
RTs (respiratory therapists), 256
RUGs (Resource Utilization Groups), 171
Rules, 347
RWJF (Robert Wood Johnson Foundation), 114,
    245

S
Safe harbor laws, 367–368
Safety, as leadership challenge, 17
Safety needs, 25
Safety stock level, 222
Satisfaction progression, 26
Schemas, 46
SCHIP (State Children's Health Insurance
    Program), 160, 172, 177
Scientific Management Theory, 28–29
Security, of healthcare data, 148
Selection of quality improvement plan, in
    FOCUS-PDCA framework, 100
Self-actualization needs, 26
Self-awareness, 7, 8t
Self-fulfilling prophecy, 44–45
Self-regulation, 7, 8t
Sensemaking, 47–51
Servant leadership, 9
Service connected conditions, veterans and, 184
Service line approach, to teamwork, 308–309
Services, upcoding, 358
Sexual harassment case study, 416–420
Sherman Antitrust Act, 364
Shewhart, Walter A., 94
Shewhart cycle, 95, 95t
Shortages, of healthcare personnel, 244, 257,
    268–269
Sick leave, 286
Simplifications, cognitive, 43–44
Situational approach to leadership, 5
Situational Assessment
    functions of, 61
    Internal Assessment (*See* Internal
        Assessment)
    Market Assessment, 61
    Mission Vision and Values, 61
    strategy identification and, 61
Situational cues, 44
Six Sigma, 101–102
Skilled nursing facilities (SNFs), 11
Skinner, B., 27–28
SNFs (skilled nursing facilities), 11
Social health insurance. See Medicaid; Medicare
Social insurance
    TRICARE, 181–183, 182t
    for veterans, military personnel and their
        families, 181
Socialized medicine, 159
Social loafer syndrome, 317

Social Security Act (SSA), Criminal-Disclosure Provision of, 360–362
Social Security Acts of 1965, 170
Social Security Trust Fund, 188
Social skills, 7, 8*t*
Software fail-safe systems, 149
SPC (statistical process control), 94, 105
"Special cause" variation, 94, 97, 98, 105
Specific identification, 223
Speech forms, in Tobert's Action Inquiry, 52
Spina Bifida Healthcare Program, for Vietnam veterans, 186
Spirituality leadership, 9, 10*t*
SSA (Social Security Act), Criminal-Disclosure Provision of, 360–362
Staffing needs
    future service volumes, 276–277
    ratio method for determining, 276
    reduction, case study of, 423–428
Staff model health maintenance organizations (HMOs), 164
Staff training, cultural competency and, 329–330
Stakeholders, involvement in strategic planning, 76
Standard operating procedures, 118–119
Standards, as information technology challenge, 151
Stark Laws I and II, 361, 365–367, 369
State Boards of Physician Quality Assurance (BPQA), 234
State Children's Health Insurance Program (SCHIP), 160, 172, 177
Statistical process control (SPC), 94, 105
Statistical process control, Continuous Quality Improvement and, 97
Statistics budget, 226
Statutes, 347
Stereotypes, 334
Storming, of teams, 312
Strategic direction, selection of, 70–71
Strategic performance, 69
Strategic plan, monitoring and control, 73, 74*f*
Strategic planning, 59–77
    Continuous Quality Improvement, 98–99
    definition of, 59
    in health care, history of, 59–60
    healthcare manager role in, 76–77
    implementation of plan, 72–73
    importance of, 60
    participants, 76

process, 60–61, 62*f* (*See also* Situational Assessment; Strategy execution)
    Strategy Identification and Selection, 70–71
    tactical plans, 71–72, 72*t*
    purpose of, 60
    resource allocation and, 60
    rollout of plan, 72
    strategy execution, 75–76
    supporting plans for, 72–73, 73*f*
Strategies, successful, 71, 72*t*
Strategy execution, 61, 75–77
Strategy identification, 70–71
Strategy Identification and Selection, 70–71
Style approach, to leadership, 5
Subordinates, responsibility for their own motivation, 34
Summary Report and Recommendations (National Commission on Nursing), 246
Supply-sensitive care, 118, 119, 120, 124
Surrogate decision makers, 351
SWOT (Strengths, Weaknesses, Opportunities, Threats) Analysis, 61. *See also* Situational Assessment
System improvement
    approaches, 111–115
        accrediting agency initiatives, 113–114
        employer-sponsored initiatives, 113
        federal government initiatives, 112–113
    goals of, 111
System interactiveness, 110
Systems perspective, of healthcare quality, 83
Systems thinking, 49
System thinking
    active *vs.* latent errors and, 109–110
    coupling, 110–111
    healthcare quality improvement and, 108–111
    interactiveness, 110

T
Tactical plans, 71–72, 72*t*
Task forces, 305
Tax Equity and Fiscal Responsibility Act (TEFRA), 170–171, 207
Tax status, of healthcare organization, 200–202, 202*t*
Teams
    benefits of, 308–309
    communication in, 315–316, 317
    conflict resolution in, 318–319